Leadership and Management

in Athletic Training

An Integrated Approach

Leadership and Management in Athletic Training

Matthew R. Kutz, PhD, ATC, CSCS

Assistant Professor of Athletic Training and Clinic Management

Clinical Education Coordinator, ATCM Program

School of Human Movement, Sport, and Leisure Studies

Bowling Green State University

Bowling Green, Ohio

Acquisitions Editor: Emily Lupash
Development Editor: David R. Payne
Product Managers: Jennifer Ajello & Erin M. Cosyn
Vendor Manager: Kevin Johnson
Manufacturing Manager: Margie Orzech-Zeranko
Marketing Manager: Christen Murphy
Design Coordinator: Teresa Mallon
Production Service: Cadmus Communications

Printed in China

Library of Congress Cataloging-in-Publication Data

Kutz, Matthew R.
  Leadership and management in athletic training : an integrated approach / Matthew R. Kutz.
      p. cm.
  Includes bibliographical references and index.
  ISBN 978-0-7817-6905-1
  1. Physical education and training—Management. 2. Leadership. I. Title.
  GV343.5.K87 2010
  613.7068—dc22

                                                                    2009009869

Care has been taken to confirm the accuracy of the information presented and to describe generally accepted practices. However, the authors, editors, and publisher are not responsible for errors or omissions or for any consequences from application of the information in this book and make no warranty, expressed or implied, with respect to the currency, completeness, or accuracy of the contents of the publication. Application of the information in a particular situation remains the professional responsibility of the practitioner.

The authors, editors, and publisher have exerted every effort to ensure that drug selection and dosage set forth in this text are in accordance with current recommendations and practice at the time of publication. However, in view of ongoing research, changes in government regulations, and the constant flow of information relating to drug therapy and drug reactions, the reader is urged to check the package insert for each drug for any change in indications and dosage and for added warnings and precautions. This is particularly important when the recommended agent is a new or infrequently employed drug.

Some drugs and medical devices presented in the publication have Food and Drug Administration (FDA) clearance for limited use in restricted research settings. It is the responsibility of the health care provider to ascertain the FDA status of each drug or device planned for use in their clinical practice.

To purchase additional copies of this book, call our customer service department at (800) 638-3030 or fax orders to (301) 223-2320. International customers should call (301) 223-2300.

Visit Lippincott Williams & Wilkins on the Internet: at LWW.com. Lippincott Williams & Wilkins customer service representatives are available from 8:30 am to 6 pm, EST.

10 9 8 7 6 5 4 3 2 1

RRS0907

This book is dedicated to everyone who models leadership effectively; and to my sons, Nathan and Jonathan, with hope and excitement about your futures.

Preface

PURPOSE

Welcome to *Leadership and Management in Athletic Training: An Integrated Approach.* As the title implies, this is a textbook devoted to integrating leadership behaviors into the practice and management of athletic training. Management and leadership are crucial components of the successful athletic training program. Now more than ever before, certified athletic trainers occupy roles and positions that require effective management skills. As these roles continue to evolve, elements of leadership (those that may or may not be distinct from management) will be critical for continued success. This book discusses the aspects of management and leadership identified in the Board of Certification (BOC) Role Delineation Study and the National Athletic Trainers' Association (NATA) educational competencies.

The chapters in the book are ordered to first introduce leadership and leadership development; these concepts are then integrated throughout the remaining chapters on the day-to-day practice and management of athletic training. This book, along with the instructor's experience and class discussions, will hopefully help produce certified athletic trainers who effectively integrate the art of leadership with the science of management.

Decades ago, certified athletic trainers rarely had formal administrative and managerial responsibilities. As the practice of athletic training and athletic training education have evolved, those days are now gone. Performing leadership and management functions is now a skill required of athletic trainers. A look at the BOC Role Delineation Study reveals quite succinctly these evolving roles. Therefore, the purpose of this book is to give the athletic training student and certified athletic trainers the tools for successful management and leadership of athletic training programs.

WHO IS THIS TEXT FOR?

This text is written with four principal audiences in mind:

1. Undergraduate athletic training students preparing for the BOC exam
2. Graduate athletic training students preparing for the BOC exam and graduate students working on a post-certification masters degree in athletic training wanting to advance their careers and the profession of athletic training
3. Certified athletic trainers who are currently practicing athletic training and wish to update or improve their leadership and management competence
4. The faculty and clinical instructors in athletic training education programs who would like a detailed road map to presenting the tasks, knowledge, and skills identified in the BOC Role Delineation Study for the *Organization and Administration* and *Professional Responsibility* performance domains and their associated competencies and content areas

DIFFERENT ROLES OF THE CERTIFIED ATHLETIC TRAINER

Leadership and management require skills and behaviors that transcend title, hierarchal structure, organizational position, or rank. In the evolving health care environment, the certified athletic trainer has created a niche in a variety of work settings. These settings range from traditional settings in high schools, colleges, or professional athletics to occupational settings, industrial settings, fitness centers, hospitals, and many others. This diversity of work environments implies the athletic trainer must develop and master skills and behaviors that transcend one setting or one organization. Learning the critical aspects of leadership theory and development is a critical skill for the successful athletic trainer. Being a successful leader or efficient manager means having transferable skills; that is, skills that are applicable in any work setting. Introducing contemporary leadership models and making an effort to understand how leadership can be developed and what leadership is can help make the management duties of the athletic trainer more fluid, and ultimately promote the profession of athletic training.

CONTENT OF THE BOOK

There are two important documents that served as the guide for this book. The first document is the BOC Role Delineation Study (RDS). The RDS outlines the critical content area for the BOC exam and presents that data as tasks, knowledge, and skills necessary for entry-level athletic training. The second document used in the development of this textbook is the NATA Educational Competencies. The competencies are divided into twelve content areas, two of which are *Healthcare Administration* and *Professional Development and Responsibility,* which are covered in this book.

This book is divided into five parts. Part I, "Foundations of Athletic Training Leadership," introduces the profession of athletic training and NATA, including a brief history of both, discusses the members of the sports medicine team and communication, and demonstrates how to prepare professionally to be a successful athletic trainer. Part II, "Leadership and Motivation," presents leadership and management theories, behaviors, and tools and discusses human resources concerns. Part III, "Information, Fiscal, and Risk Management," covers key administrative responsibilities of athletic trainers, including managing technology, record keeping, fiscal management, reimbursement and revenue, legal issues, and risk management. Part IV, "Program and Facility Management," provides information on how to form and plan an athletic training program and how to design and manage a facility. Part V, "Ethical and Global Issues," investigates professional ethics and international implications related to athletic training.

The book incorporates several special features to ensure the successful integration of leadership and management competencies:

- **Chapter contents.** An outline of headings is included at the beginning of each chapter to provide an overview of that chapter's contents.
- **RDS components and educational competencies**. Forgoing the traditional "chapter objectives," a list of the competencies, as well as the relevant knowledge areas and skill areas identified in the RDS, is included at the beginning of each chapter. This is useful for the instructor and student to know exactly what knowledge areas, skill areas, and competencies are covered in each chapter.
- **Chapter introductions.** A narrative introduction appears at the beginning of each chapter and provides an overview of the concepts and skills associated with the chapter.
- **From the Field.** This feature presents an informal, real-life story told from the athletic trainer's perspective in the first-person that illustrates or reinforces the objective of a specific chapter.
- **Key Terms.** Key terms are listed and defined at the beginning of each chapter, identified in boldface in the chapter text, and included in a **Glossary** at the end of the book.
- **Leadership Application.** This case study feature is a critical thinking exercise that helps the student to apply leadership principles into the managerial and administrative practices of athletic training via realistic scenarios and critical thinking questions.
- **Leadership Activity.** This feature is a hands-on learning assignment with the goal of engaging students in activities that will
- **Leadership Spotlight.** This special section highlights the careers and significant contributions of athletic trainers to the profession of athletic training.
- **Sample forms.** Forms are included in the text and in the appendices.
- **Chapter Summaries.** Narrative summaries at the end of each chapter provide a quick review of the chapter's contents.

PHILOSOPHY OF LEADERSHIP AND MANAGEMENT (A PERSONAL NOTE TO THE READER)

In any work such as this, the personal philosophy of the author "seeps" through and, to some extent, the author reserves that right, because it is a product of personal experience, education, and scholarship. However, every effort was made to remove or avoid overt philosophical bias.

My personal philosophy on leadership and management is that they are different expressions of similar or at least overlapping skill sets. Leadership and management are different, but not mutually exclusive of each other. There are tangible and intangible differences between management and leadership. Therefore, I spend time developing both aspects and intentionally integrate contemporary leadership theory into the practice of management as it relates to athletic training.

It is obvious from the available literature that there is little consensus on what leadership is or how it is defined, but this must not keep athletic trainers from integrating and developing contemporary awareness of leadership behaviors and skills and learning how to transfer those skills into professional practice and allied health care. There is also strong debate as to whether leadership and management are in fact different. The literature is replete with conflicting views. There are three primary tenets:

1. Leadership and management are two distinct constructs
2. Leadership and management are different names for the same thing
3. Leadership and management are different, but overlap on several areas

As already stated, I tend to lean more toward the third tenet. Suffice it to say, there is ample evidence that warrants the discussion of management and leadership as distinct.

Obviously similarities exist between these two constructs. Striving to understand both leadership and management in their proper contexts is central to advancing the profession of athletic training. I prefer to think of management and leadership as interdependent. Both leadership and management can be learned and developed by the individual. The goal of this book is then to supply the reader the necessary tools for successful management and leadership of athletic training programs.

MATTHEW KUTZ, PHD, ATC, CSCS

Acknowledgments

This book is a result of a passion for leadership that was instilled in me as a young boy and student. That passion was fostered by several people throughout the years. With the guidance and direction of many excellent teachers and a few close mentors, I came to realize that dedicated and intentional leaders can change their environment for the better. Therefore, I wish to acknowledge the colleagues, teachers, and mentors throughout the years who have contributed to my understanding and practice of leadership. There is no way that I can acknowledge each of you, but I am grateful nonetheless.

First of all, I wish to thank my family: my parents, Bob and Connie Kutz for their guidance and support. Your service, lives, and marriage have been a great example to many! To my wife, Angie, who is the consummate servant leader and my greatest encouragement during this process of writing drafts, editing drafts, rewriting, and re-editing. Thank you, Angie; you had the hardest job in all of this. I love you. To my sons, Nathan and Jonathan, although you are young, training you and guiding you these past eight years has taught me much about leadership that I suspect is difficult to learn in any other way except by being a father.

Next, I wish to thank my colleagues and friends. To my fellow faculty members and athletic trainers at Palm Beach Atlantic University, especially Sharon Borhes, Chris Balske, and Jennifer Michael, who were there when I first signed on to tackle writing a text book, thanks for your friendship and support. I especially thank my mentor, colleague, and friend from Texas State University, Dr. Jack Ransone (and Connie), for modeling leadership and professionalism and for being the first to encourage me to pursue athletic training education as a career. To the first athletic trainers I ever met and true mentors from Anderson University, Steve Risinger and Greg Williamson, you taught me what an athletic trainer was and how to be one. Thank you! To my dear friends, Randy, Max, Matt, Jason, and Tim, leaders in the true sense of the word, and men whose character and integrity are above reproach and who always help me to remember to keep things lighthearted. I thank you! To my doctoral advisor, Dr. Joan Scialli, who taught me how to be a leadership scholar, thank you. Also, to my spiritual leaders who taught me and modeled for me how to lead with a servant's heart, Dr. Norman Benz, David Noel, Tom Ray, and especially my dad and George Barrett, thank you!

I also would like to acknowledge the editorial staff at Lippincott Williams & Wilkins, especially David Payne, my managing editor, Emily Lupash, and Christen Murphy. I appreciate all the time and effort you put into this project. Finally, I would like to thank the reviewers of this text; your thoughtful critiques and recommendations made this book better.

MATTHEW KUTZ, PhD, ATC, CSCS

Reviewers

STACEY BUSER
Program Director, Athletic Training
The University of Akron
Akron, OH

DAVID KAISER
Athletic Training Program Director
Brigham Young University
Provo, UT

THOMAS W. KAMINSKI
Director of Athletic Training Education
University of Delaware
Newark, DE

LAUREN KRAMER
Department of Kinesiology
Penn State University
University Park, PA

BRETT MASSIE
Director, Athletic Training Education Program
PHS Department
Miami University
Oxford, OH

RANDY MEADOR
Athletic Trainer, West Virginia University
Morgantown, WV

CHRIS SCHOMMER
Program Coordinator Athletic Training
Bowling Green State University
Bowling Green, OH

JAMES SCIFERS
Department of Health Sciences
Western Carolina University
Cullowhee, NC

LESLEE TAYLOR
Program Director, Athletic Training
Texas Tech University Health Sciences Center
Lubbock, TX

ERIK WIKSTROM
Director, Undergraduate Athletic Training
University of Florida
Gainesville, FL

Contents

Foundations of Athletic Training Leadership

Introduction to Athletic Training and NATA

Good leadership and management skills are vital to maintain esprit de corps, teamwork, and efficiency in the modern athletic training room.

STEPHEN NELLIS

CHAPTER RATIONALE

Role Delineation Study Components

Domain VI: Professional Responsibility

- Knowledge of the Board of Certification Standards of Practice
- Knowledge of relevant policy and position statements of NATA and other appropriate organizations
- Knowledge of scope of practice of the athletic training profession

Educational Competencies

- Identify key accrediting agencies for health care facilities and describe their function in the preparation of health care professionals and the overall delivery of health care.
- Describe the role and function of the governing structures of the National Athletic Trainers' Association.
- Summarize the history and development of the athletic training profession.
- Describe the role and function of the professional organizations and credentialing agencies that impact the athletic training profession.
- Differentiate the essential documents of the national governing, certifying, and accrediting bodies.

Key Terms

Accreditation: The process of assessing the rigor of the training and education for an institution or program of study in accordance with pre-established criteria.

Ad hoc: Latin, meaning "for this purpose;" typically refers to a committee that is assembled for a specific purpose and that is disbanded once that committee's purpose is completed.

Board of Certification (BOC): The professional body that sets the standards for the practice of athletic training.

Clinical proficiencies: A common set of skills that entry-level athletic trainers should possess.

Cognitive competencies: The knowledge and intellectual skills necessary for an athletic trainer to posses.

Commission on Accreditation of Athletic Training Education (CAATE): The agency responsible for accrediting entry-level (undergraduate and graduate) athletic training educational programs.

Competency: A demonstrated behavior or skill an athletic trainer is required to possess.

Domains: One of six general practice areas in which an athletic trainer needs to have competency and proficiency.

National Athletic Trainers' Association (NATA): The membership-based professional association that represents the needs of athletic trainers and the profession of athletic training.

Policy: A written statement intended to encourage a specific behavior.

Procedure: A written course of action, usually in sequential steps, intended to accomplish a certain outcome.

Psychomotor competencies: The manipulative and motor skills necessary for an athletic trainer to posses.

Role Delineation Study (RDS): The athletic training job analysis authorized by the Board of Certification that identifies essential knowledge and skills for the athletic training profession and is used for exam development.

Standards of professional practice: A document published by the Board of Certification that outlines behavior expectations of athletic trainers.

Standing committees: Committees organized by NATA that have perpetual existence.

Stakeholders: Any person or party that has a vested interest in what is being done.

Physician extender: Any allied or health care professional who acts on the behalf of or in conjunction with a licensed physician by providing time with patients that the physician is unable to spend.

---

*I n a dynamic health care environment, leadership and management skills need to be exercised effectively. The need for leadership and management in athletic training is evident in the daily practice of an athletic trainer. Athletic trainers routinely call on leadership skills such as strategic thinking, communicating, managing crisis, innovating, showing initiative, delegating, and implementing new ideas in order to do their job effectively. Likewise, management practices such as budgeting, minimizing risk, and creating policy complement leadership and improve overall effectiveness. In any given day an athletic trainer performs leadership and management duties simultaneously and independently. At one moment the athletic trainer is a clinician, the next an administrator, then an emergency responder, later a mentor, and then perhaps a counselor. These and other roles require an athletic trainer to be proactive and responsive to changing contexts, changing needs, and the changing or even conflicting values of **stakeholders**. Stakeholders are any individuals or groups that have an interest or "stake" in what takes place. Therefore, properly integrating the necessary management practices with the appropriate leadership behaviors increases the chances of successful athletic training practice.*

In this chapter, the history of athletic training is presented. Why cover history in a leadership text? To best contribute to the development of the profession, one should understand its history. Without a context of where athletic training has come from, there is little hope to accurately plan for the future. Each generation of athletic trainers is less likely to repeat mistakes of the past and more likely to innovate when their professional history is comprehended.

Next, we will consider the current state of the profession, along with the various settings in which athletic trainers work. Finally, we will cover the primary organization of the profession, the National Athletic Trainers' Association (NATA), considering its purpose, structure, key documents, and policies and procedures.

HISTORY OF ATHLETIC TRAINING

From its inception in the late nineteenth century to the present, athletic training has grown and developed into a respected health care profession. This history includes many noted leaders, men and women, and, in particular, the organization of NATA.

Early Years

In 1881, when coaches and physicians almost exclusively handled injuries, Harvard University set a new precedent and hired James Robinson as their "athletic trainer."[5] In 1897, the University of Texas at Austin hired Tennessee native and future Longhorn Athletics Hall of Fame inductee Henry "Doc" Reeves, who was one of the nation's earliest athletic trainers (Fig. 1-1). An African American, "Doc" Reeves served as team "trainer," masseuse, and assisted with medical issues.[2] Many consider Mr. Reeves to be the first African-American "athletic" trainer. Michael C. Murphy of Yale and later University of Pennsylvania also functioned as an athletic trainer in those early days. Many consider Mr. Murphy to be the first "official" athletic trainer in the United States.[5]

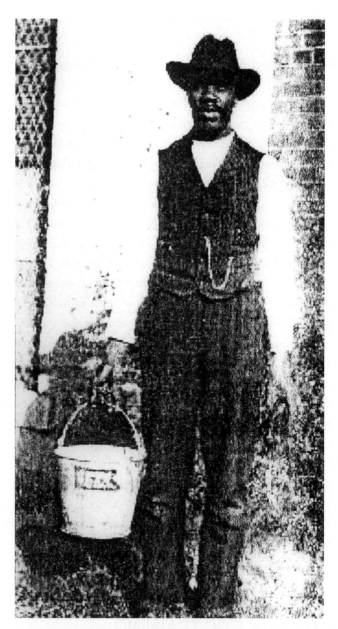

FIGURE 1-1 "Doc" Reeves, a fixture at Longhorn football games and first African-American athletic trainer and University of Texas Athletic Hall of Fame inductee. Photo courtesy of the National Athletic Trainers' Association.

However, Dr. Samuel E. Bilik is considered the "Father of Athletic Training." In 1914, Bilik entered medical school, worked as an athletic trainer at the University of Illinois, and published one of the first texts in athletic training, titled *Athletic Training*.[5] In the 1920s, the Cramer brothers, Charles "Chuck" and Frank, promoted this young profession of athletic training (Fig. 1-2). A pharmacist, Chuck Cramer founded Cramer Products Co. in 1920 (originally called Cramer Chemical Co.), which manufactured and sold liniment and other athletic training supplies. In 1932, the Cramer brothers observed the athletic training techniques used on the U.S. Olympic team and promptly began a series of traveling workshops teaching these techniques.[5]

These early athletic trainers used whatever materials were available and proved to be masters at innovation and creativity when it came to athletic training. Often without formal medical or athletic training education, these early "trainers" were driven by character, integrity, selflessness, and a passion to serve and learn. These qualities still drive athletic trainers today, but with the advantage of formal education, modern equipment, and recognition as allied health professionals. Early athletic trainers did not have the luxury of modern equipment or the use of modalities and often turned to their hands as their primary modality. Much of the early athletic trainer's job consisted of massage, soft tissue manipulation (i.e., stretching), applying ice and heat, and team management. The practice of their trade was often limited to an athletic context.

Perhaps the most significant event for athletic training in those early years occurred in 1938 with the formation of the National Athletic Trainers Association (NATA) (without the apostrophe, back then). The early version of NATA held two annual meetings, one at the Drake (west) and one at the Penn (east) Relays. The founders were William Frey from the University of Iowa and Chuck Cramer. Mike Chambers of Louisiana State University was appointed the association's first president.[5] In 1944, the infant NATA lost momentum and disbanded.

However, athletic training would not be gone forever. In 1947, regional groups of athletic trainers began to reorganize. As these local groups began to formalize, athletic training began taking on new life. In June of 1950, Cramer Chemical Co. sponsored the First National Training Clinic in Kansas City, Missouri, and the **National Athletic Trainers' Association (NATA)** as we know it today was founded with 101 members (Fig. 1-3; Fig. 1-4).

In 1955, NATA made some organizational changes and appointed William E. "Pinky" Newell as its executive secretary (Fig. 1-5). As executive secretary, Newell's duties included collecting dues, official correspondence, transacting the NATA's business, acting as spokesperson, keeping minutes for committees, planning the national program, and carrying out the Board's mandates.[5] Needless to say, Newell's responsibilities were significant. In the 13 years that Newell served NATA as executive secretary, the profession made significant strides toward credibility as a profession. In 1957, the board adopted the NATA Code of Ethics, as drafted by Newell and Howard Waite from the University of Pittsburgh. In 1965, NATA became a 1,000-member organization.

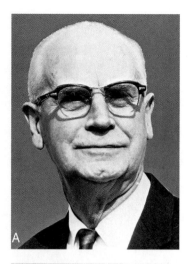

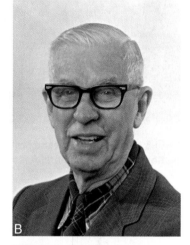

FIGURE 1-2 Cramer brothers, Charles and Frank, early fathers of athletic training and conveners of the first athletic training annual meeting. Photo courtesy of the National Athletic Trainers' Association.

Evolution of Athletic Training

In the 1970s, NATA underwent additional organizational changes and elected its first president, Robert H. "Bobby" Gunn from Lamar University. At the 1974 national convention, the board officially defined athletic training as "the art and science of prevention and management of injuries at all levels of athletic activity," and defined the athletic trainer as "one who is a practitioner of athletic training."[5] These definitions have changed over time as the profession continues to evolve.

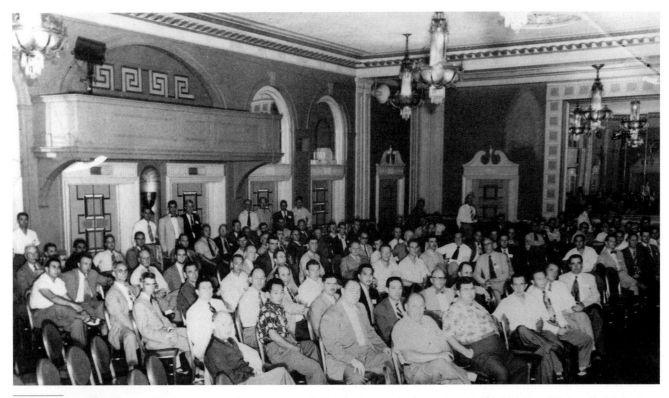

FIGURE 1-3 **Attendees at the first athletic trainers' annual meeting in Kansas City, MO in 1950.** Photo courtesy of the National Athletic Trainers' Association.

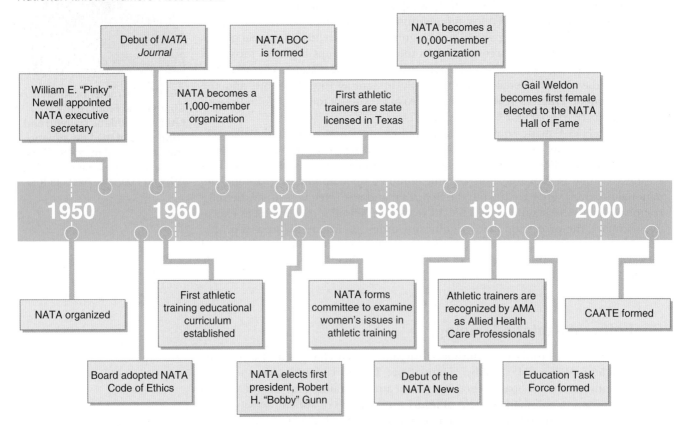

FIGURE 1-4 **Athletic training evolution timeline.**

The next two decades saw continued growth and development for NATA. In 1983, NATA officially incorporated, and three years later, it passed another significant milestone by reaching 10,000 members. Because of this growth, in 1988 NATA moved its headquarters to Dallas, Texas, where it remains today. On June 22, 1990, the American Medical Association officially recognized athletic training as an allied health profession.[4,13] The profession of athletic training continues to grow, and NATA now boasts well over 30,000 members.

Women in Athletic Training

An important part of athletic training's history is the early initiative and leadership of women. In 1956, Celester Hayden became the first female in this new profession to work as an athletic trainer during the Olympic games.[11] One decade later, Dorthey "Dot" Cohen became the first female member of NATA, and later that year, Sherry Kosek-Babagian became the second professional member and was the first woman to sit for the NATA certification exam.[11] In 1973, the NATA Board of Directors created an ad hoc committee to explore the issue of women in athletic training. Holly Wilson (Fig. 1-6) was the chair of that committee, which was charged with identifying the needs of female athletic trainers and making recommendations to NATA for the advancement of women in athletic training.[11] That ad hoc committee's first recommendation was that females be represented on all standing committees of NATA. Holly Wilson also authored the first athletic training textbook by a woman for women in this growing profession, titled *Workbook: Fundamentals of Athletic Training for Women.* During the 1970s and the birth of Title IX of the Education Amendments of 1972 (now known as the Patsy T. Mink Equal Opportunity in Education Act), women continued to gain momentum in this traditionally male-dominated profession. In 1976, Gail Weldon (Fig. 1-7) became the first female selected for the U.S. Olympic team medical staff and went on to serve as an athletic trainer for several Olympic games. Because of her work as a pioneer in athletic training, Ms. Weldon became the first female elected into the NATA Hall of Fame in 1995.[11] During the decades of the 1980s and 1990s, the female presence in NATA and in athletic training was a catalyst for much of the growth and recognition the profession enjoys today. The 1980s saw the first female district director, Janice Daniels, elected to the NATA Board of Directors, and the 1990s saw Julie Max (Fig. 1-8) become the first female NATA vice-president, Eve Becker-Doyle the first female NATA executive director, and Denise Fandel the first female president of the Board of Certification (BOC). In 2000, Julie Max went on to be the first female NATA president. Today, 49% of NATA membership is female. Athletic training can now boast that Holly Wilson's original goals and many of the goals of her predecessors have been achieved.

Education

As NATA and the profession of athletic training advanced, the education of athletic trainers needed to advance as well. Athletic training education has continually evolved throughout the history of NATA. In 1956, Pinky Newell, then chair of the Committee on Gaining Recognition, studied how to improve professionalism in athletic training. The committee recommended a national certification and athletic training education.[4] In 1959, the first curriculum was established.[4] That initial curriculum included prerequisites for entry into physical therapy school and was an important step in identifying a specific body of knowledge for the profession. However, critics of that initial curriculum pointed out a lack of athletic training–specific courses. By 1974, 14 colleges and universities offered

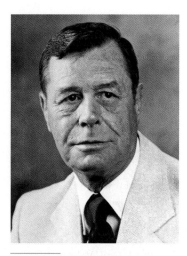

FIGURE 1-5 William "Pinky" Newell, first executive secretary of NATA and co-author of the first NATA Code of Ethics. Photo courtesy of the National Athletic Trainers' Association.

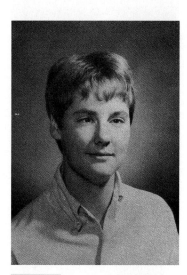

FIGURE 1-6 Holly Wilson, charter member and chair of the ad hoc women in athletic training committee and first female author of an athletic training text. Photo courtesy of the National Athletic Trainers' Association.

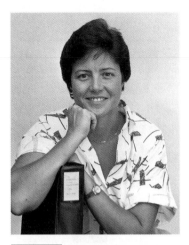

FIGURE 1-7 **Gail Weldon, first female NATA Hall of Fame inductee and first female to serve on the medical staff for the U.S. Olympics.** Photo courtesy of the National Athletic Trainers' Association.

athletic training education programs and two offered graduate programs. In 1994 the Education Task Force was formed and given purview over the educational development of athletic training educational programs. Since that time exciting changes in athletic training education have occurred and continue to occur. Part of these educational changes included the national accreditation of athletic training education programs by the Commission on Accreditation of Athletic Training Education (CAATE).

ATHLETIC TRAINING TODAY

Today athletic trainers enjoy practicing in a rich variety of settings. Athletic trainers can be found wherever people are active or injured, including high school, college, amateur, and professional sports; inpatient and outpatient physical rehabilitation clinics; hospitals; performing arts venues; the armed forces; industry; fitness facilities; and physicians' offices. Athletic trainers also satisfy many societal roles ranging from clinicians, to educators, to administrators and executives and are a recognized component of a valuable and diverse health care team.

Sports Teams

Perhaps the most traditional setting for the athletic trainer is the athletic team. Sport is certainly a unique culture, which historically is very comfortable for the athletic trainer. This setting involves the athletic trainer in preventing, treating, and managing a variety of activity-related injuries. In this environment the athletic trainer spends a majority of his or her time with athletes, coaches, parents, and athletic administrators. The duties of athletic trainers in the sport setting lean heavily toward taping and bandaging, prepping for practices and games, evaluating injuries, treating injuries, rehabilitation, traveling with teams, managing an injury referral system and records, and communicating with local physicians.

Occupational and Physician Offices

Some athletic trainers opt to work directly with a physician's practice. In this role the athletic trainer is referred to as a "**physician extender.**" A physician extender, as the name implies, increases the reach of the physician by providing time with patients that the physician is unable to spend. In this role the athletic trainer spends a considerable amount of time with the physician, the physician's patients, and other health care providers (i.e., specialty physicians, nurses, and therapists). Ideal practice settings for athletic trainers who are physician extenders include: orthopedics, osteopathy, physiatry, occupational medicine, or chiropractic. Much of the athletic trainer's time is spent one-on-one with patients explaining treatment options and performing rehabilitation and health screenings.

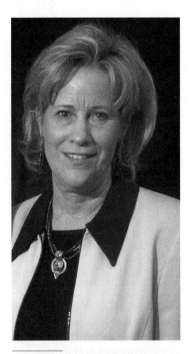

FIGURE 1-8 **Julie Max, first female NATA vice president and first female NATA president.** Photo courtesy of the National Athletic Trainers' Association.

Clinical Settings

Another common setting for athletic trainers is rehabilitation. For the most part clinical settings include sports medicine and rehabilitation clinics. This can and often does involve split responsibilities at an alternate site. A conventional model might include working mornings in the clinic rehabilitating patients, then covering practices for a local sports team in the afternoon. However, many athletic trainers do work exclusively within the clinic. In such cases, athletic trainers spend most of their time interacting with patients and other health care professionals and the duties include primarily applying therapeutic modalities, rehabilitation, and reconditioning of multiple musculoskeletal and orthopedic-related injuries.

Corporate/Industrial Settings

Industry is a unique setting where the athletic trainer is part of a diverse health care team within a factory. In this setting, the athletic trainer performs work hardening, rehabilitation, job safety, and ergonomic assessment. The objective of the athletic trainer in this setting is to increase production and decrease injuries to employees. Most of the athletic trainer's time is spent with factory employees (i.e., patients) and division or department managers.

There are many other settings in which athletic trainers can and do work. The setting is only limited to the athletic trainer's imagination and willingness to try new things. Athletic training is a very satisfying and rewarding career with unlimited potential. Regardless of the setting, athletic training has come as a very long way from the early days of being a "trainer" on the sidelines.

NATIONAL ATHLETIC TRAINERS' ASSOCIATION

As a would-be professional in athletic training, you should become familiar with the profession's national association, the National Athletic Trainers' Association (NATA). Provided below is an overview of NATA's mission, accreditation function and oversight of education, certification, corporate governance, standards of practice, and key documents and consensus statements.

Mission

Today, the mission of NATA is to enhance the quality of health care provided by certified athletic trainers and to advance the athletic training profession. NATA states in its bylaws five purposes for which it was organized:

1. To enhance the quality of health care for the physically active.
2. To advance the profession of athletic training through education and research in the prevention, evaluation, management, and rehabilitation of injuries.
3. To safeguard and advance the interests of its Members by presenting the profession's viewpoints, concerns, and other important information to the media and to appropriate legislative, administrative, regulatory, and private sector bodies and by developing a working relationship with appropriate governmental and private sector not-for-profit and for-profit entities.
4. To advance Members' levels of knowledge through the collection, interpretation, and dissemination of information on subjects appropriate to the profession.
5. To engage in any lawful act or activity for which a corporation may be organized under the Texas Non-Profit Corporation Act.[10]

Accreditation

In June 2006, the **Commission on Accreditation of Athletic Training Education (CAATE)** (formerly the Joint Review Committee on Educational Programs in Athletic Training) began accrediting entry-level athletic training education programs. Before CAATE, athletic training education programs were accredited by the Commission on Accreditation of Allied Health Education Programs (CAAHEP).

✎ From the Field

The athletic training profession offers many rich and diverse settings for professionals to practice. This was not always the case. As a student in the early 1990s, I remember attending student workshops where athletic trainers were presenting proposals and ROI (return on investment) projections to work in industrial settings. I remember realizing the significance and impact athletic training could have on health care outside of sports. That realization was so acute that after the workshop I interrogated our head athletic trainer as to why we (as a profession) stigmatized ourselves to athletics, with the title "athletic trainer." Since then I have grown much and have been fortunate to work as an athletic trainer is multiple settings, from high schools, clinics, and hospitals, to colleges and fitness centers. I have worked with several types of patients and handled a variety of injuries, illnesses, and disorders. I no longer consider it a stigma to be an "athletic" trainer. In fact, it is a point of pride, and athletic trainers should be proud of their profession, its name, and their credentials no matter where they practice.

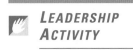

LEADERSHIP ACTIVITY

Pick a historical aspect of athletic training that interests you and research it on the internet or at the library. For example, find out who the first athletic trainer in your state or region was and some biographical details about him or her. Alternatively, you could find out what methods or techniques were used by early athletic trainers and how practices have changed over the years. Finally, you could pick a particular sport or even team from history and learn about how the introduction of an athletic trainer impacted the sport or team. After you have gathered the information, write a brief, 250-word summary of your findings and present it to the class.

Accreditation is a process by which an external agency reviews and assesses the curriculum of an academic institution that offers education or training in a specific discipline to verify that it is in full compliance with the minimum acceptable educational standards.

The purpose of CAATE is to develop, maintain, and promote appropriate minimum standards of quality entry-level athletic training education programs. CAATE is supported and sponsored by several other professional organizations, including the American Academy of Family Physicians, the American Academy of Pediatrics, the American Orthopaedic Society for Sports Medicine, and NATA.[3]

Graduate Education

Athletic training education has evolved dramatically since its inception. Today athletic training education includes bachelor's degrees, master's degrees (both entry-level and post-certification), and doctorates in athletic training. Curricula have evolved from primarily internships to competency-based curriculums.

Since the inception of the first athletic training curriculum, graduate-level education has been distinct from entry-level education. Post-certification master's degrees in athletic training are a necessary route to advanced-practice standing within the profession of athletic training. Post-certification master's programs in athletic training are accredited by NATA based on a recommendation from the NATA Education Council. Post-certification graduate education in athletic training must include the following six principles:[6]

1. Mastery of subject matter
2. Critical thinking
3. Theoretical understanding
4. Proficiency in research and/or creative activities
5. Service orientation
6. Diverse representation of perspectives

One issue coming to the forefront in athletic training education is advanced-practice (i.e., post-professional) athletic training. In 2005, NATA formed the Post-Professional Education Committee (PPEC), charged with developing and promoting formalized athletic training education beyond the entry level. Because entry-level certification is only the beginning of an athletic trainer's professional preparation, the PPEC is responsible for developing an educational structure that prepares certified athletic trainers to become advanced-practice clinicians and develop specialized knowledge that prepares clinicians as leaders and researchers for advanced roles or settings within allied health care.[7]

The overall mission of post-professional master's degree programs in athletic training is to "expand the depth and breadth of the applied, experimental, and propositional knowledge and skills of entry-level certified athletic trainers, expand the athletic training body of knowledge, and to disseminate new knowledge in the discipline."[6] Offering post-certification masters' degrees in athletic training helps the profession solidify its standing as a credible and reputable profession and allows athletic trainers who have earned such recognition greater influence and leadership opportunities.

Board of Certification

Because of the need for respected and validated credentials of the growing profession, in 1971, the National Athletic Trainers' Association **Board of Certification (BOC)** was officially created and the first certification exam was given. The Mission of the BOC is to certify athletic trainers and to identify for the public quality health care professionals through a system of certification, adjudication, standards of practice, and continuing competency programs.[2]

To determine what content should be tested in its certification exam, the BOC conducted the **Role Delineation Study (RDS)**. The RDS is an empirical investigation to identify an athletic trainer's responsibilities and the knowledge and skill areas required to perform them. The RDS delineates six practice **domains**. The domains are:

Domain 1: Prevention

Domain 2: Clinical Evaluation and Diagnosis

Domain 3: Immediate Care

Domain 4: Treatment, Rehabilitation, and Reconditioning

Domain 5: Organization and Administration

Domain 6: Professional Responsibility

Based on the findings of the RDS, the Professional Education Committee published **competencies** for entry-level practice of athletic training, which were included in the original 1983 *Guidelines*. Competencies are the skills and abilities that are essential to perform certain tasks. Currently the *Athletic Training Educational Competencies* is in its fourth edition and was released in 2006. The credibility gained from the BOC's RDS and the resulting educational competencies served the profession by paving the way for licensure at the state level. Currently 46 states have some government regulation of the athletic training profession, with 36 states now offering licensure. This book and subsequent chapters are organized around the educational competencies and the RDS' findings for Domains 5 and 6. Each chapter's content corresponds to certain competencies, which are identified at the beginning of each chapter.

Corporate Governance

NATA is a non-profit organization governed by an eleven-member, elected Board of Directors, one member from each of the 10 NATA regional districts (Table 1-1), and a president. A vice-president and a secretary/treasurer are nominated from among the members and elected by the Board. The Board of Directors hires an executive director, an executive assistant to the executive director, and staff to help operate the daily activities of NATA.

Any certified-regular or certified-student member is eligible to be elected to the board of directors by their respective district. Members of the board of directors serve three-year terms, which begin immediately after the NATA annual meeting. Elections of board members are staggered so that at no time does the entire board consist of new members, allowing for smooth transitions and little to no break in board activity and momentum. Committees designated by NATA may be **ad hoc** or **standing committees** (ad hoc is a Latin phrase meaning "for this purpose"). Members and officers of ad hoc committees are appointed by the president or the Board. Once the ad hoc committee's purpose has been accomplished, it is disbanded. Standing committees (Box 1-1) are permanent and have a perpetual existence, and their composition, purpose, and duties are described in the NATA Policies and Procedures Manual. For example, the Career Assistance Committee's purpose is to "provide advice and counsel to members on the employment process and opportunities." Its duties are three-fold:

1. Oversee and administer the operations of the NATA Career Center at the annual meeting.
2. Provide up-to-date employment information to members.
3. Promote effective employment-seeking practices.[9]

TABLE 1-1 NATA Regional Districts

District #	District Name	Web Site	States/Regions in That District
1	Eastern Athletic Trainers' Association	http://www.eatad1.org/	Connecticut, Maine, Massachusetts, New Hampshire, Rhode Island, Vermont, Quebec, New Brunswick, Nova Scotia
2	Eastern Athletic Trainers' Association	http://www.natad2.org/	Delaware, New Jersey, New York, Pennsylvania
3	Mid-Atlantic Athletic Trainers' Association	http://www.maata.org/	Maryland, North Carolina, South Carolina, Virginia, West Virginia, District of Columbia
4	Great Lakes Athletic Trainers' Association	http://www.glata.org/	Illinois, Indiana, Michigan, Minnesota, Ohio, Wisconsin, Manitoba, Ontario
5	The Mid America Athletic Trainers' Association	http://maata.net/	Iowa, Kansas, Missouri, Nebraska, North Dakota, Oklahoma, South Dakota
6	The Southwest Athletic Trainers' Association	http://www.swata.com/	Arkansas, Texas
7	The Rocky Mountain Athletic Trainers' Association	http://www.rmata.org/	Arizona, Colorado, New Mexico, Utah, Wyoming
8	Far West Athletic Trainers' Association	http://www.fwata.org/	California, Nevada, Hawaii
9	Southeast Athletic Trainers' Association	http://www.seata.org/	Alabama, Florida, Georgia, Kentucky, Louisiana, Mississippi, Tennessee, Puerto Rico, U.S. Virgin Islands
10	Northwest Athletic Trainers Association	http://www.nwata.net/	Alaska, Idaho, Montana, Oregon, Washington, Alberta, British Columbia, Saskatchewan

Each standing committee is outlined in the NATA Policy and Procedure Manual with can be accessed by NATA members at http://www.nata.org.

Documents

There are four primary sources which publish regulatory documents pertaining to athletic training. These organizations are the National Athletic Trainers' Association (NATA), NATA Board of Certification (BOC), NATA Education Council, and Commission on Accreditation of Athletic Training Education (CAATE). When developing an athletic training program in any setting or when developing policies and procedures for the operation of an athletic training facility, it is paramount to consult these different publications.

NATA serves its members by striving to enhance the quality of the care athletic trainers provide. NATA publishes position statements, a Code of Ethics, Educational Competencies and Proficiencies, and marketing materials that should be used in the development of policy and procedure manuals as well as in strategic planning. The

BOX 1-1   NATA Standing Committees
Clinical & Emerging Practices Athletic Trainers' Committee
College/University Athletic Trainers' Committee
Convention Program Council
Council on Revenue
District Secretaries/Treasurers Committee
Education Council
College/University Athletic Training Students' Committee
Continuing Education Committee
Post Professional Education Committee
Professional Education Committee
Ethics Council
Ethnic Diversity Advisory Committee
Federal Legislative Project Team
Finance Committee
Governmental Affairs Committee
Honors and Awards Committee
International Council
Journal Council
National Athletic Training Students' Committee
National Legal Review Group
Outcomes Advisory Panel
Post Professional Education Review Committee
Pronouncements Committee
Public Relations Committee
Secondary School Athletic Trainers' Committee
Strategic Implementation Team
Young Professionals Committee

BOC's mission is to protect the public. This is done by identifying and credentialing competent athletic training practitioners. The BOC publishes the Standards of Professional Practice and the Role Delineation Study. The NATA Education Council (NATAEC) serves as a "think tank" for educational issues.[12] The NATAEC publishes educational standards and guidelines for post-certification masters' programs and guidelines for technical standards in entry-level athletic training education. CAATE is responsible for establishing the standards and guidelines that govern the establishments of entry-level athletic training education programs. CAATE publishes the Standards for the Accreditation of Entry-Level Educational Programs for the Athletic Trainer. The documents published by these organizations and committees help guide and facilitate strategy, planning and policy making processes. Table 1-2 lists many of these documents and their web addresses.

Athletic Training Educational Competencies

The Athletic Training Educational Competencies outline the specific skills and abilities that each certified athletic trainer must be proficient at performing. Educational competencies are arranged into 12 content areas (Box 1-2) based on the six universal domains identified by the RDS. Each content area is organized into **cognitive competencies**, which represent knowledge and intellectual skills; **psychomotor competencies**, which are manipulative and motor skills; and **clinical proficiencies**,

TABLE 1-2 Web Site Addresses of Important Athletic Training Documents

Document Name	Published by	Web Address
Code of Ethics	NATA	http://www.nata.org
Standards of Professional Practice	BOC	http://www.bocatc.org
Entry-Level Educational Standards and Guidelines	CAATE	http://www.caate.net
Post-Certification Educational Standards and Guidelines	NATAEC	http://www.nataec.org
State Regulatory Acts	Individual states	http://www.bocatc.org
Guideline Technical Standards for Entry-Level Athletic Training Education	NATAEC	http://www.nataec.org

which represent decision-making and application of skill. Also included in the athletic training educational competencies is a listing of *foundational behaviors of professional practice*, the core values of the athletic training profession that are intended to permeate every aspect of the athletic training program and practice. These foundational behaviors include:

1. Primacy of the patient
2. Teamed approach to practice
3. Legal practice
4. Ethical practice
5. Advancing knowledge
6. Cultural competence
7. Professionalism

Standards of Professional Practice

All professionals are expected to comply with certain **standards of professional practice**. The standards represent the minimal requirements essential for the practice of their profession. Standards for the practice of athletic training have been set forth by

---

BOX 1-2   Content Areas for Athletic Training Education

1. Risk Management and Injury Prevention
2. Pathology of Injuries and Illness
3. Orthopedic Clinical Examination and Diagnosis
4. Medical Conditions and Disability
5. Acute Care of Injuries and Illness
6. Therapeutic Modalities
7. Conditioning and Rehabilitative Exercise
8. Pharmacology
9. Psychosocial Intervention and Referral
10. Nutritional Aspects of Injuries and Illness
11. Health Care Administration
12. Professional Development and Responsibility

the BOC. The BOC Standards of Professional Practice are divided into two sections. Section one is *Practice Standards* and section two is the *Code of Professional Responsibility*. The Practice Standards are mandatory standards that establish the practice expectations for all athletic trainers. There are seven practice standards intended to help the public understand what to expect from an athletic trainer, help the athletic trainer understand the responsibility that comes with carrying the athletic trainer certified (ATC®) credential, and delineate expectations for quality of care.

The Code of Professional Responsibility outlines six codes that are aimed to ensure that credential holders act in a responsible manner whenever providing athletic training services. The BOC requires that every athletic trainer comply with every code. The BOC reserves the right to discipline any athletic trainer for breach of the code. The entire BOC Standards of Professional Practice can be accessed at http://www.bocatc.org.

An important use of these publications is as a reference for the creation of policies and procedures. Regardless of the type or setting of the athletic training program being operated it is likely that the data contained in these publications will be necessary for a thorough policy and procedure manual. For example, consulting these documents can help in deciding topics to include and appropriate language in policy and procedure manuals.

ACCREDITING AND REGULATORY AGENCIES

Often times external accrediting and regulatory agencies affect an institution's policies, procedures, and practices. Accreditation is desirable for some organizations because it means the service provider has passed an in-depth review of its services. It is meant to protect the patient or the receiver of the service. It is assurance that the service provider meets pre-established guidelines for service and quality. These agencies, like CAATE (mentioned above), give an endorsement that the service provider has met pre-established service standards. There are several other agencies that can have an influence on athletic training **policies** and **procedures**. Some of those agencies are discussed below.

Commission on Accreditation of Rehabilitation Facilities

The Commission on Accreditation of Rehabilitation Facilities (CARF) is an accreditation agency setting guidelines and quality service standards for facilities offering rehabilitation services. CARF is an international agency that accredits 38,000 rehabilitation and human service organizations in the United States, Europe, and Canada.

Occupational Safety and Health Administration

The Occupational Safety and Health Administration (OSHA) is a U.S. government agency sponsored by the U.S. Department of Labor and regulates, among other things, workplace safety. Complying with OSHA regulations is the responsibility of every employer in just about any industry. Perhaps more relative to athletic training, OSHA sets the regulations in areas of ergonomics and universal precautions.

Joint Commission on the Accreditation of Healthcare Organizations

The Joint Commission on the Accreditation of Healthcare Organizations (JCAHO) was founded in 1951 and established guidelines on how hospitals ought to operate

TABLE 1-3 Accrediting Agencies Affecting Athletic Training

Agency Name	Agency Web Address
Commission on Accreditation of Athletic Training Education	http://www.caate.net
Commission on Accreditation of Rehabilitation Facilities	http://www.carf.org
Joint Commission on Accreditation of Healthcare Organizations	http://www.jcaho.org
Occupational Safety and Health Administration	http://www.osha.gov

to ensure quality care of patients. JCAHO is considered the "gold seal of approval" for health care providers.[8] JCAHO has roots that reach back to 1926, when the first manual of hospital standards was published by the American College of Surgeons. In 1951, the Joint Commission on Accreditation of Hospitals was formed as a not-for-profit organization to oversee the care given at hospitals. Today it is an agency that accredits over 17,000 ambulatory health care facilities and offers disease-specific certifications for health care providers.

Table 1-3 presents a list of these and other agencies, with their addresses for references. Once a program is accredited by any of these agencies the agency then monitors the respective programs to ensure compliance. Oftentimes these agencies require the submission of self-study reports and evaluations and perform inspections.

CHAPTER SUMMARY

Athletic training involves a significant level of leadership and requires implementing different management techniques. In order to be an effective leader and manager, understanding the origins and working structure of athletic training is important to

Leadership Application

You are an athletic training student at State University, a CAATE-accredited program. Frank is the head athletic trainer and your assigned clinical instructor for the fall. Frank graduated from the same university in 1989 with a degree in athletic training, but the athletic training program was not accredited at that time. You arrive for your first day with Frank as your supervisor and Frank states that athletic training competency is best acquired through hands-on experience. Frank then reminisces that back in his day he had accumulated over 3,000 hours of athletic training experience as a student and that "trial and error" was, in his opinion, the "only" way to become a competent athletic trainer. After a week of working with Frank, you are frustrated with your clinical experience and perceive that Frank had little appreciation or patience for students needing close supervision. You then ask Dr. Jones, the clinical coordinator, if you can be reassigned to another clinical instructor. If you cannot be reassigned, you are contemplating dropping the athletic training major.

Critical Thinking Questions

1. Who is responsible for speaking to Frank about his "educational philosophy?"
2. Would having a better appreciation of the history and growth of athletic training education and practice benefit Frank? If so, how?
   a. What specific aspects might be the most beneficial?
3. What responsibility, if any, do you have regarding speaking to Frank?
4. If you were Dr. Jones, how might you approach Frank about this situation?

guide the profession into the future. In this chapter the history of athletic training was outlined beginning with the pre-NATA days of the late-1800s up until the advent of NATA in 1950. The evolution of NATA and the athletic training profession included the creation and implementation of a code of ethics, standards of professional practice, educational competencies, a nationally recognized educational curriculum, formal athletic training, graduate education, and the inclusion of women into the profession. As a result, athletic training is now a respected allied health care profession with professionals practicing in a wide range of settings. This recognition has been a catalyst for NATA and the profession that helped spawn graduate and CAATE accreditation standards, the Board of Certification, the NATA Education Council, and other agencies with a vested interest in athletic training.

Leadership Spotlight

MARJORIE J. ALBOHM

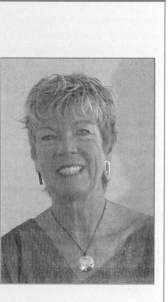

Education:
BS, Valparaiso University, 1972; MS, Indiana State University, 1973

Current job:
Manager of Fellowships and Customer Education, Ossur Americas; Consultant

First athletic training job:
Graduate Assistant, Indiana State University, 1972–1973

Professional interests/research focus:
Female athlete

Athletic training–related awards/honors:
- NATA Hall of Fame
- Distinguished Athletic Trainer
- Tim Kerin Award

Athletic training–related involvement:
- NATA President
- NATA Board of Directors
- NATA REF President

Q & A

What first inspired you to enter the athletic training profession?

Being injured as an intercollegiate field hockey player and realizing there was no one to care for injuries occurring among female athletes.

How would you define leadership in athletic training?

Being the best professional you can be, in every situation, and having a vision for where our profession should go to allow athletic trainers to be all that we can be.

Who is the most influential athletic trainer in your professional life, and why?

Really too many to name. My first head athletic trainer, Bob Young (no longer in the profession), opened doors for me that started my career and enabled me to learn so much.

What is the best advice you ever received from another athletic trainer?

Know that you can't solve all of the problems but you can positively influence most of them.

What has been the most enjoyable aspect of athletic training?

Sharing the information that we know as health care professionals with people of all ages, who desperately want and need it.

What has been the least enjoyable aspect or your biggest challenge in athletic training?

None!

What advice would you give a first-year athletic training student?

Learn everything you can from everyone you come in contact with. Ask questions and take initiative to learn more.

What advice would you give a brand new BOC-certified athletic trainer who is deciding between taking that first professional job or entering graduate school to pursue a master's degree in athletic training, and why?

Determine which opportunity best further develops your skills and gives you the opportunity to be exposed to new information and skills. Where you can learn the most is the key, and that includes professional growth.

What other interests outside of athletic training have you pursued?

Personal fitness—spinning! Outdoor biking.

Where do you think (or hope) athletic training will be in the next 10 years?

Athletic training will be recognized as a highly respected and valued health care profession, providing care to people of all ages. Athletic trainers will be in high demand in a variety of settings.

References

1. Anonymous. (2006, February). Voices from the past: How the NATA and Athletic Training Grew. *NATA News February 2006*: 12–15.

2. Richardson S. (2003). *Tales from the Texas Longhorns*. Champaign, IL: Sports Publishing, LLC.

3. Commission on Accreditation of Athletic Training Education. *Standards for the accreditation of entry-level athletic training education programs*. Dallas, TX: NATA, 2005.

4. Delforge G, Behnke R. The history and evolution of athletic training education in the United States. *J Athletic Training 1999; 34*(1):53–61.

5. Ebel R. *Far beyond the shoe box*. Toronto, ON: Forbes Custom Publishing, 1999.

6. Graduate Review Committee. (2002). Standards and guidelines for post-certification graduate athletic training education programs. Available at: http://www.nataec.org/documents/downloads/graduate/pcgestandards12.pdf. Accessed January 18, 2006.

7. Hunt V. (2006, January). Education continues to evolve: Post-professional work expands. *NATA News January 2006*: 14–19.

8. Joint Commission on Accreditation of Healthcare Organizations [corporate brochure]. 2003. Available at: http://www.jcaho.org/about+us/corporate_brochure.pdf. Accessed May 6, 2005.

9. NATA Policies and Procedures Manual. 2006. Available at http://www.nata.org/members1/documents/policy_procedures_manual.pdf

10. National Athletic Trainers' Association, Inc. 2004 Bylaws. Available at: https://www.nata.org/downloads/documents/101Bylaws%200504.pdf. Accessed May 7, 2005.

11. Shingles RR. *Women in athletic training: Their career and educational experiences* [dissertation]. Michigan State University, UMI # 3036748; 2001.

12. Starkey C. The athletic training triad: NATA, JRC-AT and NATABOC. *NATA News July 2001*.

13. Weidner T, Henning J. Historical perspective of athletic training clinical education. *J Athletic Training 2002; 37*(4S):S222–S228.

Chapter 2

The Sports Medicine Team and Communication

"The strength of the team is each individual member…the strength of each member is the team."

PHIL JACKSON

CHAPTER RATIONALE

Role Delineation Study Components

Knowledge of Various Effective Communication Styles and Techniques

Educational Competencies

- Differentiate the roles and responsibilities of the athletic trainer from those of other medical and allied health personnel who provide care to patients involved in physical activity and describe the necessary communication skills for effectively interacting with these professionals.
- Identify the objectives, scope of practice, and professional activities of other health and medical organizations and professions and the roles and responsibilities of these professionals in providing services to patients.
- Describe the theories and techniques of interpersonal and cross-cultural communication among athletic trainers, patients, administrators, health care professionals, parents/guardians, and other appropriate personnel.

Key Terms

Agreement: The ancient belief that dialogue, and not sharing a common opinion, was the most important aspect of working together.

Co-acting teams: Teams with members who function with a high degree of autonomy.

Collaborative teams: Teams that share common values and goals but have diverse experiences and backgrounds.

Communication: The use of a variety of different means to convey information.

Conflict: A state of disagreement or incompatibility between two or more people or groups of people.

Groupthink: A social phenomenon in which members of a team remain silent when a point is open for discussion and debate out of the assumption that everyone either already knows or shares a similar opinion.

Homogeneous teams: Teams that are composed of individuals who share common experiences and backgrounds.

Interdependent teams: Teams whose members rely heavily on other members of the team for accomplishing goals and objectives.

Minutes: Notes or the records from the proceedings of a meeting.

Psychological barriers: Barriers in communication that result from skepticism or cynicism.

Rapport: A relationship of mutual understanding and trust.

Semantic barriers: Barriers in communication as a result of industry-specific jargon and personal or cultural meanings.

Social loafing: When members of a team significantly decrease their effort, forcing other members to "pick up the slack."

Synergy: The compounding impact of group effort, which results in more being accomplished than what individual efforts might have produced.

Team: An interdependent group formed for an express purpose that must rely on mutual collaboration and insist on accountability.

Teamwork: An action of a group who have agreed to work together for the sake of a common goal.

Technological barriers: Barriers in communication as a result of a lack of face-to-face interaction.

Tolerance: Acknowledging others' differences of opinion, values, and beliefs without allowing those differences to affect team dynamics or productivity.

A s organizations and society continue to evolve, more responsibility is being delegated to teams rather than individuals.[16] Athletic training is no exception. As athletic training evolves, collaborative effort should replace individual production. Teamwork is a universal value and a critical leadership behavior within health care.[4,13] Part of effective teamwork outlined for health care professionals includes working interdependently, conveying mutual respect, trust, support, and appreciation of each discipline's unique contributions to health care."[13] This type of team collaboration requires agreement. Perhaps no other team-based concept has transcended time or culture like agreement. In ancient times "*agreement*" was determined based on on the willingness to assemble or meet together for dialogue.[1] Interestingly, the ancient concept of agreement did not presume everyone needed share a common opinion in order to "agree." Therefore, agreement as formerly understood is a valuable concept that includes both working together and communication.

In this chapter we will develop the concept of team and describe effective teamwork as well as the disadvantages and advantages of teams. We will endeavor to discuss the different types of teams that exist and their characteristics. Next, we will identify common members of the sports medicine team and their roles, as well as outline some strategies to establishing relationships. Next, we will examine how conflict arises on teams and offer some strategies on how to handle conflict. Following that we will discuss communication in general and in the athletic training context, including written and verbal communication and appropriate use of body langage. Finally, we will discuss common barriers to communication and how to overcome those barriers.

TEAMS

The concept of a functional team is a paradox. For example, a team's progress is often a result of individual effort. On the other hand, people who are not able or willing to contribute on their own can substantially contribute when part of a team. Therefore, the proverbial statement that "a team is often greater than the sum of its parts" has significance, while "a team is only as strong as its weakest link" is also valid.

Definitions of team are wide and varied. Instead of attempting to delineate one agreed-upon definition, many authors and leadership scholars simply try to describe different types of teams. There are certainly many different types of teams and varied reasons to form them. However, this does not negate the need to have a concise definition. A suitable definition of **team** is a group formed for an express purpose that must rely on collaboration and insist on accountability throughout the entirety of its existence.[2,3]

It is important to note that all teams are groups, but not all groups are teams.[3] **Teamwork**, on the other hand, occurs when a group intentionally agrees to work together for the sake of a common goal. The concept of team implies longevity, unselfishness, and an established relationship; teamwork on the other hand may be very short-lived, may be egocentric, and may not exist outside of the work context.

An example of short-lived and egocentric teamwork in sports might be the "all-star" team. Typically, all-star teams consist of rival team members. These rivals are supposed to put individual differences and rivalries behind them and work together. Often, getting these "all-star" rivals to display teamwork is an obstacle to their success. Typically, coaches (i.e., leaders) have to spend a disproportionate amount of time on developing teamwork compared to task-specific skills. Part of the difficulty in this case is that these individual team members have been tremendous individual contributors on their other teams. It is difficult for these former team standouts to assume a different, perhaps less prominent role, for the sake of the group.

Another example of teamwork within a sports team can be seen when different members of the team are asked to change their roles based on the circumstances. An illustration of this is the application of offense and defense. No serious team leader would consider substituting an offensive line for a defensive secondary; they are simply not suited to perform the expected tasks. More specifically, it would be selfish for a runningback to insist that he get the ball on a third-and-12 situation, when that situation obviously calls for a pass. Likewise, it would be selfish for a wide receiver to insist that the quarterback throw him the ball on a second-and-two situation. Team members who show such little appreciation of the team concept quickly alienate themselves.

Barriers to Effective Teams

Working on teams requires self-sacrifice and willingness to depend on others' competence. This interdependence presents many challenges for team members and team leaders. Some of the disadvantages and barriers to teams include the following points:[2,3,8,11]

1. There are occasions when individuals can handle a situation better and more efficiently.
2. Team development takes time.
3. Teams tend to evolve into bureaucratic committees.
4. Team decisions take time.
5. Teams can not always be assembled or consulted in emergency decisions.
6. Team members run the risk of **groupthink**. Groupthink is assuming everyone either already knows or shares your opinion and usually manifests by refusing to "state the obvious," which can be devastating to a team's ultimate goal.
7. Team members run the risk of **social loafing**. At times members of a team will significantly decrease their effort, forcing other members to "pick up the slack." Social loafing can demoralize and sabotage team members who always have to pick up the slack.
8. Teams develop communication barriers.
9. Combining different personalities can foster conflict.

Another disadvantage of team is the time required to develop a comfort level or familiarity with the personalities of the other members. The personality of these members is often based on their individual values and experiences. Having a rich mixture of values and experiences can be advantageous, but can be difficult for a team to filter through and appreciate. Then there is the personality of the collective group. Finally, the organization has a personality (culture) of its own. It is an important skill for team members to be able to diagnose and assimilate these different "personalities."

Because of diverse personalities, teams may self-destruct if objectives and missions are not clear, if cliques or unhealthy competition is fostered between members, when internal politics or hidden agendas are propagated, or when organizational support is poor.[11] Unwillingness to accept or creating barriers to new team members or new ideas can also destroy a team.[7] In spite of the effort it takes to keep teams productive, once established, teams can be very beneficial. A leader who is willing to take these risks can establish practices that reduce the potential barriers to teams.

Advantages of Teams

While the risks of teams can seem severe, the advantages far outweigh any negative aspect of team or teamwork. There are several key advantages associated with teams:[3,11]

1. Teams offer new and different perspectives. Past failures and success of members can be valuable contributions to teams.
2. Teams offer a greater sum total of expertise. Once a team decides to collaborate, the collective total of expertise increases exponentially.
3. Teams create **synergy**. Synergy is the compounding impact of group effort that results in more being accomplished than what individual efforts might have produced.
4. Teams often foster higher morale.
5. Teams foster creativity. Team members often evaluate each other's thinking and logic, which cultivates different ways of strategic thinking.
6. Team offers increased flexibility and reduces dependence on certain individuals.
7. Team involvement often results in higher employee retention.

Arguably one of the greatest strengths of teams is the many types that can be formed. Teams come in various shapes and sizes. Creating a culture where different types and styles of team can be expressed is a strength. The beneficiaries of that added strength may be the organization as a whole, stakeholders, and the individual team members.

Types of Teams

Teams can be collaborative or homogeneous. **Homogeneous** teams consist of members with similar or equal experiences, backgrounds, or abilities. For example, a group of athletic trainers working at the same school, or from the same school, with similar or identical backgrounds are homogeneous. **Collaborative** teams are made up of individuals with varied backgrounds and areas of expertise, e.g., the sports medicine team, which consists of athletic trainers, physicians, athletes, coaches, administrators, and other allied health care professionals.

Within these two constructs teams can be classified as either co-acting or interdependent.[16] **Co-acting teams** are essentially groups in which individual members retain a high level of autonomy. The work of individual members within a co-acting team needs little coordination. On the other hand, **interdependent teams** rely heavily on other individuals and require a high level of coordination. Examples of co-acting teams include wrestling or gymnastics. While these are "team" sports, their success is based on the accumulative total of individual performances. Each member is expected to do their part for the team, but individual performances may not be enhanced by the actions of others. On the other hand, soccer or basketball would be examples of interdependent teams. It can be said of interdependent teams that the team is only as strong as its weakest link. There are many other types and descriptions of teams; Table 2-1 contains a list and description of those teams. Every team has inherent characteristics that enable a team to function effectively. In the next section, we will briefly explore those team characteristics.

Characteristics and Behaviors of Teams

Teams characteristically have all the knowledge, skills, and experience necessary to fulfill its mandate resident within the team members.[11] Exploiting some of these characteristics is a challenge to some organizations. The organization (or leader) can create an atmosphere that promotes or hinders these behaviors. These characteristics and behaviors include

1. Self-governing
2. Promoting innovation
3. Being credible
4. Behaving ethically
5. Managing internal conflict quickly.

Self-governing implies the ability to monitor and police its own activities and establish its own set of criteria on which to base performance. Promoting innovation (i.e., new ideas) requires challenging member's ideas or confronting long-standing techniques or traditions. The team's first challenge to creating a culture of innovation may be a history of past success or a culture built to protect the status quo. Teams can overcome either of these obstacles with deliberate and focused dialogue. Credibility is ideal, and ultimately enhances the overall effectiveness and authority

TABLE 2-1 Types of Teams	
Type of Team	**Description**
Functional Teams	Functional teams are created by higher authority for a specific purpose and function and therefore have little control over their mission or objectives. Once team objectives are met, the team is normally dissolved. Functional team members typically have similar areas of expertise and have a strong team leader.
Cross-Functional Teams	Cross-functional teams are very similar to functional teams. However, there is typically a much greater diversity in expertise of individual members.
Self-Managed Teams	Self-managed teams have very little control over their teams' overall objectives; typically they are assigned. However, this type of team has very high autonomy over its work procedures and no strong internal leader directing its activities. Self-directed teams typically will have little diversity in members' expertise.
Executive Teams	An executive team has a very high control over its own mission and objectives, has a strong internal leader, has high autonomy of its work procedures, and has a high level of diversity among members' experience and expertise.
Self-Defining Teams	A self-defining team has a high control over its own mission and objectives, but does not have a strong internal leader. It has high autonomy of its work procedures and the diversity among members' experience and expertise is varied depending on the team's purpose.

Reprinted with permission from Yukl G. (2002). *Leadership in organizations*. 5th ed. Upper Saddle River, NJ: Prentice Hall.

of the team. Credibility is gained when actions are repeatedly perceived and trustworthy, reliable, and useful. Credibility garners authority from a positive track record and a history of trustworthiness. Teams must also demonstrate stringent ethical standards, which are self-imposed and based on organizational culture and professional responsibility. Finally, effective teams address conflict as soon as it arises.

Once a team has matured, a healthy team exhibits the following behaviors:[6]

1. All members contribute what they are thinking.
2. Decisions and actions are made on consensus, not a vote.
3. A member's value is judged by the merit of the idea and not on personal issues.
4. Appropriate priorities are reflected as time spent on the different agenda items.
5. Members understand, know, and appreciate each other.
6. Members are objective about approaching their goals and tasks.
7. Rewards and criticisms are shared.
8. Information is fed to all members.
9. Individuals are respected as members of the team regardless of contribution.

Once a team is producing positive outcomes and facilitating necessary changes, they must continue to be vigilant and proactive. One way to do this is to recruit a diversity of team members. In the next section we will discuss the sports medicine team and how to handle conflict that may arise within this team.

THE SPORTS MEDICINE TEAM

The sports medicine team is varied and diverse and consists of many professions and trades. The diversity within the sports medicine team is one of its strengths. Often the team draws on the expertise and experience of the other members to build the best treatment intervention possible for the athlete or patient. Tables 2-2 and 2-3 list some of the members who may participate on the sports medicine team. It is important to realize not every team member will always contribute and of those who do contribute, all do not contribute equally.

The athlete or patient is often the central focus of the sports medicine team. Within the larger sports medicine team there is usually a core group who has frequent communication with the athlete or patient. In the traditional athletic training context, these core individuals are the team physician, the athletic trainer, and the coach. It is the team or referring physician who has the highest authority within this matrix (Fig. 2-1). However, the athletic trainer typically serves the coordinating role

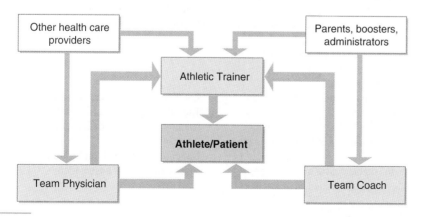

FIGURE 2-1 Sports medicine team matrix

TABLE 2-2 Members of the Sports Medicine Team

Discipline	Description	Respective Professional Association(s)
Athlete/patient	The central member of the sports medicine triad.	
Athletic Administration	Athletic Director or administrator	National Association of Collegiate Directors of Athletics
Athletic Trainer/ Therapist	An allied health care provider capable of performing immediate and emergency injury management, injury assessment, and rehabilitation.	National Athletic Trainers' Association World Federation of Athletic Trainers and Therapists Canadian Athletic Therapists' Association
Biomechanist	An exercise scientist educated and trained in the mechanics of human movement and providing evaluation, assessment, and recommendation of body mechanics.	British Association of Sport and Exercise Sciences
Sport Coach	The person in charge of the preparation of an athlete or a team.	National Collegiate Athletic Association
Exercise Physiologist	A professional who monitors and assesses cardiovascular and metabolic effects and mechanisms of exercise.	American Society of Exercise Physiologists American College of Sports Medicine
External Stakeholder	A booster, attorney, community member, or parent.	NA
School Counselor	A professional who helps all students in the areas of academic achievement, personal/social development, and career development.	The American School Counselor Association
Massage Therapist	A practitioner trained to apply manual massage techniques with the intention of positively affecting the health and well-being of the client.	American Massage Therapy Association
Nutritionist	A health professional with special training in nutrition who can offer help with the choice of foods a person eats and drinks. Also called a dietitian.	American Dietetic Association
Pharmacist	A health professional who practices pharmacy. A pharmacist typically takes an order for medicines from a physician in the form of a medical prescription and dispenses the medication to the patient.	American Pharmacists Association
Physical Therapist	A trained health professional who performs and teaches exercises and other physical activities to aid in rehabilitation and maximize physical ability with less pain.	American Physical Therapy Association
Physician Assistant	A physician assistant (PA) practices medicine under the supervision of physicians and surgeons. A PA is formally trained to provide diagnostic, therapeutic, and preventive health care services, as delegated by a physician.	American Academy of Physician Assistants
Registered Nurse	A nurse is a health care professional responsible (with others) for the safety and recovery of acutely ill or injured people, health maintenance of the healthy, and treatment of life-threatening emergencies in a wide range of health care settings.	American Nurses Association
Sports Psychologist	A terminally degreed/licensed psychologist who specializes in sports performance.	American Psychological Association The American Board of Sport Psychology
Strength Coach	A professional who deals with the strength (weight lifting) and conditioning (muscular and aerobic) needs of athletes.	National Strength and Conditioning Association National Academy of Sports Medicine
Team Physician	A team physician is the medical director of the sports medicine team and is a board-certified, licensed physician (MD or DO).	American Medical Association
Technician	A medical tech, x-ray tech, phlebotomist, lab tech, or pharmacy tech	NA
Athletic Training Student	A student enrolled in an entry-level CAATE-accredited athletic training education program.	NA

TABLE 2-3 Specialty Physicians

Specialty Physician (area of focus)	Professional Association
Chiropractor (spine)	American Chiropractic Association's Council on Sports Injuries and Physical Fitness
Dentist (teeth, mouth, and jaw)	American Dental Association
Obstetrician/Gynecologist (pregnancy, childbirth, female reproductive conditions)	American College of Obstetricians and Gynecologists
Oncologist (cancer)	American Society of Clinical Oncology
Ophthalmologist (eyes)	American Academy of Ophthalmology
Optometrist (eyes, vision)	American Optometric Association
Orthopedist (musculoskeletal issues)	American Academy of Orthopaedic Surgeons
Pediatrician (children and adolescents)	American Academy of Pediatrics
Physiatrist (physical medicine and rehabilitation)	American Academy of Physical Medicine and Rehabilitation
Podiatrist (foot and ankle)	American Podiatric Medical Association
Psychiatrist (brain and mental disorders)	American Psychiatric Association

for much of the team's activities and communications. In order to have a good working relationship within this team, it is important to establish solid relationships and manage conflict effectively.

Establishing Relationships

Establishing meaningful relationships with other members of the sports medicine team is a wise behavior and critical function of the savvy athletic trainer. Team formation includes clearing up role confusion and eliminating dissatisfaction that results from a lack of trust. As resolution is achieved, roles are clarified, and trust is established, productivity of the team increases (Fig. 2-2).

Creating **rapport** is often an important factor in building meaningful and lasting relationship with other health care professions. Rapport is having mutual understanding and a foundation of trust between two or more parties. The cornerstone to establishing professional relationships is consistently demonstrating competent, professional, and ethical behavior.

The following practices are helpful in establishing rapport.

1. When making a first impression, do not be too casual; refer to an individual by their appropriate title and full name.
2. Be aware of the feelings and values of others.
3. Listen intently, take genuine interest in them and their topic.
4. Exhibit self-confidence and professional behavior.
5. Exhibit ethical standards of practice professionally and personally.

Ultimately, having good rapport in the community as a health care professional promotes athletic training. Once relationships are developed it takes energy and time to sustain them. Often if that energy is not given conflict emerges.

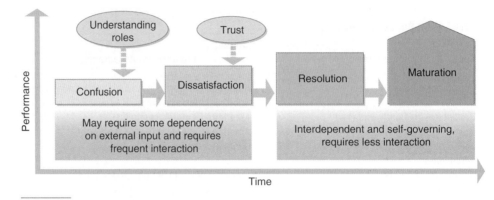

FIGURE 2-2 Team formation strategies

THE NATURE OF CONFLICT

Teams will experience conflict. **Conflict** is a state of disagreement or incompatibility between two or more people or groups of people. Conflict is an inevitable consequence of cooperative action.[10,14] Managers and leaders can spend up to 40% of their day dealing with some form of conflict.[15] Although unpleasant, conflict that is managed correctly can end up strengthening the team. Sometimes, conflict can end complacency, initiate dialogue, facilitate action, foster innovation, and demand participation.[5,7] However, most leaders and managers still prefer to prevent conflict.

Types of Conflict

Conflict can be interpersonal or organizational. Interpersonal conflict is a result of two or more competing values emerging within a group and is typically described as a clash between personalities. Organizational conflict develops when there is a difference in opinion and practice between the values or culture of the organization and an individual or team. Both types of conflict have a negative influence on group members and can even affect external stakeholders. Ultimately, if unable to be resolved, either type of conflict may require intervention.

Causes of Conflict

Sources of conflict are many and varied. However, conflict is fundamentally about two or more competing values. For example, the organization or organization's representative (i.e., the coach) values winning above all, but the student athlete (or parents) values education above all, and the athletic trainer values health of the athlete. Obviously all three team members want to win, but in the heat of competition these values compete to be in the top spot. Valuing winning, the coach may suggest playing an injured athlete; valuing the overall health of the athlete, the AT resists the coach, resulting in a conflict. Adding to conflict is the parent or athlete who is already upset because there is an exam first period the next morning, and is frustrated because a game was scheduled the night before an exam. With these three group members (coach, athlete, ATC) each valuing something different, it is easy to see how conflict can be introduced. The causes of conflict are often associated with:

1. Poor communication
2. Unclear expectations

3. Loss of trust or credibility due to unethical or illegal behavior
4. Unresolved disagreements
5. Perception of excessive ego
6. Failure to compromise
7. Fear of being taken advantage of

Once the source of the conflict has been identified, strategies can be formulated to help manage and prevent future conflicts.

Managing Conflict

The difficulty with conflict lies in the underlying assumptions, values, or beliefs made by the different parties involved in the conflict. Team members should take strides toward understanding other member's values. It is sound practice to seek to understand each party's point of view and frame of reference when bringing up potentially volatile issues, which necessarily requires a thorough awareness of your own perspective, biases, and values. Few other strategies are as important or likely to be as effective in resolving conflict as knowing your own biases, beliefs, and values.

Tolerance is an important behavior in managing and preventing conflict. **Tolerance** has evolved to imply more than what it originally meant, which was "the capacity to endure."[12] The concept of tolerance is not synonymous with acceptance nor is it the absence of disagreement. Tolerant behavior inherently acknowledges there are other views, behaviors, and beliefs; it does not mean one must accept those views or beliefs as correct or valid (or else there would be nothing to tolerate). A tolerant athletic trainer is willing to acknowledge that any opposing philosophy or value has little influence on overall competence or the ability of the team to accomplish its mission. A truly tolerant team can vehemently disagree on personal and organizational levels, but it sets aside those differences and pursues productive dialogue on the relevant issues in a non-threatening fashion. Because tolerance is an ideal that is difficult to practice, it is incumbent on teams to understand how people cope with conflict.

Coping with conflict often includes one of the following behaviors: collaborating, controlling, compromising, avoiding, or accommodating.

1. Collaborators assert their viewpoint, but welcome and encourage feedback. Collaborating is referred to as the "win-win" situation and often requires innovation and creativity. True collaboration can be time consuming, but is often invigorating and morale building to the team.
2. Controllers tend to discourage disagreement and are unwilling to entertain the input of others. Those given to controlling often demonstrate very little tolerance of other's viewpoints.
3. Compromisers tend to believe each party should be required to give something up. While not always a bad strategy, compromising runs the risk of promoting self preservation, which undermines teamwork. Compromising has been referred to as lose-lose because no one gets exactly what they wanted.
4. Avoiders are those who just ignore or divert attention from a problem.
5. Accommodators accept other's viewpoints at the expense of their own opinion. Accommodating can be good if one does not feel strongly about his or her opinion.

Because conflict is a certainty, there several behaviors and practices that can be used to prevent or resolve conflict. Competencies that can help curb conflict include:

1. Effective communication
2. Active listening
3. Global and cultural literacy
4. Critical thinking
5. Empathy

Practices that can help prevent or limit conflict include:

1. Separating the people from the problem. Do not allow different viewpoints to overly influence how you value someone else's contribution. Focus on intended outcomes, not personal positions or values.
2. Disseminating expected outcomes. Clearly state team missions, goals, and milestones in advance of a team initiative or project.
3. Giving the benefit of the doubt. Preserve and promote the ideal that each member of the team is as committed or more committed to the ultimate goal or mission as everyone else.
4. Establishing parameters for disagreement. Every team will have disagreements. Establish guidelines and policies for handling conflicts before the team is formed.
5. Honoring confidentiality of team members. Team members interact as part of the formal team with everyone present and outside of the formal team meeting. Do not disclose information that is given in confidence regardless of where interaction occurs.
6. Identifying underlying values and interests of team members. Understanding someone's view is not the same as agreeing with it. Seek to understand the viewpoint of others. This may include moral, religious, socioeconomic, or ethnic backgrounds.
7. Telling the truth. Honesty is the cornerstone of credibility.

Many of these strategies and competencies required for effective teamwork and conflict management depend on effective communication. Communicating is arguably one of the most important skills for any leader, management role, or position. In the next section we will discus the various applications of communication.

COMMUNICATION

Clear and effective **communication** is the single most important aspect of any successful team and one of the most important skills of any leader.[11] Communication is the act of conveying information. Often, effective communicators are leaders within an organization.[3] Communication that is effective must be timely, from a credible source, comprehensive, objective and factual, and multidirectional.[11]

For example, effective communicators often plan and time the release of information. Information that is released too far in advance or too late in the action process can sidetrack or disable others' efforts. Furthermore, information must be from a reliable source. Information that is not from a credible source is often given a low priority or ignored. Lastly, it is important that information be shared with supervisors, subordinates, and peers. Keeping as many people as possible informed of actions and decisions facilitates teamwork and raises morale.

Three aspects of communication have been identified as important leadership behaviors within athletic training practice:[9]

1. Written communication
2. Verbal communication
3. Body language

Written Communication

Written communication includes information that is conveyed through any written or typed medium. It is necessary for written correspondence to be concise, articulate, and convey meanings that will be understood by the receiver. Written communication takes several forms, including memorandums, e-mails, letters, proposals, scholarly papers, newsletters, medical records, and reports. Grammar, punctuation, sentence structure, and writing style are important even if communicating informally. It is important to realize that using e-mail abbreviations, text messaging, and other informal forms of written communication, while convenient, can undermine the importance of the intended message and may not be appreciated or understood by all recipients.

Written correspondence should meet these minimum standards. (Keep in mind that an individual company or department may have additional standards.)

1. Clearly identify who this message is intended for.
2. Clearly identify who the message is from.
3. Include the date the message was generated.
4. Include a clear, concise subject line or heading. Be sure that title or contents of the message are clearly distinguishable very early on.
5. The body of the message should be concise and free from redundancy.
6. Identify any other person who also received a copy or "carbon copy" (i.e., cc).
7. Include an acceptable closing (i.e., sincerely, respectfully, regards, etc).

Finally, once the document is drafted, proof read and edit carefully. Make sure the tone is appropriate and any ambiguous language clarified.

Verbal Communication

Compared to written communication, verbal communication requires a different level of skill and comfort to convey ideas and establish rapport. Verbal communication includes conveying information through speaking and includes speeches, presentations, formal and casual conversations, and report giving. Sign language is also considered a form of verbal communication. Tone of voice, comfort, sound level (volume), and awareness of personal space are important issues to consider when speaking to others.

There are several valuable strategies that can help improve verbal communication skills:

1. Be aware of your volume and intensity. Be careful to not speak too loudly or too softly.
2. Take the time and speak slowly, even if in a hurry or there is a sense of urgency.
3. Animate your voice, do not use a monotone. Fluctuate the volume and pitch of your words.
4. Do not mumble, enunciate all your words.
5. Make eye contact with the intended recipients.

6. Be aware of others involved. Use occasional pauses, being sure to allow someone to interject when you sense they want to speak or if they become fidgety.

It is not uncommon to experience anxiety when preparing to speak to groups. It is important to realize that even though there may be evidence to the contrary, people who experience a lot of anxiety before speaking to others (especially in a public setting) tend to avoid communicating verbally in general. The avoidance of public communication is perceived as a leadership weakness. Therefore, it is important to be intentional about verbal communication. To curb speech anxiety, remember the following tips:

1. Be prepared, know your speech and the content.
2. Have a list of key points, be ready to consult the list if necessary.
3. Know the audience.
4. Control your breathing.
5. Practice, practice, practice: rehearse your speech in front of friends.

In addition to practicing the above strategies, good communicators also must be prepared to listen carefully.

Listening

Listening is also an important aspect of verbal communication. Listening conveys respect and is a sound strategy for building rapport and gaining trust. Good listeners are perceived by others as leaders. Listening requires that the hearer be attentive and responsive to the one speaking. Effective listening includes not ignoring or being distractive when someone else is speaking, letting someone completely finish their thought before you interject a comment or response, and making eye contact with the speaker. Another aspect of listing includes formulating a response. Good listeners do not use the time when someone else is speaking to formulate or think of a response. The best listeners listen the entire time they are being spoken to, and wait until the speaker's point has been made before formulating their response.

In its most simple form listening is critically appraising what was communicated. The hearer must keep in mind that what is being communicated often times includes more than the actual words spoken. Dye and Graman[4] outline several listening behaviors for health care professionals that can enhance overall communication.

1. Feedback. When communicating, expect to receive feedback. When finished speaking expect a reply or rebuttal, do not presume the final word; after all, you just engaged someone in dialogue. The listener must be careful to not be formulating their rebuttal while being spoken to. Listen first, rebut later.
2. Develop a clear, active listening posture. Listening is more than just being quiet while someone else is speaking. Make sure you eliminate condescending gestures or sounds, make and maintain eye contact, turn your shoulders toward whoever is speaking, and frequently acknowledge their points by nodding or a gentle smile.
3. Summarize. Paraphrase what was communicated back to the speaker. Do not simply repeat what was said; after all, what was said may not be what was communicated. Take a moment to reflect and analyze, then summarize key points or ideas, being sure to give the speaker a chance to confirm of disconfirm.
4. Ask probing questions. Follow up questions can be a tremendous asset for effective communication. They can spawn new ideas, clarify points or positions, and ultimately reduce the risk of miscommunication.

5. Monitor emotions. Emotional reactions on the part of the hearer will derail the hearer and the speaker. The hearer needs to be aware of emotions such as anger, frustration, elations, shock, or boredom and take intentional measures to project the correct listening posture.

Communication also includes appropriate use of gestures and body language.

Body Language and Nonverbal Communication

Appropriate use of body language is an important behavior for athletic training practice.[9] Body language can influence communication dramatically. Body language includes employing appropriate facial expressions, gestures, eye contact, and use of personal space. Effective athletic trainers use non-verbal cues and body-language when communicating to others. Nonverbal communication is enhanced when:

1. Posture is erect. Slouching and slumping send signals of disinterest and lack of respect.
2. Appropriate physical contact is used. Lightly tapping someone on the shoulder or a firm hand-shake.
3. Eye contact is maintained. Keep eye contact with other parties at all times and keep a relaxed smile when being spoken to.
4. Appropriate gestures are used. Subtly nodding your head in agreement when appropriate. Furrowing your brow, squinting your eyes, turning your back, or inquisitive facial expressions, or crossing your arms can send signals of mistrust or unbelief.

Lastly, non-verbal communication is also dramatically effected by appearance. Appropriate hygiene and grooming is essential to sending clear and credible messages. Having clean, pressed shirts, polished shoes, clean fingernails, clean shaven or tightly trimmed mustache or beard, well groomed hair, reasonable jewelry (not gaudy), absence of body odor, and clean teeth are all essential. Failure in any of these areas of communication may lead to barriers in communication.

Barriers to Communication

There are three primary barriers to effective communication: technology, semantics, and psychological. **Technological barriers** are a result of the loss of face to face communication skills due to emails, memos, voice mails, fax machines, instant messages, text messaging, and the like. While technology certainly facilitates communication and makes access to others easier, it does not necessarily enhance communication. In fact, never communicating face to face can be construed as barriers to learning interpersonal communication techniques. While it is important to take advantage of technology, it should not be substituted for personal interaction, appropriate body language, and articulating an idea or thought clearly and concisely. Another barrier can be semantics.

Semantic barriers are those breakdowns that occur because of the many hats athletic trainers wear in a given day. Semantics is the meaning speakers give to their words. Semantics are always interpreted in conjunction with body-language, values, and context. Therefore, it is possible to say one thing and mean another. For example, saying to an injured athlete "I think you are going to be OK" while simultaneously grimacing, looking away, and winking at a near-by student athlete, means something different than saying the same words in a very affirming, assuring voice, with direct eye contact. However, body language is only one aspect of semantics. Semantic barriers include the assumptions made based on different definitions and view of the world. Each of us has different experiences on which we frame our

> ### From the Field
>
> *Meetings are usually an important part of athletic training programs; even if you are not the one who convened the meeting, you will likely be required to attend many of them. If I had to guess, I'd say the following example has happened in dozens of meetings I have either attended or convened. This case in point is more general than some of the others, deals with several issues, and is about the ineffectiveness of vague language, team strife, as well as a failure to redirect and manage a meeting effectively.*
>
> *I can remember an incident when there was disagreement between two members of the athletic training staff (we'll call them Fred and Bill) over the how a specific incident was handled. The disagreement was ultimately over preferences, and not about something done incorrectly or incompetently. Bill thought it would have been better to do "XYZ" instead of "ABC." "ABC" was exactly what Fred did. Unfortunately, Bill did not speak to Fred about the situation directly. During the next staff meeting Bill used innuendo and implied that Fred's actions were wrong, but did not explicitly cite Fred or the specific action. When it came time for Bill to have the floor, he used his time to jump on his personal "soap box," stating that anytime this particular situation arises, XYZ should always be the automatic procedure for handling it. Most of us in the room could immediately feel Fred bristle and knew that Bill's comments were a reaction to Fred's recent handling of that situation. However, some of the others in the room were not privy to what Fred had just done, therefore had no frame of reference for the comment. Having no frame of reference and not caring personally, they verbally supported Bill's XYZ procedure. Before anyone else could offer a suggestion, Fred reacted to the suggestions and a controlled but hostile and uncomfortable "discussion" over how this specific situation should be handled ensued; needless to say, not much else was discussed and the meeting was very unproductive.*

communication. The speaker must be careful not to assume or generalize that everyone has the same experiences. There is also professional jargon, organizational culture, and "trade-ese" (i.e., the terms or phrases unique to a profession) that change meanings of words or ideas. Being aware of semantic barriers (those meanings unique to a certain culture) can help eliminate communication barriers.

Psychological barriers can be the most harmful. These barriers include blaming, interrupting, inappropriate joking, threatening, or patronizing. It also includes making statements or gestures of apathy or indifference. These cues invariably send signals of disrespect and demonstrate a total lack of teamwork. Classic examples of putting up a psychological barrier include statements such as, "I do not know" (without offering to help find out); "That is not my problem;" "That is not our policy;" or "I can not help right now."

Incorporating all the aspects of communication can be effectively demonstrated by facilitating a meeting. While it is not likely that new athletic trainers will convene and facilitate many meetings, understanding how to manage and lead a meeting is a valuable skill. In the next section we will see that facilitating and planning meetings can be an effective way to communicate.

Managing Team Meetings

In general, people tend to dislike meetings. Many times a leader's or manager's reputation is demonstrated in his or her ability to run a meeting. In spite of their reputation, meetings are great vehicles for disseminating important information, and if run properly can help in fostering team dynamics. Meetings also provide a platform for training and development, updating and reminding, problem solving, explaining changes, friendly debating, conveying thanks and gratitude, and reviewing procedures. Because meetings can meet so many needs they are essential. However, because they take significant time and energy to organize and administrate, and because many people do not appreciate meetings, leading them takes skill and thoughtful planning.

Facilitating a meeting smoothly requires addressing several considerations, including the selection of competent minute takers. The **minutes** are notes or the records of the proceedings from the meeting, which should include discussion points relevant to agenda items and action items and assignments. Nothing is as frustrating as a great comment or discussion that no one can remember. Getting the minutes distributed after the meeting is just as important, if not more important, than the meeting itself.

Meeting facilitators may need to organize table or room set-up. While King Arthur's fabled "round table" fosters ownership and equality, which is also very important to facilitate, at times a rectangle table is best. The traditional rectangular table, with a designated "head" establishes a leader. When agenda items are expected to be hotly debated, having a clear head can help facilitate getting through the entire agenda. However, if "hot topics" are expected, the chairperson might also consider organizing the seating. It is to everyone's best interest not to seat rivals next to or facing each other; it will only end up as a distraction and ultimately detract from the team's purpose for meeting.

The most important aspect of any meeting is setting the agenda. The agenda is a powerful tool and the person who controls the agenda ultimately controls the meeting. The agenda indicates what is going to be discussed, the priority of topics, and how much time will be spent on a topic. It is a wise leadership practice to offer a chance to participants to add items to the agenda. Not every submission needs to be added, but there might be issues raised by other team members that do need a place on the agenda.

Once the agenda is set, distribute it a few days before the meeting. This helps those attending prepare for the meeting and gather and organize their thoughts about agenda items. It is also important to identify the expected outcome of each agenda item in the topic. For example, sample agenda items might include:

1. "to discuss" the problem of recurrent equipment theft.
2. "to decide" how to handle recurrent equipment theft.
3. "to recommend" how to handle recurrent equipment theft.
4. "to report" on recurrent equipment thefts.

Each of the outcomes, to "discuss, decide, report, or recommend" implies a different purpose. Identifying the topics in this fashion may help the facilitator's and participant's frame of mind for the meeting or topic discussion. If participants know in advance the purpose is to "discuss" rather than "decide," it helps set them in the correct frame of mind for the meeting. A valuable resource to anyone who convenes or facilitates meetings is Robert's Rules of Order. Robert's Rules of Order (originally published in 1876) delineates rules for ordering a meeting, setting an agenda, accepting motions or nominations, debating, voting, gaining or giving the floor, and taking minutes. It is an exhaustive set of guidelines that covers any situation that can arise in a meeting. Meetings usually follow a prescribed sequence that includes:

1. Calling the meeting to order by a presiding member.
2. Approving the minutes. This is for clarifying and ratifying proceedings from the previous meeting.
3. Hearing reports from standing and special committees. This allows committees to update the group on activities since the last meeting. If there are no reports then the meeting immediately goes to discussing the issues for which the meeting was assembled (i.e., agenda items)

4. Discussing Old Business. This is for discussing or deciding on issues that were not closed at the previous meeting.

5. Introducing New Business. Including "new business" in a meeting agenda can take two forms. First, the items are submitted in advance to the meeting chair and included at the chair's discretion. Second, open the floor for new business. Opening the floor is only recommended if the team is cohesive and mature, otherwise this could be a volatile move.

Robert's Rules of Order clearly establish that a presiding chair take control of the meeting, one who will maintain order and decorum, and keep to the agenda at hand. Running a smooth meeting with clear objectives enhances the perception of leadership ability. Ultimately, a smooth meeting can also add to the chemistry of the team, make each individual feel like a contributing member, and prevent the perception that the meeting was a waste of time.

CHAPTER SUMMARY

Agreement, the willingness to enter into productive dialogue, is an important aspect of effective teamwork. The teamed approach to health care is vital to a successful athletic training program, and requires intentional integration of diverse medical and health care professionals. As teams develop and grow, it is likely that conflict will arise. To manage conflict effectively it is important to listen carefully to what team members are trying to communicate and to value that contribution. Effective teams not only deal with conflict quickly, but also communicate effectively. One of the greatest sources of conflict among teams is poor communication. Athletic trainers need to be excellent verbal, non-verbal, and written communicators. Effective communicators make every effort to speak and write clearly and concisely, avoid common communication barriers, and use body language and gestures appropriately.

 Leadership Application

One morning, you're having coffee with three other athletic trainers and the strength coach at your university. After a few minutes one of your colleagues begins to talk about an incident at practice between a coach and athlete that occurred the previous day. During the incident the coach, who is of Indian origin, began to yell at an athlete about his performance and effort during practice. The athletic trainer telling the story starts to imitate the coach's accent and exaggerate his facial gestures and body language. The others begin to laugh and at that moment the athlete who was being scolded by the coach walks into the athletic training room.

Critical Thinking Questions

1. What would you do...
   a. If you were the athlete entering the room?
   b. If you were another coach entering the room?
   c. If you were the coach and found out about the athletic trainer's morning coffee talk?
2. How could the situation affect the coach?
3. How might this affect the relationships involved?

References

1. Brown F, Driver SR, Briggs CA. (1952). *A Hebrew and English lexicon of the Old Testament.* New York: Oxford University Press.

2. Clegg S, Kornberger M, Pitsis T. (2005). *Managing and organizations: An introduction to theory and practice.* London: Sage Publications.

3. Dubrin, A. (2004). *Leadership: Research findings, practice, and skills.* 4th ed. New York: Houghton Mifflin Co.

4. Dye C, Garman, A. (2006). *Exceptional leadership: 16 critical competencies for healthcare executives.* Chicago: Health Administration Press.

5. Dye, C. (2000). *Leadership in healthcare: Values at the top.* Chicago: Health Administration Press.

6. Gangel K. (1997). *Team leadership: Using multiple gifts to build a unified vision.* Chicago: Moody Publishers.

7. Haraway D, Haraway W. (2005). Analysis of the effects of conflict-management and resolution training on employee stress at a healthcare organization. *Hospital Topics 83, 4*:11–17.

8. Kowalski K. (2003). Building teams through communication and partnership. In: Yoder-Wise P. *Leading and managing in nursing.* St. Louis: Mosby; 323–347.

9. Kutz M. (2006). *Importance of leadership competencies and content for athletic training education and practice: A Delphi technique and national survey* [dissertation]. Boca Raton, FL: Lynn University.

10. Liebler J, McConnell C. (2004). *Management principles for health professionals.* Boston: Jones and Bartlett.

11. McConnell C. (2006). *Umiker's management skills for the new health care supervisor.* Boston: Jones and Bartlett Publishers.

12. Merriam-Webster. (2003). *Merriam-Webster dictionary.* 11th ed. Springfield, MA: Merriam-Webster.

13. Pew Health Professions Commission. (1998). *Recreating health professional practice for a new century.* The Center for the Health Professions. Available at: http://www.futurehealth.ucsf.edu/pdf_files/recreate.pdf. Accessed on August 8, 2007.

14. Porter-O'Grady T. (2004). Constructing a conflict resolution program for health care. *Health Care Management Review 29, 4*:278–283.

15. Thomas R. (2002). *Conflict Management systems: A methodology for addressing the cost of conflict in the workplace.* Available at: http://www.mediate.com/articles/thomasR.cfm#. Accessed August 22, 2007.

16. Yukl, G. (2002). *Leadership in organizations.* 5th ed. Upper Saddle River, NJ: Prentice Hall.

Chapter 3

Professional Preparation

"Success always comes when preparation meets opportunity."

HENRY HARTMAN

CHAPTER RATIONALE

Role Delineation Study Components

Knowledge of:

- Resources for continuing education
- The credentialing process and laws for athletic trainers

Educational Competencies

- Describe the process of attaining and maintaining national and state athletic training professional credentials.
- Describe the current professional development requirements for the continuing education of athletic trainers and how to locate available, approved continuing education opportunities.
- Describe the role and function of the professional organizations and credentialing agencies that impact the athletic training profession.
- Summarize the current requirements for the professional preparation of the athletic trainer.
- Summarize the principles of planning and organizing workshops, seminars, and clinics in athletic training and sports medicine for health care personnel, administrators, other appropriate personnel, and the general public.

Key Terms

Altruism: An approach in which an individual is more concerned with benefitting others than himself or herself.

Certification: A form of credential that is awarded by a national association or organization.

Continuing education: Education and or training activities earned by a certified or licensed professional that are acquired post-credential in order to maintain that credential.

Credentials: Official statement or recognition of a governing body that an individual has demonstrated pre-established competency in an area.

Education: The process of equipping an individual to perform undefined functions in unpredictable situations.

Egoism: Behaviors based solely on self-interest and personal gain.

Exemption: A type of state regulation that allows a professional to practice without having to comply with the standards of practice of other professionals.

Licensure: A form of credential that is awarded by a state or federal agency. Licensure is often more restrictive than certification.

Profession: An organized body of educated people who have specialized knowledge.

Professional: An individual who has acquired a highly specialized education within a defined body of knowledge.

Registration: A form of state credential that protects the public by requiring professionals to notify the state of their intent to practice.

Training: The process of preparing individuals to perform a specific task within a defined or predictable situation.

T he athletic training profession has experienced tremendous numerical growth and continues to gain a reputation as a rigorous and desirable profession. Before 1950 "trainers" as they were commonly known, handed out water and massaged athletes' sore muscles. Today "athletic trainers" (as they are correctly called) have become a respected and diverse group of allied health care professionals, with a specialized body of knowledge and clinical expertise. Athletic training's growth has occurred, in part, because of professionalization and because the profession's leaders insist on professionalism from all new athletic trainers. Ensuring athletic training's continued growth and respect depends on athletic trainers who understand and can conceptualize the importance of professional preparation. Truly, professional behavior and a strong sense of professionalism are leadership behaviors that will continue to foster the growth of athletic training.

In this chapter we will outline the professional preparation of the athletic trainer. First, we will conceptually address professional behavior and describe what it means to be a professional. Next, we will elaborate on the credentialing process for athletic trainers, including how to maintain credentials. Last, we will discuss professional responsibilities, such as social and community sustainability, giving specific strategies for planning a workshop or community event.

PROFESSIONALS AND PROFESSIONALISM

Gaining recognition as an allied health care profession was a key milestone in athletic training's development. This milestone was a major catalyst for change within athletic training. Maintaining status as an allied health care profession continues to provide impetus for innovation and growth in athletic training practice and education. A strong sense of duty and responsibility should accompany the designation as a "profession." Professionals and those engaged in professional education are obligated to behave professionally. It is precisely this obligation, accompanied by a sense of duty to the profession that is a catalyst for growth within athletic training.

Expectations of Professionals

All professions, regardless of their industry, have certain expectations placed on them by society. These societal expectations vary according to profession. However, for the most part, professions are expected to ensure ethical conduct of their members, credential their members for the purpose of protecting the public (or stakeholders), and contribute some good to society.

When discussing professionalism, it is important to first define "professional" and "profession." A **professional** is an individual who has acquired a highly specialized education within a defined body of knowledge and has demonstrated a minimal set of predetermined competencies within that body of knowledge. A **profession** is an organized body of educated people with specialized knowledge. As implied in the definition, a profession is larger than any individual. A profession (i.e., the group as a whole) is obligated to promote and disseminate its specialized knowledge to other members, other professional associations, and to society. Within athletic training,

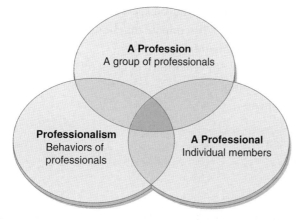

FIGURE 3-1 Relationship of a professional and his or her profession

the certified (and in many cases licensed) athletic trainer is a professional and "athletic training" is the profession (Fig. 3-1).

Expectations of a professional can be further delineated by a comparison between different types of preparation, i.e., education and training. **Education** is the process of equipping an individual to perform undefined functions in unpredictable situations.[5] The intended outcome of education is ultimately to prepare individuals to think critically, appraise different situations, integrate multiple stimuli, and make appropriate decisions for any number of circumstances. On the other hand, **training** prepares individuals how to do a specific task or job in predictable or defined situations.[5] Training results in technical knowledge and produces a technician. For example, athletic trainers are educated in six broad practice domains and at least twelve content areas in addition to any content required by the school or university that educates them (Table 3-1). This breadth of education is then intended to be assimilated by the athletic trainer to make informed clinical decisions.

Characteristics of Professions

Reputable professions typically have all or most of the following characteristics:[4]

TABLE 3-1 **Practice Domains and Core Content Areas Required in all CAATE-Accredited Athletic Training Education Programs**	
Practice Domains	**Core Content Areas**
1. Prevention	1. Risk Management and Injury Prevention
2. Clinical Evaluation and Diagnosis	2. Pathology of Injuries and Illnesses
3. Immediate Care	3. Orthopedic Clinical Examination and Diagnosis
4. Treatment, Rehabilitation and Reconditioning	4. Medical Conditions and Disabilities
5. Organization and Administration	5. Acute Care of Injuries and Illnesses
6. Professional Responsibility	6. Therapeutic Modalities
	7. Conditioning and Rehabilitative Exercises
	8. Pharmacology
	9. Psychosocial Intervention and Referral
	10. Nutritional Aspects of Injuries and Illnesses
	11. Health care Administration
	12. Professional Development and Responsibility

1. Specialized body of knowledge and skills
2. Scholars who discover and disseminate that body of knowledge
3. Socialization of student members
4. Licensure/certification (or other form of credential)
5. Professional associations
6. Governance by peers
7. Social prestige
8. Service to society
9. Code of ethics
10. Autonomy
11. Equivalence of members
12. Special relationship with clients

In addition to the above attributes, there are certain ideals to which all professions and professionals should aspire. These ideals (i.e., values) also form the foundation of ethical behavior. The values of professionalism include: altruism, accountability, duty, integrity, and respect.[4]

Altruism is the unselfish concern over the needs and values of others. It is the practice of putting others first in spite of self interests. An example of altruism is demonstrated when an athletic trainer places their patient's needs and desires before his or her own, such as staying late for treatments in spite of personal obligations, because the well-being of the athlete is of primary importance. Altruism is the antithesis of egoism. **Egoism** (not to be confused with *egotism*) is behavior predicated on self-interest and personal gain. An example of egoism includes staying late to treat the same athlete for no other reason than to eliminate personal guilt, avoid a confrontation with a coach or administrator, or to have something to hold over the coach or athlete by getting them to "owe you one."

Accountability is also innate within an authentic profession. Accountability involves taking responsibility for actions in light of commitments and expected outcomes. Athletic trainers are accountable to their patients, the community, their employer, their peers, other professionals, and their profession. Accountability is closely related to duty.

Duty in a professional sense is different from duty in the legal sense. In a professional sense, duty implies a commitment to serving the profession, collaborating with colleagues, and life-long learning. Athletic trainers often exhibit duty by serving on community committees or working on committees such as the American Red Cross or Emergency/Disaster Relief Teams. In other words, the athletic trainer feels a sense of obligation to offer his or her specialized knowledge to a greater cause and humanitarian-based efforts. Integrity is another aspect of professionalisms that includes adhering to personal and professional codes and commitments, and remaining truthful at all times. Finally, professionals are respectful, which is demonstrated by esteeming and honoring patients, their families, and all colleagues. The athletic trainer should make every effort to practice all the above values and in so doing model the epitome of professional behavior.

The ABCs of Professionalism

Relative to a profession, professionalism requires a conceptual understanding. Professionalism is similar to leadership in that it is easily recognized but difficult to define. Some authors have cited as many as 90 elements of professionalism.[3] Professionalism in medicine and health care has been defined as "those attitudes and behavior that serve to maintain another's interest above self-interest,"[1] and "displaying values, beliefs and attitudes that put the needs of another above your personal needs."[2] Based on these descriptions, professionalism is rooted in attitudes and behaviors that put other's feelings or needs above self (i.e., altruism). The principle of denying self for the good of the client or society is fundamental to professionalism. Professionalism (or the lack of it) is most likely to be demonstrated in a stressful or unplanned situation. When in the midst of a stressful or unplanned situation, it can help to remember and self reflect on the ABCs of professionalism: attitude, behavior, and character.

Attitude

Attitude is a disposition to act or behave in a certain way. In a trying or stressful situation, ask yourself, "Am I having a good attitude about this?" If the answer is "no" or "not sure," it is likely that professionalism is lacking. Attitude can either be "bad" or "good." A good attitude is demonstrated by a predisposition to act positively or optimistically in any number of different situations. Often athletic trainers are asked or expected to go above and beyond the call of duty (i.e., late hours, early mornings, multiple errands). Often these "requests" come without proper recognition or are unwritten expectations. While it is important to not let oneself be taken advantage of, deciding in advance to respond positively no matter what situations arise is a sign of a good attitude.

Behavior

Behavior is the action or reaction of a person. When considering behavior, it is important to ask, "What is the right thing to do, regardless of what seems to be fair?" When taking this perspective it is easier to behave professionally. In a professional context, appropriate behaviors are often purposeful; inappropriate behavior is often a result of a thoughtless reaction. While in an emergency or life-threatening situation, it is important for athletic trainers to "react" with accuracy and precision. These reactions are based on years of education and purposeful rehearsing. Thoughtless reactions to other individuals are often detrimental. Ultimately, professionalism is a result of appropriate behaviors regardless of what appears to be "fair."

Character

Character is fundamentally based on effective self-reflection. Ensuring character involves asking yourself, "Have my attitudes and behaviors been correct?" Individuals with character regularly reflect on their attitudes and behaviors then adjust them if necessary. Having character does not mean mistakes will never be made or that one must always admit guilt in a conflict or misunderstanding. On the contrary, people with great character can make major mistakes. It is, however, because of character that they admit their mistake and immediately take steps to rectify the outcome and change their behavior. Ultimately, owning up to poor attitudes or improper behavior is a sign of great character and is an important attribute of professionalism and a hallmark of leadership. Ultimately, every professional should routinely engage in critical self reflection.

Foundations of Professional Behaviors

The National Athletic Trainers' Association (NATA) educational competencies outline specific professional behaviors that are intended to permeate every aspect of an athletic trainer's practice of his or her profession.[6] These professional behaviors are outlined by NATA in their educational competencies manual. Furthermore, there

The next time you are surfing or browsing the World Wide Web, log onto the BOC website (at http://www.bocatc.org), familiarize yourself with the site, and search for the information listed below. Be prepared to bring the information you find to class and discuss it with classmates and faculty.

1. The BOC Candidate Handbook.
2. BOC policies regarding acquiring and maintaining approved provider status.
3. A list of ten (10) BOC approved CE providers.
4. A list of 10 upcoming CE events.
5. Find the link on the BOC website to your specific state regulatory agency and if applicable print your state's athletic training practice act.

From the field

As an undergraduate, I was both an athlete and an athletic training student (ATS). At certain times this created a unique predicament for me. It was not always clear to me how to handle these two roles, especially when I was with my teammates. As part of a small accredited athletic training education program, there were times when I was present in the athletic training room when my teammates were being treated. This can lead to a professional or even ethical dilemma (i.e., conflict of interest). On one occasion, I was in the athletic training room during open clinic hours and one of my teammates came in for an ultrasound treatment. Another ATS performed the treatment, but I could not resist joking around with my teammate even though my official capacity at that time was as an ATS. It just so happened (unbeknownst to me) that the school's chief nurse was in a meeting in an adjoining room to the athletic training room. She heard me say something inappropriate to this patient and was mortified at my behavior. First thing the next day I received a private invitation to meet with her and the head athletic trainer. I did not know why I was summoned and did not make the connection until the scene was replayed for me by the school's nurse. Needless to say, I was disciplined... and I deserved it. I had never considered how my joking might be perceived by other professionals or by other patients. She did not know that patient was a teammate of mine, but it did not matter. I was a young professional student, with a patient receiving treatment, and I behaved unprofessionally. I had not yet realized the distinction between my role as an ATS and my other roles. She was understanding and graceful, but it was made clear to me in no uncertain terms not to let it happen again.

are six codes of professional responsibility outlined by the Board of Certification, Inc. (BOC). These codes span six content areas including responsibility to patients, expected competency levels, professional involvement, conducting research, how to behave toward society, and expectations for business practices. These codes are listed in Box 3-1. While there are additional behaviors that are implied or expected from society or stakeholders, these behaviors are athletic training specific and are mandated by the profession of athletic training.

CREDENTIALING ATHLETIC TRAINERS

Every new profession must fight for proper recognition. Fighting for recognition certainly has been true for athletic training. Once a profession is recognized, there are different forms of regulation to help validate the profession and protect the public's interest. In athletic training, validation and regulation include credentialing. **Credentials** are an official statement or recognition, supported by a larger governing body that validates the holder as competent to perform certain tasks or demonstrate knowledge. Having some form of credentials implies that the holder can be trusted.

Professions have a responsibility to the public to credential their professionals. The Board of Certification (BOC) is the entity that credentials athletic trainers on the national level. In addition to national credentials, many states also credential athletic trainers. This dual credentialing model is desirable and lends to increased credibility of athletic training. Currently, 46 states regulate the profession of athletic training in some fashion. For a list of states that regulate athletic training, visit the BOC website at http://www.bocatc.org. There are three forms of credentials used to regulate athletic training: licensure, certification, and registration.

BOX 3-1   **BOC Codes of Professional Responsibility**

CODE 1: PATIENT RESPONSIBILITY

The Athletic Trainer or applicant:

1.1 Renders quality patient care regardless of the patient's race, religion, age, sex, nationality, disability, social/economic status or any other characteristic protected by law

1.2 Protects the patient from harm, acts always in the patient's best interests and is an advocate for the patient's welfare

1.3 Takes appropriate action to protect patients from Athletic Trainers, other health care providers or athletic training students who are incompetent, impaired or engaged in illegal or unethical practice

1.4 Maintains the confidentiality of patient information in accordance with applicable law

1.5 Communicates clearly and truthfully with patients and other persons involved in the patient's program, including, but not limited to, appropriate discussion of assessment results, program plans and progress

1.6 Respects and safeguards his or her relationship of trust and confidence with the patient and does not exploit his or her relationship with the patient for personal or financial gain

1.7 Exercises reasonable care, skill and judgment in all professional work

CODE 2: COMPETENCY

The Athletic Trainer or applicant:

2.1 Engages in lifelong, professional and continuing educational activities

2.2 Participates in continuous quality improvement activities

2.3 Complies with the most current BOC recertification policies and requirements

CODE 3: PROFESSIONAL RESPONSIBILITY

The Athletic Trainer or applicant:

3.1 Practices in accordance with the most current BOC Practice Standards

3.2 Knows and complies with applicable local, state and/or federal rules, requirements, regulations and/or laws related to the practice of athletic training

3.3 Collaborates and cooperates with other health care providers involved in a patient's care

3.4 Respects the expertise and responsibility of all health care providers involved in a patient's care

3.5 Reports any suspected or known violation of a rule, requirement, regulation or law by him/herself and/or by another Athletic Trainer that is related to the practice of athletic training, public health, patient care or education

3.6 Reports any criminal convictions (with the exception of misdemeanor traffic offenses or traffic ordinance violations that do not involve the use of alcohol or drugs) and/or professional suspension, discipline or sanction received by him/herself or by another Athletic Trainer that is related to athletic training, public health, patient care or education

3.7 Complies with all BOC exam eligibility requirements and ensures that any information provided to the BOC in connection with any certification application is accurate and truthful

3.8 Does not, without proper authority, possess, use, copy, access, distribute or discuss certification exams, score reports, answer sheets, certificates, certificant or applicant files, documents or other materials

3.9 Is candid, responsible, and truthful in making any statement to the BOC, and in making any statement in connection with athletic training to the public

3.10 Complies with all confidentiality and disclosure requirements of the BOC

3.11 Does not take any action that leads, or may lead, to the conviction, plea of guilty or plea of *nolo contendere* (no contest) to any felony or to a misdemeanor related to public health, patient care, athletics or education; this includes, but is not limited to: rape; sexual abuse of a child or patient; actual or threatened use of a weapon of violence; the prohibited sale or distribution of controlled substance, or its possession with the intent to distribute; or the use of the position of an Athletic Trainer to improperly influence the outcome or score of an athletic contest or event or in connection with any gambling activity

3.12 Cooperates with BOC investigations into alleged illegal or unethical activities; this includes but is not limited to, providing factual and non-misleading information and responding to requests for information in a timely fashion

3.13 Does not endorse or advertise products or services with the use of, or by reference to, the BOC name without proper authorization

CODE 4: RESEARCH

The Athletic Trainer or applicant who engages in research:

4.1 Conducts research according to accepted ethical research and reporting standards established by public law, institutional procedures and/or the health professions

4.2 Protects the rights and well being of research subjects

4.3 Conducts research activities with the goal of improving practice, education and public policy relative to the health needs of diverse populations, the health workforce, the organization and administration of health systems and health care delivery

CODE 5: SOCIAL RESPONSIBILITY

The Athletic Trainer or applicant:

5.1 Uses professional skills and knowledge to positively impact the community

CODE 6: BUSINESS PRACTICES

The Athletic Trainer or applicant:

6.1 Refrains from deceptive or fraudulent business practices

6.2 Maintains adequate and customary professional liability insurance

Licensure

Licensure is a credential awarded by a state. A state licensing board oversees who is licensed in their state and enforces state regulations on licensees. Of all the types of regulation, licensure is typically the most restrictive. This is because the state is responsible for the public's safety. As the most restrictive, licensure is often the most coveted form of credentialing by a profession. Currently 36 states offer licensure for athletic trainers. Typically athletic trainers must be BOC certified before they are state eligible for licensure. Furthermore, many states often restrict the use of the title "athletic trainer" to those who are licensed. However, each state has its own set of rules and regulations regarding who can be licensed and how licenses are attained.

Certification

Certification is form of credentialing awarded by a national association or organization. Certification is awarded when an individual demonstrates a predetermined level of competency. Standards for demonstrating minimal competency are left to the certifying agencies. However, certifying agencies must also undergo rigorous scrutiny to further protect the public and potential certificate holders. The National Commission for Certifying Agencies (NCCA) is a federal entity that accredits certifying agencies. The BOC is accredited by the NCCA. Competency is also demonstrated by graduating from an accredited university or college, often with regional and programmatic accreditation. Regional accreditation is for the entire institution. Programmatic accreditation is only for specific programs.

Within athletic training, an individual may not be considered a "professional" until certification is awarded by the BOC. The BOC owns the trademark on the ATC® credential. Therefore, it is the BOC (and not NATA) that administers the national exam and grants the ATC credential to those who successfully pass the national exam. In general, certification is not as restrictive as licensure, however most states only grant a license to an individual with BOC certification.

In the case of athletic training, graduating from a CAATE-accredited athletic training education program does not in and of itself satisfy standards to practice as an athletic trainer. However, it is the only avenue that qualifies someone to sit for the BOC exam. Once certified by the BOC, in most states, you are not yet qualified to practice as an athletic trainer; one hurdle remains. That hurdle is the state-level credential (i.e., the license). Only after being credentialed by the state may an individual use the title "athletic trainer" and practice in that state as an athletic trainer. Figure 3-2 is chain-of-events map that depicts the steps required to practice athletic training. Note that there are exceptions to this process and that specific regulations vary from state to state.

Registration

Registration is a third form of professional credentialing that helps to regulate professions. Like licensure, registration operates at the state level. Registration offers protection for the profession by not allowing those not registered to use the title "athletic trainer." However, guidelines for registering in a state may be as simple as notifying the state of your presence and demonstrating that you are a practicing member of a profession or there may be a more rigorous process. In any case, athletic training registration requires evidence of BOC certification.

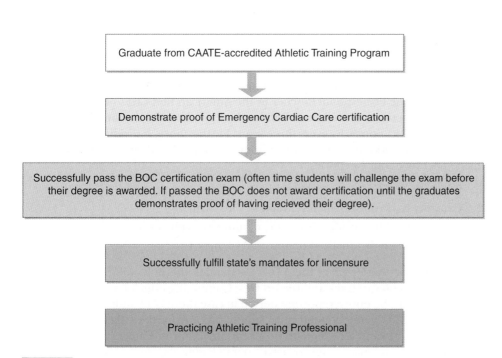

FIGURE 3-2 Chain-of-events map to athletic training practice

Exemption

Exemption is an additional form of regulation (not a credential) that allows athletic trainers to practice athletic training. Exemption is granted to professions so that they do not have to comply with the practice acts or scope of practice standards that a state may enforce on other professions. Exemption is not standard free. Athletic trainers in states that offer exemption still must meet specific guidelines to practice, such as demonstrating the appropriate educational degree and BOC certification. Furthermore, exempted athletic trainers are required to follow the standards and scope of practice outlined by their professional association or credentialing body. Currently three states offer exemption for athletic trainers and four states have no regulation for athletic trainers. Once a credential is acquired, the recipient has some obligation to the profession and the state.

PROFESSIONAL RESPONSIBILITY

Professional responsibility of athletic trainers is less about professional behavior (although professional behavior is a responsibility) and more about what it takes to promote their profession and maintain involvement in their profession. Membership within the athletic training profession is not determined solely by being a member of NATA per se, although that is a part. Membership within the profession is based on three fundamental issues:

1. Attaining the appropriate credentials.
2. Maintaining those credentials through continuing education and committment to life-long learning.
3. Engaging in activities that promote the profession's knowledge.

Continuing Education

Attaining the ATC® credential requires commitment and sacrifice. Maintaining the credential once it is earned requires life-long commitment and sacrifice. This includes maintaining a posture of life-long learning and involvement in continuing education.

Athletic trainers must continually maintain emergency cardiac care certification (e.g., CPR for the Professional Rescuer by the American Red Cross or Basic Life Support by the American Heart Association) and accumulate and document 75 hours of Continuing Education (CE) every three years. Furthermore, individual state practice acts may require additional CE contact hours. Within athletic training CE hours are divided between four categories.

1. Category A – BOC approved provider programs
2. Category B – Professional development (50 CE max.)
3. Category C – Post-certification college/university coursework
4. Category D – Individualized options (20 CE max.)

After an athietic trainer earns the ATC® credential, the BOC will provide detailed information on how to track and record CEs. Continuing education documentation must be kept for the entire reporting period in case there is an audit. In the event of an audit, the ATC being audited must supply proof from the CE-event sponsor of attendance. For example, adequate proof for any event in Category A is typically a certificate of attendance, letter, or event name badge that includes the attendee's name and license, certification, or member number.

BOX 3-2 **List of the NATA Position, Official, and Consensus Statements**

POSITION STATEMENTS

- Emergency planning in athletics
- Exertional heat illnesses
- Fluid replacement for athletes
- Head down contact and spearing in tackle football
- Lightning safety for athletics and recreation
- Management of asthma in athletes
- Management of sport-related concussion
- Management of the athlete with Type 1 Diabetes Mellitus

OFFICIAL STATEMENTS

- Automated external defibrillators
- Commotio cordis
- Communicable and Infectious Diseases in Secondary School Sports
- Community-acquired MRSA infections
- Full-time, on-site athletic trainer coverage for secondary school athletic programs
- Steroids and performance enhancing substances
- Use of qualified athletic trainers in secondary schools
- Youth football and heat-related illness

CONSENSUS STATEMENTS

- Appropriate medical care for secondary school-age athletes
- Recommendations on emergency preparedness and management of sudden cardiac arrest in high school and college athletic programs
- Inter-association task force on exertional heat illnesses
- Prehospital care of the spine-injured athlete
- Sickle cell trait and the athlete

Engaging in professional activities that promote athletic training knowledge is also a professional responsibility. Examples of this include research, scholarly presentations and writing, and community education. Usually research and scholarship are done by graduate students or the profession's scholars; community education is the responsibility of all athletic trainers. Other ways to promote athletic training include celebrating national athletic training month (which is annually recognized in March); writing articles for local newspapers or other publications; or hosting community educational workshops or sponsoring a booth at local health fairs. Another important way practicing professionals can promote athletic training knowledge is by educating parents, coaches, patients, and other community members on the role and education of athletic trainers, as well as disseminating the profession's knowledge such as common injury recognition and prevention techniques or ensuring that NATA's position statements are being followed. Box 3-2 is a list of the NATA position, official, and consensus statements.

Planning a Seminar or Community Event

Part of the athletic trainer's responsibility is to serve as a liaison to the local community. One way to promote athletic training and foster professional relationships is to organize and administrate educational events. This may take on several forms, from a small local seminar to a larger regional conference. Obviously planning a regional conference is more involved. Conferences typically serve the needs of a diverse group of professionals, attract people from different geographical locations, and have multiple educational tracks. On the other hand, seminars or symposia are usually topic focused, serve the needs of a specific group, or have a narrow geographical draw. The planning process involves the following phases and steps and some may require advanced planning of up to 18 months.

1. **Conduct a needs analysis.** Determine what group(s) the conference or seminar will target. This may consist of identifying the educational needs or interests of a

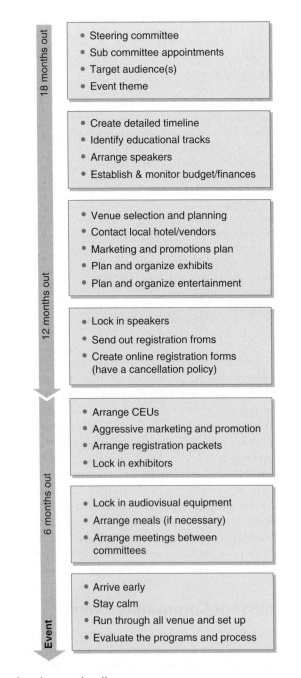

FIGURE 3-3 Educational event timeline

specific audience or audiences (i.e., coaches, athletes, physicians, athletic trainers, etc). For smaller seminars another approach is to identify an area of interest or expertise to which you (or others) are able to present.

2. **Develop a planning committee**. Once the target audience is identified and their needs identified, create a team (or teams) who can organize the event. Separate from the organizing (or Steering Committee) there needs to be sub-committees created to manage different aspects of the conference. Sub-committee examples:

    a. Finance Committee. To manage the conference budget including all revenue and expenses.
    b. Venue Committee. To manage the conference location (i.e., parking, traffic flow, exhibits, room capacity, access to local restaurants, local attractions). Several of these aspects may require their own sub-committee (for example, exhibits),
    c. Educational Committee. To manage educational tracks, speaker's invitations, speaker's schedules, technology for presentations, and CEUs for participants.
    d. Registration Committee. To manage all registrations, travel and accommodations.

    Obviously, these committees need to work together closely. Some committees will have to stay in closer contact than others. Also, these sub-committees may also create a special needs task force, (e.g., one for technology). The overall planning committee needs to stay abreast of committee actions and needs. Do not underestimate the value of having a team member or consultant who is experienced at planning and organizing seminars and conferences.

3. **Develop a timeline for implementation**. Finally, it is critical to have a realistic timeline to convene a conference. It may take as much as 18 months to plan and organize a large conference. A small seminar may only require a few months of planning.

It is important when planning seminars to consider your target audience. Consider the time of year, holidays, vacations, cost of travel, venue, and attractions. All of these factors influence desirability of the event. Figure 3-3 is a sample timeline for planning a large educational event. A well-planned and organized event goes a long way to placing a positive light on the profession and is an excellent demonstration of professional leadership.

CHAPTER SUMMARY

Professional students and young professionals need to be aware of where their profession came from and have a grasp of the obstacles that were overcome to gain professional status. Furthermore, professionals must maintain and adhere to a high standard of excellence and engage in critical self reflection to ensure professional attitudes, behaviors, and character. Understanding the credentialing process, including the differences between licensure, certification, and registration within athletic training is important. Athletic trainers must understand that practicing professional behavior strengthens the athletic training credential, promotes the profession, and demonstrates leadership. Finally, taking professional responsibilities seriously by promoting and disseminating athletic training's unique knowledge is critical. This can be accomplished by partaking in continuing education, or offering or hosting educational opportunities for other members or for the community.

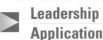

Leadership
Application

You are the director at a small rehabilitation clinic in a rural part of the state. John is the only staff athletic trainer and carries a huge patient load and is responsible for providing athletic training services to the local high school. John arrives to work one morning and he is worried and preoccupied. You notice John's behavior and are concerned, so you ask him what is wrong. John's reply is that he received a letter from the BOC stating that his continuing education cycle is coming to end in 8 weeks and he has not yet reported any CE activity; if he does not meet the stated CE requirements, his certification will be revoked. John is worried because he has completed some CE activity, but has lost the documentation, and he fears he will be a few hours short of what is required.

Critical Thinking Questions

1. As his clinical director, what is the first bit of advice you would give to John?
2. Where and how can John attain some CE's in the next 8 weeks?
3. What can you do to help John verify the CE activity he claims he has completed?
4. How will you prevent this situation from happening in the future?

References

1. American Board of Internal Medicine. (1995). *Project Professionalism*, ABIM Committee on Evaluation of Clinical Competence, Philadelphia.

2. Beardsley RS. (1996). Chair report of the APhA-ASP/AACP-COD Task Force on Professionalization: Enhancing professionalism in pharmacy education and practice. *Am J Pharm Educ 60*:26S–28S.

3. Craig D. (2006). Learning professionalism in athletic training education. *Athletic Training Education Journal* 1(1):8–11.

4. Hammer DP. (2000). Professional attitudes and behaviors: The "A's and B's" of professionalism. *American Journal of Pharmaceutical Education 64*:455–464.

5. Johnson M. (1967). Definitions and models in curriculum theory. *Educational Theory 17*(2):127–140.

6. National Athletic Trainers' Association. (2006). *Athletic training educational competencies*. NATA; Dallas, TX.

Leadership and Motivation

Chapter 4

Leadership and Management Theory

"The key to successful leadership today is influence, not authority."

KENNETH BLANCHARD

CHAPTER RATIONALE

Role Delineation Study Components

Domain V: Organization and Administration

- Knowledge of leadership styles
- Knowledge of management techniques
- Task D of Domain V states, "Manage human and fiscal resources by utilizing appropriate leadership, organization and management techniques to provide efficient and effective healthcare services."

Key Terms

Authority: The degree to which power is accepted or acknowledged by a subordinate.

Counterpower: Influence that a subordinate has over a supervisor.

Empathy: Awareness of someone's feelings from remembering or imagining being in similar circumstances.

Influence: The ability to affect the behavior of others in a particular direction.

In-group: A supervisor–subordinate relationship based on trust, respect, close interaction, and mutually developed objectives.

Leadership: The ability to facilitate and influence superiors, peers, and subordinates to make recognizable strides toward shared or unshared objectives.

Management: The ability to use organizational resources to accomplish predetermined objectives.

Moral agent: An individual who takes personal responsibility for actions and is genuinely committed to other's wants, needs, aspirations, and values.

Out-group: A supervisor–subordinate relationship based on predefined roles, job descriptions, and formal contracts.

Power: The degree to which influence is exercised by an individual.

Submission: The voluntary yielding to the authority of another person.

Zone of indifference: The tolerance of or adherence to commands or requests because they fall beneath an individual's threshold of what is consequential.

Regardless of context or role, athletic trainers need to use effective leadership behaviors. The Board of Certification Role Delineation Study (RDS) states explicitly that athletic trainers need to utilize leadership and have knowledge of leadership styles.[4] Leadership can help position athletic training as a competitive health care profession. The construct of leadership has hundreds of nuances, anecdotes, gradations, and theories. So much literature exists on leadership and development that it is difficult to sort through and implement. Leadership is beneficial nonetheless and is a worthwhile pursuit for all athletic trainers.

The popularity of leadership as a stand-alone discipline is evolving. In the past, many of the concepts and ideas concerning organizational effectiveness and motivation focused solely on management techniques. Recently there has been a clear swing toward leadership competencies as a means of achieving organizational effectiveness and employee motivation. It is clear that management and leadership, whether independent of each other or in combination, are necessary within the health care and sports industries.[22]

In this chapter we will discuss the evolution and development of leadership theory. We will begin by discussing the differences and similarities between leadership and management. Next, we will delineate why leadership is important and how it can be learned, and then discuss several specific leadership theories. After that, we will examine leadership-related constructs, such as power and authority. Next, we will begin to discuss the evolution of management science by looking at the contributions of management thinkers and practitioners. We will follow this with a discussion of specific management techniques that the athletic trainer can integrate into his or her practice of athletic training to increase leadership effectiveness.

LEADERSHIP AND MANAGEMENT

The athletic trainer assumes many responsibilities. These responsibilities are likely to require managerial acumen as well as leadership ability. While management often tends to be a formal role related to a title or position, leadership can be formal or informal and practiced regardless of a context or specific role. Table 4-1 is a list of common leadership roles the athletic trainer may be expected to perform.

There are primarily three schools of thought concerning the similarities and differences between leadership and management. The first is that the two constructs are the same. The second is that both constructs overlap to some degree.[16,19,33] The third is that they are completely different.[27] There is less consensus for views one and three; most of the consensus seems to indicate that leadership and management are different, but have overlapping characteristics and behaviors. Because the aim of this text is to "integrate" leadership and management, we will adopt the second viewpoint.

TABLE 4-1 Common Leadership Roles[9]

Leadership Role	Description
Figurehead	Involved in ceremony and ritual
Spokesperson	Internal and external reporting and answering
Negotiator	Making deals for needed resources
Coach	Recognizing achievements and giving feedback
Team Builder	Hosts meeting and parties, encourages morale
Team Player	Appropriate conduct and assistance
Technical Problem Solver	Expert and advisor
Entrepreneur	Expected to be innovative and creative
Strategic Planner	Coordinates and carries out input, sets vision and goals

TABLE 4-2 Differences in Leaders and Managers

Leader's Tendencies	Manager's Tendencies
• Proactive	• Reactive
• Focus on long-term	• Focus on short-term
• Change agent	• Protect status quo
• Defines & creates vision	• Implements vision
• Risk taker	• Avoids risk
• Identifies opportunities	• Identifies obstacles
• Idea and person-centered	• System and plan-centered
• Inspires loyalty	• Can create resentment
• Shares information freely	• Shares "need to know" information
• Uses interpersonal skills to handle conflict	• Uses precedent, policy, procedure to handle conflict
• Places emphasis on team accomplishments	• Places emphasis on individual performance
• Works to prevent conflict or problems	• Works to solve existing conflict or problems

Both leadership and management motivate, both deal with people, both use the different types of power, and both have to set and accomplish goals and evaluate outcomes. In spite of these similarities, there are general differences. Table 4-2 outlines some of the differences that have been identified between leaders and managers.

While it is popular to separate leadership from management, both are needed for the effective operation of the athletic training room.[22] Athletic trainers often use management techniques in the administration of their facilities for record keeping, budgeting, making clinical decisions, and controlling risk. On the other hand, integrating different leadership styles and motivational techniques is required when working with a diversity of patients and community interests, as well as interacting with peers, team members, subordinates, and supervisors. Despite using common techniques, managers and leaders in general are different types of people. Generally speaking, managers tend to use transactional techniques, data, policy, and positional power to accomplish tasks and motivate subordinates. Leaders tend to use personal power, intuition, and charisma to accomplish similar goals.[19]

Furthermore, it can be argued there is a philosophical difference in how each uses influence and power. Managing tends to focus on accomplishing activities, maintaining order and status quo, consistency, and mastering routines, while leading focuses on influencing others, creating vision, and implementing change.[3]

The irony is that every organization needs consistency and change, status quo and vision. Therefore, it is important for the athletic trainer to integrate management and leadership. Leaders are not automatically managers and managers are not automatically leaders.[19] The athletic trainer may often have to change hats between management and leadership. Figure 4-1 is the leadership–management matrix, which shows how increasing levels of leadership skill combined with increasing levels of managerial skills can improve overall performance.

Perhaps the most compelling reason for delineating any differences between leadership and management involves when and where each tends to be enacted. Leadership is often exercised in crises when there is no established precedent for handling or solving the problem, which requires innovation and creativity. Management, on the other hand, is exercised when problems reoccur and there is established precedent, policy, or formula to address the problem. Furthermore, leadership is often context free, can be exercised in multiple roles or settings, and is often expressed outside of the formal work context in other civic or social roles. On

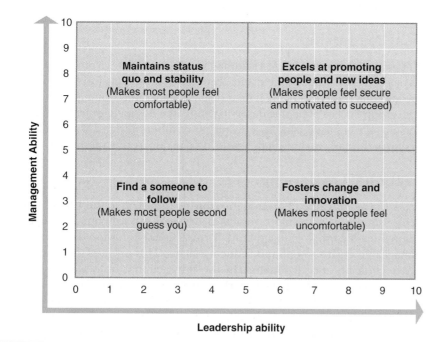

FIGURE 4-1 Leadership/management matrix

the other hand, management is often context-specific. In other words, management is rarely exercised outside of the work environment. Stated another way, when changing jobs or careers, leadership ability is transferable and can be put to use immediately, whereas specific management techniques or policies may have to be unlearned then new ones relearned for a different work environment or context.

In summary, while there are some similarities in leadership and management outcomes, they are arguably different constructs. Next we will examine how leadership theory evolved through the millennia compared to the relatively recent phenomena of management. Leadership theory and practice has undergone some dramatic transformations in the recent past.

EVOLUTION OF LEADERSHIP THEORY

Leadership and fascination with it date back to antiquity. Leaders and what makes them leaders has been a topic of interest since the beginning of recorded history.[1] There are four major leadership ideologies based on beliefs about leadership at that time:[1] classical, transactional, visionary, and organic.

Individuals and organizations often use one of these leadership ideologies as the lens through which to evaluate leadership "effectiveness." For example, athletic trainers educated within a transactional framework (1950s to 1980s) may have a bias toward management and prefer a structured hierarchy. This is in contrast to some recently certified athletic trainers who hope for a more fluid hierarchy and less emphasis on linear authority. This helps to explain generational differences. Generational differences are perhaps less a condition of culture and technology as one might presume. The dominant leadership ideology can be a polarizing aspect of professional socialization. The wise athletic trainer will recognize what leadership ideology peers, supervisors, and subordinates operate under and tailor his or her behavior appropriately.

Classical Leadership

Classical leadership is by far the longest standing ideology and dates from antiquity to the 1970s.[1] As such, it is a commonly held and deep rooted ideal. Classical (or trait) leadership is the idea that leaders were great men (usually men, rarely women) who were part of a special group or class of people deserving and often destined for leadership. Classical leadership ascribes leadership as a divine gift or inherent right. Much of the study of leadership in the early to mid-1900s was devoted to uncovering these traits.

Transactional Leadership

Transactional leadership came to prominence during the 1970s to the 1980s.[1] It is most often demonstrated as a formal transaction between subordinate and supervisor. Transactional leadership is management. Transactional behaviors center on creating a manageable environment and reducing chaos. This involves the leader being an expert technician and negotiator. In the transactional framework, leadership research focused on identifying ideal work environments, appropriate use of resources, and other controllable factors. Transactional leadership was expressed in the exchange of the employee's time and effort for a pre-defined reward, such as salary or benefits, and manifested in the form of a contract or other formal agreement between parties.

Visionary Leadership

Visionary leadership gained popularity form the mid-1980s up to 2000.[1] Exploration into visionary leadership takes into consideration the volatile conditions where lead-

---

▶ Leadership Application

Imagine you are the brand new assistant athletic trainer at XYZ University. You have only been certified for a few months (you passed the BOC exam in April and now are starting your new job in August) and came from an accredited entry-level masters athletic training education program. The head athletic trainer is an "old school" athletic trainer from an internship program. He has no advanced athletic training education and only had a handful of athletic training–specific courses, but learned athletic training from over 4000 hours of "observation" and was certified back in the early 1970s. He hired you because he liked your enthusiasm and work ethic, especially the fact you "worked" (his terminology) instead of "covered" (your terminology) football for a D-I institution in your last year of graduate school. He is the head football athletic trainer, and he assigns you cross-country, rehab coordinator, and soccer. If there is nothing going on Saturday evening, he expects you to be on the sideline of the football game. Furthermore, because you are a master's degree–prepared athletic trainer (albeit entry-level), you have to assist the program director by teaching laboratory courses within the CAATE-accredited undergraduate program.

Critical Thinking Questions

1. What might be some of your fears and apprehensions about interacting with the head athletic trainer?
2. What issues might any confrontation likely be over?
3. How might you foresee your first confrontation playing out?
4. What concessions might you be willing to give and what concessions might you expect from the head athletic trainer?

ership is played out and is called upon in turbulent times. Visionary leadership also popularized the notion that leaders can be anywhere in the organization, not just at the top. Often visionary leaders can be found at any level in an organization and often transcend a specific context. Research tended toward charismatic, inspiring, and transformational attributes of leaders. Visionary leaders tend to clearly articulate what they need and also have the ability to inspire people to change.

Organic Leadership

The final leadership ideology is *organic leadership* and dates from 2000 and extends into the future.[1] Organic leadership sees the organization as a living entity capable of growing on its own. Leaders are seen primary as facilitators and are often identified and developed internally. Research in organic leadership tends to fall toward the "leaderless" organization relying instead on shared or revolving leadership (i.e., leadership by a group of peers), cross-functional teams, self-managed or self-led groups, knowledge management, and cultural diversity.[1] The main impetus behind organic leadership is the growing concern over how to motivate and reward a highly specialized and educated work force.

▶ Leadership Application

Who in your circle (perhaps other athletic training students) do others look to for approval of decisions? Within groups there are often one or two individuals who the others intentionally or unintentionally look to in order to frame their reaction. For example, a new announcement is made to all athletic training students that seems unfair, but after a quick (perhaps subconscious) scan of the room you notice one or two other students nodding their heads in agreement. You instantly (perhaps subconsciously) reevaluate your position on the issue and conclude it must not be that unfair after all. This is influence in action. You were not necessarily looking to be influenced, you may not even care for this other person, but he or she has influence over you.

Critical Thinking Questions

1. Who influences you?
2. Do you influence those around you?
3. In what way(s) do you influence others?

DEFINING LEADERSHIP AND INFLUENCE

The literature is clear that leadership involves the ability to influence. Influence is easily identified but very difficult to measure and understand. **Influence** is the ability to affect the behavior of others in a particular direction.[18] The exciting aspect of influence is that it transcends roles, job title, and hierarchy.

Defining Leadership

Defining leadership has proven to be a very difficult task. The difficulty rests, in part, because perceptions of important leadership behavior changes constantly and because thousands of leadership-related attributes have been identified. In spite of this, it remains necessary to define and describe leadership as it applies to athletic training. Therefore, **leadership** is the ability to facilitate and influence superiors, peers, and subordinates to make recognizable strides toward shared or un-shared objectives.

Within this definition several subtle aspects emerge, which warrant explanation. "Ability to facilitate" includes skills such as organizing, administrating, motivating, and a host of interpersonal communication skills. Another aspect is leadership's ability to transcend hierarchy, therefore having influence with superiors, peers, and subordinates. The aspect of outcomes is demonstrated in delineating "recognizable strides." This implies a measure of objectivity, but also allows for subjective measures of improvement. Lastly, "shared or un-shared objectives" implies team objectives (where a team exists), but also includes a leader's ability to align different people (even antagonists) in recognizing and even embracing a new way of thinking or a different behavior. Now that we have described leadership it is important to ask, why is leadership important?

Why is Leadership Important?

Leadership is important because employers of athletic trainers desire applicants and new hires to have leadership skills.[15] Furthermore, knowledge of leadership styles is important for entry-level practice[4] and preparation for leadership roles should be a distinguishing characteristic of advance-practice athletic training education.[13] In addition to knowing that leadership is desirable for a well-rounded education and employment, what else is there about practicing leadership that is beneficial? In general, the outcomes of leadership include: increased leadership in others, greater credibility, lasting and new relationships, greater consensus among groups, a more motivated workforce, higher morale, dedication of followers, learning, mutual respect, empowerment, critical thinking, positive change, innovation, creativity, a sense of direction and hope for the future, and greater satisfaction and contentment.[1,18,31,32] Because demonstrating leadership is important, how does one become a leader?

Learning to Lead

Can someone learn to lead? It is widely accepted that, yes, one can learn to lead. However, there still remains the issue of deciding, what is it about leadership that can be taught? Tubbs & Schulz[30] contend that there are three factors that influence the development of leadership ability. Those three factors are personality, values, and leadership behaviors. Personality is set at an early age and is influenced little by the leadership development process. Likewise, the formation of values seems resistant to the leadership development process. However, leadership behaviors are likely to emerge or change as a result of leadership development efforts.[30] These leadership behaviors are typically called competencies, which are the characteristics that lead to success on a job or task.[30] Developing leadership competencies typically involves a combination of three aspects: trial and error; formal education; and observation.[6]

Trial and Error

Job experience and assignments are important ways in which leadership is learned. In hindsight, having tried something and failed is often better than never having tried at all. Often after failing a resilient person will try again; this ability to persevere often eventually results in successful attempts. Failure can be the best teacher when an effort is made to learn from mistakes. For example, a rookie athletic trainer may perform poorly during their first solo road trip, but the next road trip probably will

TABLE 4-3 Summary of Common Leadership Theories, Management Techniques, and Their Characteristics

Expectancy Theory	Decision making process of subordinates and employees based on individual factors, such as personality, experience, knowledge, skills, and abilities.
Human Resource Management	Understands the importance of appropriate motivational techniques, rewards and evaluation procedures (360-degree feedback, balanced scorecard and other evaluation tools) in the morale and performance of subordinates and team members.
Leader-Member Exchange (LMX) Theory	Addresses leadership as the process centered between the leader and follower. It makes the relationship of central concern. Relationships focus on trust, respect, and reciprocal influence.
Management By Objective (MBO)	Aims to increase organizational performance by aligning goals and subordinate objectives throughout the organization. Ideally, employees get strong input from managers/leaders in identifying individual objectives, including: time lines for completion, etc. MBO includes ongoing tracking and feedback in the process of reaching objectives.
McGregor's X and Y Motivational Theory	This theory is that individuals either: X – dislike and will avoid work; or Y – think work is as natural as play and will show self-discipline and effort for the benefit of the organization. X and Y motivational theory asserts managers adopt one of these two philosophies of people and use motivational techniques based on their philosophy of people.
Servant Leadership	The leader is not self-serving and puts others' desires and needs before his or her own. Emphasizes listening in problem solving and typically inspires trust by being trustworthy. Provides ample tools to employees and participates in the work of subordinates.
Situational Leadership Theories (contingency and path-goal)	Leader analyzes and adjusts behaviors and reactions to specific situations based on the premise and different situations and individuals require a different style of leadership and motivation. Analyzes the "variables" inherent in the circumstance (i.e., individual or group characteristics and the demands of the task) and charts delineated path to a desired goal.
Team Leadership	Where collaboration, coordination, and conflict resolution are priorities in the accomplishment of goals and objectives. Power is vested in the team and not an individual per se, creating interdependence among the leaders. This style also can manifest as dual or rotating authority/responsibility.
Total Quality Management	(TQM) is management technique using strict metrics in the management of quality. Quality can be managed if outcomes are strictly measured and ALL parties involved in production or outcomes adhere to these standards
Trait/Great Man Theory	Innate qualities or "traits" were believed to contribute to what made "great" social, political, or military leaders. Trait theory explores what those traits may be.
Transactional Leadership	Top-down hierarchal structure of governance where authority is vested in the organizational position. Use of incentives to influence behaviors and use of penalty to influence behaviors. There is a heavy emphasis on avoiding mistakes.
Transformational (Charismatic)	Attends to needs and motives of followers, empathizes to a high degree with subordinates. Leaders are often self-sacrificing and take on personal risks. Leader displays optimism and encourages and creates an environment of creativity. Leaders help people understand the need for change and involve people in transcending self-interest.

not be as bad as the first, and so on. Eventually the athletic trainer will know how to prepare for and perform on road trips. Not being afraid to fail and trying again after failure is a must when it comes to developing leadership. The proverbial school of hard knocks is a great teacher, but is not the only teacher.

Formal Education

While it has become commonly accepted that everyone has some ability to lead, it is not as clear how to turn that ability into reality. Formal programs and classes can inform about leadership theories, styles, communication, organizational skills, stress reduction, and coping skills, which can help one become a better leader. However, these formal courses do not make one a leader, they can only make one leader literate. Leadership literacy is a necessary precursor to effective leadership, but it is not leadership. Ultimately, formal education must be tested by practice.

Observation of Others

The old paradigm of "knowledge is power" may hold truth, but true power lies in sharing knowledge.[10] Relationships with leaders often are the critical keys to successful leadership development. Being told how to do something is important, but then having the ability to watch someone do it, then later have them watch you do it is critical. The concept of being a protégé, mentoring, or even being an apprentice has transcended culture and time and is still today a trusted and reliable competency development model.

LEADERSHIP STYLES AND THEORIES

There are many theories and styles of leadership. To attempt to describe them all in this text would be futile. In this section we will review some of the more prominent leadership theories and styles and relate them to athletic training. The savvy athletic trainer will take what is appropriate for his or her circumstances from each of the styles and theories and integrate them into his or her own style. Table 4-3 is a summary of the common leadership styles, management techniques, and characteristics.

Situational Leadership

Situational leadership has been revised several times. In its simplest form, the situational leader changes his or her behavior based on the follower's response and action. The premise is that different situations and different employees require different leadership. The skill required by the situational leader is correctly identifying the situation and choosing the most appropriate leadership style. Situational leaders base their behavior on the developmental level of the subordinate. For example, the head athletic trainer of a university may use one style when leading certified staff and another style when leading athletic training students, and still another style when working with coaches.

Leadership behavior is based on the motivation (willingness) and skill (ability) of the subordinate. The leader changes the degree to which he or she is directive and supportive based on that motivation and skill. For example, a follower who is not motivated and has no skill (i.e., unwilling and unable) requires specific direction, as opposed to a follower who is willing and able.

TABLE 4-4 Key Traits and Values of Transformational Leaders[25]	
Traits of Transformational Leaders	**Values of Transformational Leaders**
• Creates shared vision	• Dignity
• Communicates the vision	• Respect
• Builds relationships	• Deals with social injustice
• Develops a supporting structure	• Altruism
• Guides implementation	• Fairness
• Exhibits character	• Justice
• Achieves results	• Liberty
	• Human rights
	• Honesty
	• Integrity
	• Equality

Directive behaviors include:

1. giving directions
2. establishing goals
3. defining roles
4. evaluations

Supportive behaviors include:

1. using two-way communication
2. giving emotional and social support
3. asking for input
4. sharing personal stories
5. offering praise for good work

In addition to directive and supportive, situational leadership may also require coaching style, which combines elements of direction and support. A fourth style that can be implemented is delegation, which is used when the follower is highly motivated and skilled. This behavior calls for little direction and little support. Delegation is used more often when workers are educated professionals, like in athletic training.

Transformational Leadership

Transformational leadership is perhaps the most popular of contemporary leadership styles. Much of the current research and literature on leadership juxtaposes transactional and transformational leadership. Followers prefer transformational leaders. Transformational leaders recognize and exploit the needs of followers, exhibit charisma, look for potential motives in followers, seek to satisfy follower's higher needs, and engage the full person.[7] Transformational leaders convert followers into leaders and make leaders into "moral agents."[7] Burn's[7] idea of a **moral agent** is someone who takes personal responsibility for actions, commitments, and is genuinely committed to the follower's fundamental wants, needs, aspirations, and values. Transformational leaders excite and transform followers by heightening motivation and instilling a sense of purpose.[7] Transformational leaders tend to be results oriented. They place a high premium on delegating the appropriate level of authority with assigned responsibility. Table 4-4 lists the values and seven elements of transformational leadership.

Laissez-Faire

Perhaps more a personality issue than leadership style, laissez-faire is a philosophy or practice characterized by a deliberate abstention from direction or interference. This style of leadership is intentionally absent in decisions or directions. Most all decisions are left to the workers with little to no input from a supervisor. The benefit of this style is that workers and employees are left alone to determine the best course of action based on their experience and knowledge, which is only good if the follower is highly skilled and motivated. The major weakness to this style is that there is virtually no direction. Morale is often very low under this style of leadership because feedback is often insufficient.

Emotional Intelligence

Emotional intelligence (EI), while not a specific leadership theory, is a critical leadership behavior that includes awareness of self and others and the ability to handle

**Leadership
Application**

Scenario A

You are the head athletic trainer at XYZ University and your athletic director informs you that you are hosting the conference championship basketball tournament and that you are in charge of all medical aspects of the tournament. You are relieved to find out that all the teams that will be arriving for the tournament will be bring their own certified athletic trainers and other medical personnel, as an extra bonus your conference has budgeted enough money so you can hire an additional four athletic trainers to help cover the medical needs of the tournament.

Scenario B

Your university is hosting a Winterfest basketball tournament as a revenue generator for the athletic department. Your athletic director has appointed you to be the medical director of the tournament. The athletic director has announced to the other teams that all medical coverage will be provided by the host institution. That means you, the two other staff athletic trainers, and 19 athletic training students will be providing all of the medical coverage.

Critical Thinking Questions

1. What might be some the main leadership difference between administrating these two events?
2. What are some of the differences between leading a group of certified athletic trainers versus a group of athletic training students?
3. What situational leadership style do you adopt for each scenario?

---

emotions and relationships.[5] The term emotional intelligence was taken from social intelligence, defined as "the ability to understand and manage [people]…to act wisely in human relations."[5] EI is based on the leader's emotional quotient (EQ) which is a play on IQ (intelligence quotient). EQ is often associated to be highly developed in transformational leaders. Having expertise and technical knowledge is not a substitute for EQ. A high IQ, low EQ ratio typically is perceived by subordinates as arrogance, inflexibility, inability to adapt to change, and distain for collaboration and teamwork.[11]

Goleman[12] identified four key elements of emotional intelligence: self-awareness, self-management (both are internal factors) and social awareness and social skill (both are external factors). The *self-aware* leader can read and understand their own emotions and recognize their emotion's impact on the performance of others. Realistic self-assessment and the ability to critically self-reflect is also a part of being self-aware. The second aspect of EI is *self-management*, which includes self-control, trustworthiness, adjusts to change and obstacles well, has an internal drive for excellence, and takes initiative to seize opportunities. The third aspect of EI is *social-awareness* which includes empathy and organizational awareness, networking effectively, navigating organizational politics, and a focusing on the needs of others. The last aspect of the emotionally intelligent leader is *social-skill.* These abilities include inspiring others, developing and promoting others, persuading, initiating new ideas, getting others to think in new directions, building teams, and cultivating relationships.

Servant Leadership

Servant leadership occurs when the leader's primary responsibility is to serve the employee and assist him or her in any way that is ethical to accomplish goals and objectives. The servant leader spends most of his or her time in learning about and understanding their subordinates to better serve their needs. Servant leaders demonstrate good empathy and listening skills. **Empathy** is experiencing what others feel because you experienced it yourself or imagine yourself in the same circumstance. A servant leader also has a very powerful ethical dimension. This ethic is seen most potently in that ethical decision-making takes a precedent over personal or financial interests of the organization. Finally, the servant leader uses his or her power to promote, support, and empower in an altruistic fashion. Trustworthiness of the leader is established via consistency of servanthood, honesty, and openness. The focus on the follower takes precedence over the organization, which is what makes servant leadership distinct from transformational leadership.[24,29]

Path–Goal Leadership

The path–goal theory of leadership relies heavily on what motivates employees. The stated goal of this theory is to "enhance employee performance and employee satisfaction by focusing on employee motivation."[23] Morale and productivity of the employee is the goal of the leader. The leader does what is necessary to delineate or outline a specific path to a stated goal for a group member so that the employee can accomplish that goal with a high degree of satisfaction. This is a common leadership style utilized by athletic trainers in rehabilitation of injured athletes. The objective is getting the subordinate to understand the payoff and believe they can accomplish the task.

Path–goal is centered on three key assumptions: 1) subordinates must believe they can do what they are being asked to do; 2) subordinates need to believe their effort will have a desirable outcome; and 3) the outcome will be worthwhile. The leader's role in the path–goal model is to help subordinates overcome obstacles by removing them, clarifying paths (directives), providing support, and defining goals.

Leader Member Exchange (LMX)

Leader member exchange (LMX) is a popular expression of a dyad leadership model which emphasizes how a relationship is developed and maintained between leader and follower.[8,28] The leader's and follower's roles evolve through three stages, role-taking, making, and routinization.

1. Role-taking: leaders and followers begin to understand how the other perceives respect.
2. Role-making: a level of trust is determined and subsequently the level of influence.
3. Role-routinization: social exchange patterns are identified and behaviors that are typically associated to that pattern become routine. The social exchange patters are formed from self identification into one of two groups.

These groups include in-groups and out-groups. **In-groups** are those relationships where responsibilities and roles are mutually-developed by the leader and follower. In-group relationships have a strong bond and share many common values and therefore allows for greater interaction between leader and follower. **Out-groups** are those relationships where leader-member relationship is based on defined roles, job descriptions, and formal contracts.

Regardless of the style, the use of power becomes an important consideration in the practice of leadership. No matter which theories, styles, or combinations of leadership are practiced the leader has a responsibility to ethically and non-coercively use power. In the next section we will discuss the concept and types of power. In the next chapter we will discuss important leadership behaviors for athletic trainers to implement.

POWER

Power can be as difficult to define as leadership. Many of the synonyms for power (i.e., influence, control, and authority) are also synonyms for leadership. **Power** can be considered the degree or level to which influence is exercised. Power transcends the concept of leadership in that different leaders possess greater and lesser amounts of power. Historically power has been understood on two levels, supernatural and governmental. A supernatural power influences nature, the elements, and illnesses. A senator, king, or governor had governmental power over a region or city. The ancient Greeks integrated these two concepts of power in the form of an ambassador or one who was "sent out" as a delegate. This delegate carried a recognized formal governing authority and therefore had the power to act as if they themselves were the very voice or a literal extension of the original source of power. In this sense power was understood to be delegated and was therefore, highly respected. In athletic training this is similar to the physician extender role of many athletic trainers. As the name implies, a physician extender is acting in behalf of or as a representative of the physician, and as such has certain influence that might not be present normally.

Today the concept of delegated power has lost its potency. Generally, those who have greater power are viewed with skepticism and cynicism. Contemporary concepts of power are based on having a decision-making position with little accountability to others.

From a leadership perspective, power comes in two forms, and can be vested in people and positions. Positional power comes from a position or title and is also called assigned leadership. For example, the head athletic trainer or athletic director has power because of his or her title; the power is only intact as long as he or she occupies that position. The head athletic trainer can make decisions about the budget because of his or her position; once out of that position they no longer have power over the budget.

Personal power is recognized to be resident in the person with the most influence and ironically is typically not the person with the highest ranking title and is also called emergent leadership. Emergent leaders have power based on who they are, their history or experience, or their personality, and is given by followers or peers. For example, a former clinical instructor may continue to have a significant role in a former student's life as an advisor or mentor long after graduation. In athletic training a majority of the leadership activity falls within the realm of personal power. Northouse[23] identified five behaviors of emergent leaders. Emergent leaders are:

1. verbally involved in dialogue
2. informed of issues and trends
3. interested in other's opinions
4. actively pursue new ideas and concepts
5. firm in their convictions, but flexible.

Informational Power

Informational or expert power is influence that is based on the possession of and access to information.[32] Those who hold information that is necessary for others to do their work operate in this form of power. Athletic trainers operate with a high degree of informational power. For example, injury records, knowledge of prognoses, knowledge of physiology and anatomy, scholarly activity, and originating the "injury report" are examples of how the athletic trainer has or uses informational power. In terms of injuries athletic trainers have power over many athletes because they presumably know the prognosis and can manipulate the circumstances and outcomes surrounding the injury and the athlete's recovery.

Counterpower

Counterpower is defined as influencing superiors.[32] Having and using counterpower is critical in athletic training because often the athletic trainer acts in a staff role. In spite of the staff role there is significant influence because of the athletic trainer's expertise. This expertise manifests with supervisors. Often the role of the athletic trainer requires the use of counterpower to influence those with positional power.

Coercive and Reward Power

Coercive power is ability to punish or interfere in the progress of someone's work.[5] An athletic trainer's decision to deny or delay treatment to an incompliant athlete is an example of coercive power (this is also unethical). Use of coercive power is the manipulation of rewards and punishment and is usually limited to threats and punishments. **Reward power** is the authority to give awards for compliance, such as bonuses or time off and is directly opposite of coercive power. These two forms of power are components of positional power.

Legitimate Power

Legitimate power exists because of a lawful right to make a decision and expect compliance[9] and fits within the scope of positional power and the concept of jurisdiction. This is seen in sports through the officials and referees. The game's officials have the power over the match despite disagreement of coaches, athletes, and fans, but make authoritative decisions nonetheless, typically not considering the input of these other stakeholders.

AUTHORITY

Authority is very similar to power. Like power, the concept of authority is based on knowledge (i.e., expertise) and delegation. The subtle differences between power and authority involve the buy-in of the subordinate. **Authority** is limited to the degree it is accepted by the subordinate.[2] The subordinate must accept the command as authoritative. For this acceptance to take place, four conditions must be met simultaneously:

1. The subordinate can and does understand the command.
2. The subordinate believes (at the time the decision is made) that the decision is consistent with the purpose of the organization.
3. The subordinate believes (at the time the decision is made) that the decision is compatible with personal interests.
4. The subordinate is able mentally and physically to comply.[2]

Furthermore, authority has its basis elsewhere. There is no authority unless the organization, society, or culture confers it. Central to the practice of authority is the idea of the zone of indifference.[2] The **zone of indifference** is a conceptual "zone" where

> ### *From the Field*
>
> As a graduate assistant certified athletic trainer, I had a confrontation with a coach over how fast an athlete was recovering from her injury. I and the rest of the staff were doing all we knew to do to treat the injury, but, the coach was just not sure if I should be doing something more. So she decided to approach the team physician about the injury, without any of the athletic training staff's knowledge. When the coach confronted the team physician, he assured the coach that I had his full support and more he had 'full faith in my ability to treat the athlete.' He expressed to the coach that he trusted my judgment and ability to treat this athlete. After this 'meeting,' the coach did not question my ability any further on this or any other issue. In the eyes of the coach authority was delegated to me verbally by the physician and again by his support. The coach now knew there was no going over my head and violating my authority in this area. The beauty of this is that the effect carried over into the rest of my time as a GA. This also served to promote me in the eyes of the coach and athletes as I was no longer merely a GA, but an ATC, something that could only of have been given to me by a higher authority, such as our team physician.

> ## BOX 4-1 Henri Fayol's 14 Principles of Management
>
> 1. **Division of labor**. Specializing encourages continuous improvement in skills and the development of improvements in methods.
> 2. **Authority**. The right to give orders and the power to exact obedience.
> 3. **Discipline**. No slacking, bending of rules. The workers should be obedient and respectful of the organization.
> 4. **Unity of command**. Each employee has one and only one boss.
> 5. **Unity of direction**. A single mind generates a single plan and all play their part in that plan.
> 6. **Subordination of individual interests**. When at work, only work things should be pursued or thought about.
> 7. **Remuneration**. Employees receive fair payment for services, not what the company can get away with.
> 8. **Centralization**. Consolidation of management functions. Decisions are made from the top.
> 9. **Chain of superiors** (line of authority). Formal chain of command running from top to bottom of the organization, like military.
> 10. **Order**. All materials and personnel have a prescribed place, and they must remain there.
> 11. **Equity**. Equality of treatment (but not necessarily identical treatment).
> 12. **Personnel tenure**. Limited turnover of personnel. Lifetime employment for good workers.
> 13. **Initiative**. Thinking out a plan and doing what it takes to make it happen.
> 14. *Esprit de corps*. Harmony, cohesion among personnel.

all requests that fall within this zone are complied to without question, because consequences are deemed unsubstantial or convictions of the subordinate are not challenged. However, commands that fall outside this "zone" are questioned, ignored or outright disobeyed.[2] Each subordinate has their own "zone of indifference." This means that authority levels differ with each subordinate.

Validating Authority

The authority of a leader is limited to the degree he or she is supported by others. Unlike influence or leadership, which can be context free, authority is typically only valid when acting as an agent of an organization. Realms of authority pertain only to those areas one has control over (this is similar to the concept of legal jurisdiction). For example, the head athletic trainer has authority over the condition of the athletic training room and therefore has authority to ask athletic training students or staff to keep it clean. However, the head athletic trainer cannot tell those same students to go and clean the school cafeteria, because the cafeteria is outside the athletic trainer's realm of authority.

Legitimate authority is supervisory in nature, meaning authority is worthless unless there is something or someone over which to exercise. Illustrating this point is an old Chinese proverb which states, "If you think you are a leader and have no one following you, you are only out for a walk." Accrediting agencies such as Commission of Accreditation of Athletic Training Education (CAATE), Commission on Accreditation of Rehabilitation Facilities (CARF), the Southern Association of Colleges and Schools (SACS), and state regulatory and practice acts hold authority of legitimacy. For example, completing an entry-level athletic training degree from a non-CAATE accredited school is illegitimate, meaning there is no authority (or credibility) behind the credential.

Submission

Submission is an essential concept of legitimate authority, which benefits both the "leader" and the subordinate. "The determination of authority always lies with the subordinate individual."[2] Therefore, **submission** is the voluntary yielding to the control of another. Submission is a paradox in that authority is not realized unless submission is given. Because submission can be withdrawn at any time it is a potent form of power for the subordinate. Therefore, submission has a two-fold benefit it is a vehicle to confer authority to an individual as well as a way to empower a subordinate.

MANAGEMENT EVOLUTION AND THEORY

Compared to the study of leadership, management is a relatively new phenomenon. Management theory was formulated as a tool to help organizations combat chaos and introduce order. Management is the ability to get things done through other people. Early concepts of management dealt almost exclusively with coercive and reward power. **Management** is working effectively with resources to accomplish organizational outcomes. Several management techniques and theories have emerged that shape contemporary understanding of management and how it relates to leadership. The following sections are brief descriptions of management practitioners and theorists followed by several management techniques.

Frederick W. Taylor

The man credited as the father of scientific management was Frederick W. Taylor. Taylor published *The Principles of Scientific Management*, which suggested that sole responsibility of the organization rested with the manager. Therefore, it was only the manager who needed to be concerned with working conditions and outcomes. Employees were tools for the manager to implement. According to Taylor, a manager's responsibility was to provide detailed and specific instructions on how to do the assigned task. Taylor believed that the organization was more important than the individual.[20,26] Scientific management's basic tenet was that monetary payment was the only motivation employees needed. Scientific management is not a popular model in today's organizations, however, remnants of scientific management can be seen in bureaucratic and transactional behaviors. Eventually scientific management was rejected, but Taylor's contribution to management practice has contributed to where it is today.

Henri Fayol

Approximately five years after Taylor's book was published, Henri Fayol wrote a book titled *General and Industrial Management*. Fayol outlined five functions of management, which are still the foundational tenets of management theory. Fayol's five functions of management included:

1. Planning (exploring the future and creating a vision and plan of action)
2. Organizing (establishing a framework for completing actions plans and securing necessary resources)
3. Commanding (organizing personnel to execute plans)

BOX 4-2   Example of S.M.A.R.T. Objectives

1. To increase overall departmental revenue by 10% through the acquisition of athletic training contracts by the end of the fiscal year 2008.
2. To complete the daily injury report for Coach Jones by 8:00 am, so it is under her door before she arrives to the office every day during the season.
3. To personally meet the parents of all the athletes on the volleyball team before week 4 of the season.

---

4. Coordinating (conforming to the organization and demanding efficiency)
5. Controlling (confirming plans and instructions are followed).

Fayol's ideas became known as "command and control" style of management. Box 4-1 summarizes Fayol's 14 management principles, which expand on his five functions of management. Basically, Fayol's ideas of management were that labor needed to be divided and a government centralized,thereby establishing a clear hierarchy. Individual interests were to be discarded for the good of the company. Fayol still has many supporters today and in fact several organizations, including the military and emergency response organization, operate within Fayol's "command and control" system. The strengths of Fayol's ideas are the clear lines of communication and command.

Leadership Application

Consider Jane Smith, ATC, the head athletic trainer of a small, private, religious, very expensive liberal-arts university in a white-collar city. Jane has an excellent record-keeping system in place with which she tracks every injury observed in the athletic training room. She automatically syncs this information to her PDA and produces injury reports for every coach precisely at 8:00 am every morning. She has emergency action plans established and rehearses them monthly. Her capital expenses and supply budget are balanced to the penny. The athletic training students are respectful, on time for practices, and in dress code everyday. Jane uses the available technology to its fullest potential and has intricately planned and time-managed the activities of each day. She has mastered her budget to maximize every penny, and her policies and procedures are in place and enforced. In 20 years, she has never been named in a lawsuit, and she has her state license displayed for all to see. By all accounts, Jane is an excellent manager and occupies a leadership role.

One afternoon she is invited to travel for three weeks in the summer as the head athletic trainer with a culturally and religiously diverse group of elite athletes touring four different counties. She now has the responsibility to work with a group of athletes who have never seen her (or each other), each having different, cultural, ethnic, and religious backgrounds, and traveling to four different countries, none of which Jane has ever been to.

Critical Thinking Questions

1. What management skills will Jane need for this trip?
2. How might success be measured differently by this international team versus at her university?
3. What leadership skills are needed by Jane to make this a smooth transition?
4. What skills might be needed by Jane that she does not need (or use) at her university job?

Mary Parker Follett

Mary Parker Follett is perhaps the single greatest contributor to how management practice and theory is understood today. Follett was a political scientist and is credited with beginning a democratic style of management. Follett was a "management philosopher" and believed that an organization was a microcosm of society.[20,26] Follett placed a large emphasis on the individual and believed they define their own roles and shapes their lives. Her ideas flew in the face of scientific management principles and she became the first great thinker to introduce theories about what eventually became known as human resource management.[20,26]

Follett believed that communication should flow up and down (vertically) and not merely with coworkers and peers (horizontal). Follett believed that leadership is not only found in the tops of organizations, but leaders can be anywhere within the hierarchy. She also suggested that leadership could be learned, and anyone who did not learn leadership would always remain in a subordinate position. Leadership to Follett was getting people to realize the necessity of the instructions and not merely getting people to follow instructions. Follet saw success as a result of practice and she encouraged managers to practice and experiment with new things or ideas.

Max Weber

Max Weber is credited with introducing the bureaucratic model of management. Even though Weber advocated a bureaucratic model he had the foresight to warn of the potential for the organization to dominate policy and individuals. Bureaucratic structures are formal, centralized, have a firm hierarchy, and divide labor between specialists.[9] Bureaucracy is a form of managing where standardized rules are established in the forms of policy and procedure. The benefit to this is that there is a reference point for action and variability is minimized. However critics of bureaucratic management point out that minimized variability is not as effective with today's knowledge workers.[9] Weber believed bureaucracy to be a set of official functions bounded by rules with a clear division of labor, a clearly defined hierarchy, qualification as the basis for any selection (and not favoritism), and finally systematic discipline and control of work. Bureaucracy, as Weber introduced it, leveled the playing field and increased social equality.

Elements of bureaucratic management will always be with us, but it is the responsibility of the leader to ease the "burden" often and perhaps unduly attributed to bureaucratic management. Bureaucratic management is still a strong force in contemporary healthcare. Competent athletic training managers are needed to navigate this system effectively. Bureaucracy, as it is today, has evolved from Weber's original intents, however, it still may have uses. Among other things it is contemporary bureaucracy that necessitates state licensure, coding, billing, reimbursement procedures, and facility accreditation that many athletic trainers are thankful for today.

MANAGEMENT TECHNIQUES

While Taylor, Fayol, Weber, and Follet are credited as being some of the early forerunners of management thinking, their ideas, writings, and practices have spawned several management techniques, which are used to motivate and accomplish goals. Following are a few of the more popular management techniques used today.

Management by Objective

Peter Drucker introduced the concept of Management by Objective (MBO), which was the idea that pre-established objectives should be used in the appraisal of every aspect of an organization. MBO relies on defining objectives for each employee and assessing those objectives (or goals). MBO requires collaboration, strategic planning, and goal setting.[21] MBO takes seriously employee buy-in and participative decision-making for departmental or organizational objectives. It is not uncommon that MBO managers allow and even require the employee to devise their own action plan for implementation of these agreed-upon objectives.

MBO objectives must be S.M.A.R.T. (specific, measurable, achievement oriented, realistic and time oriented). Box 4-2 outlines some sample of SMART objectives common in MBO style. Finally, MBO requires appraisal. Appraisals are routine and involve the assessment, clarification and progress toward any previously agreed upon goals and objectives. It is typical to identify and address any obstacles that may be keeping the employee from accomplishing their objectives and creating new ones for those objectives that have been met. MBO is a technique often adopted by transformational leaders. Figure 4-2 shows a framework of management by objective.

Total Quality Management

W. Edward Deming is credited with the concept of Total Quality Management (TQM). Originally embraced in Japan, it was not until the 1980s when the United States was facing increased global competition, that TQM initiatives flourished.[31] TQM is based on Deming's 14 points of quality management:

1. Create consistency of purpose for the improvement of product and service.
2. Adopt the new philosophy.
3. Cease dependence on inspection to achieve quality.
4. End the practice of awarding business on the price tag.
5. Improve constantly and forever the systems of production and service.
6. Institute training on the job.
7. Institute leadership.
8. Drive out fear.

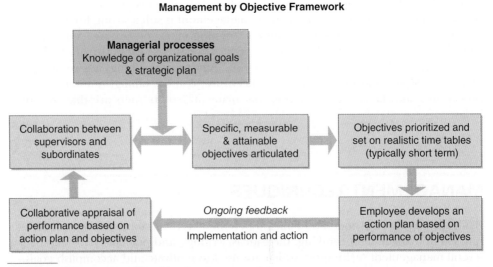

Management by Objective Framework

FIGURE 4-2 Management by objective framework

9. Break down barriers between departments.

10. Eliminate slogans, exhortations, and targets for the workforce.

11. Eliminate numerical quotas for the workforce and numerical goals for management.

12. Remove barriers that rob people of pride and workmanship.

13. Institute a vigorous program of education and self-improvement for everyone.

14. Put everyone in the company to work to accomplish the transformation.[31]

In athletic training, TQM and variations of it are seen routinely. Deming's twelfth point, "Remove barriers that rob people of pride and workmanship" is one of the things athletic trainers do with athletes. Rehabilitation protocols, facility design, and layout are also based on TQM principles. Variations of TQM include basing decisions for improvements on measurable outcomes and making those decisions based on data (e.g., evidence-based medicine). Athletic trainers then use outcomes to evaluate the effectiveness and essentially the quality of our programs. In the end, it is the patient or athlete that ultimately determines the quality. Using tools that assess patient input then using that input to publish outcomes can be one way to implement TQM in athletic training.

Knowledge Management

Knowledge management (KM) is purely a contemporary phenomenon and highly relevant to athletic trainers. It is based on the premise that professionals often know more, or at least as much, as their supervisors. In many athletic training settings this is certainly the case. This being true, special skills and behaviors are required by managers to keep motivation and momentum high. A fundamental aspect of knowledge management is that knowledge and information are changing and accelerating at an alarmingly fast pace. Therefore, keeping pace with new trends and knowledge is left to the subordinate, thus requiring a very high level of trust by the supervisor. Because of the athletic trainer's clinical competence and athletic training's accelerating knowledge-base knowledge management creates a unique dynamic within the power structure of the athletic trainer's work environment. Managing this unique dynamic requires managers who intentionally develop their leadership skills and understand the knowledge-based diversity within the health care industry.

CHAPTER SUMMARY

Knowledge of leadership styles and management techniques are the beginning steps to practicing leadership effectively. Leadership skills are critical to the practice and advancement of athletic training. Athletic trainers need to be able to identify their own leadership style and adopt the appropriate style for a given situation. Leadership skills transcend the athletic trainer's roles and job responsibilities and can be put to use outside the context of athletic training, wherever the athletic trainer has influence. Management techniques tend to be more context-specific and often need to be relearned for each new role or setting the athletic trainer assumes. There are several leadership styles, theories, and management techniques that the athletic trainer must be able to identify and adopt. The ability to use these leadership styles and management techniques when called upon will promote the profession and the individual athletic trainer's career.

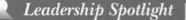

Leadership Spotlight

PETER KOEHNEKE

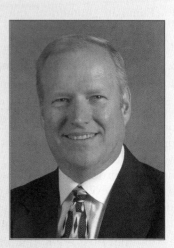

EDUCATION:

MS, Adapted Physical Education, Indiana State University, 1975

BS, Physical Education (Minor Health Education Specializations: Athletic Training and Adapted Physical Education), Indiana State University, 1974

CURRENT JOB:

Professor and Director of Athletic Training Education Program, Canisius College, Buffalo, NY

FIRST ATHLETIC TRAINING JOB:

Rhode Island College

PROFESSIONAL INTERESTS/RESEARCH FOCUS:

Athletic Training Accreditation and Board of Certification

ATHLETIC TRAINING–RELATED AWARDS/HONORS:

- NATA Hall of Fame, 2002
- NYSATA Hall of Fame, 2004
- NATA Distinguished Athletic Training Educator, 2000
- NATA Most Distinguished Athletic Trainer, 1998
- William E. "Pinky" Newell Keynote Address EATA, 2005
- NYSATA Thomas J. Sheehan Award, 1994
- Indiana State University Distinguished Alumni Award, 1998

ATHLETIC TRAINING–RELATED INVOLVEMENT:

- Chair of JRC-AT
- JRC-AT Member
- NATA Professional Education Committee
- World Task Force Athletic Training NATA
- BOC Board of Directors
- NYSATA Nominations Committee
- NYSATA District Representative
- NATA District 2 Executive Council

Q & A

What first inspired you to enter the athletic training profession?

A high school Cramer First Aider and home study course. Also, a local physician encouraged me to engage in medicine.

How would you define leadership in athletic training?

Willingness to serve while keeping the big picture in mind.

Who is the most influential athletic trainer in your professional life, and why?

Mel Blickenstaff defined what involvement was as an educator, national leader, mentor, and clinical athletic trainer.

What is the best advice you ever received from another athletic trainer?

To maintain life balance while knowing that the grass is not always greener on the other side of the fence.

What has been the most enjoyable aspect of athletic training?

Friendships made and seeing the profession and our students soar.

What has been the least enjoyable aspect or your biggest challenge in athletic training?

Administrative aspects that have grown tremendously.

What advise would you give a first year athletic training student?

Make yourself visible to others through your positive attitude and actions. Relish every minute and take it all in.

What advise would you give a brand new BOC-certified athletic trainer who is deciding between taking that first professional job or entering graduate school to pursue a master's degree in athletic training, and why?

Evaluate what is the best for you and do not let others make the decision for you. I have seen external influences create decisions that have resulted in either discouragement or failure. Only the individual can decide what is best for himself or herself while weighing the input from others.

What other interests outside of athletic training have you pursued?

Travel, novels, and golf.

Where do think (or hope) athletic training will be in the next 10 years?

Having advanced in status and economic viability through recognition by all health care providers as an equal partner.

References

1. Avery G. (2005). *Understanding leadership.* London, England: Sage Publications.
2. Barnard CI. (1968). *The functions of the executive.* Cambridge, MA: Harvard University Press.
3. Bennis W, Nanus B. (1997). *Leaders: Strategies for taking charge.* New York: Harper Collins.
4. Board of Certification, Inc. (2004). *Role delineation study.* Omaha, NE: BOC, Inc.
5. Bolman LG, Deal TE. (2003). *Reframing organizations.* San Francisco, CA: Jossey-Bass.
6. Brown L, Posner B. (2001). Exploring the difference between learning and leadership. *22(6)*:272–280.
7. Burns, JM. (1978). *Leadership.* New York: Harper & Row.
8. Drury S. (2006). *Leader-Member Exchange Theory (LMX): In-group/out-group.* Accessed March 21, 2006 from http://www.drurywriting.com/sharon/4.LMX.in.group.out.group.htm
9. DuBrin AJ. (2004). *Leadership: Research findings, practice, and skills.* New York: Houghton Mifflin Co..
10. Fagiano D. (1997). Managers vs. leaders: A corporate fable. *Management Review 86:*10, 5.
11. Fullan M. (2001). *Leading in a culture of change.* San Francisco, CA: Jossey-Bass.
12. Goleman D. (2000). Leadership that gets results. *Harvard Business Review 78*(2):78–90.
13. National Athletic Trainers' Association Graduate Review Committee. (2005). *Standards and guidelines for post-certification graduate athletic training education programs.* Accessed April 13, 2005 from http://www.nataec.org/LinkClick.aspx?fileticket=VF2HZV5TQ9E%3D&tabid=97&mid=503

14. Indvik J. (1986). Path-goal theory of leadership: A meta-analysis. *AOM Proceedings;* 189–192.

15. Kahanov L, Andrews L. (2001). A survey of athletic training employers' hiring criteria. *JAT; 36*(4):408–412.

16. Kotter JP. (1998). What leaders really do. In: *Harvard Business Review on leadership.* Cambridge, MA: HBS Press;37–60.

17. Mahar C, Maher T. (2006). *Emergent leadership: Toward an empirically verifiable model.* Accessed March 27, 2006 from http://www.cda-cd.forces.gc.ca/cfli/engraph/research/pdf/41.pdf

18. Maxwell JC. (1993). *Developing the leader within you.* Nashville, TN: Thomas Nelson.

19. McLean J. Management and leadership: Dispelling the myths. The British Journal of Administrative Management. 2005;Oct/Nov:16.

20. Miller T, Vaughan B. (2001). Messages from the management past: Classic writers and contemporary problems. *S.A.M. Advanced Management Journal 66*(1);4–20.

21. Muczyk J, Reimann B. (1989). MBO as a complement to effective leadership. *The Academy of Management Executive 3*(2);131–138.

22. Nellis S. (1994). Leadership and management: techniques and principles for athletic training. *JAT 29*(4):328–335.

23. Northouse P. (2001). Leadership: Theory and application. London, England: Sage Publication.

24. Patterson K. (2003). *Servant leadership: A theoretical model.* Accessed March 21, 2006 from http://www.regent.edu/acad/global/publications/sl_proceedings/2003/patterson_servant_leadership.pdf

25. Pielstick DC. (1998). The transforming leader: A meta-ethnographic analysis. *Community College Review 26*(3):15–35.

26. Robinson D. (2005). Management theorists: Thinkers for the 21st century? *Training Journal:* 30–31.

27. Roof J, Presswood K. (2004). Is it leadership or management? *College and University Journal 79*(4):3–7.

28. Schriesheim C, Castro S, Cogliser, C. (1999). Leader-member exchange (LMX) research: A comprehensive review of theory, measurement, and data-analytic practices. *Leadership Quarterly 10*(1):25–40.

29. Sendjaya S. (2003). *Development and validation of Servant Leadership behavioral scale.* Accessed March 21, 2006 from http://www.regent.edu/acad/global/publications/sl_proceedings/2003/sendjaya_development_validation.pdf

30. Tubbs S, Schulz E. (2006). Exploring a taxonomy of global leadership competencies and meta-competencies. *The Journal of American Academy of Business 8*(2):29–34.

31. Yoder-Wise PS. (2003). *Leading and managing in nursing.* St. Louis, MO: Mosby.

32. Yukl GA. (1981). *Leadership in organizations.* Englewood Cliffs, NJ: Prentice Hall.

33. Zaleznik A. (1998). Managers and leaders: Are they different? In: *Harvard Business Review on Leadership.* Cambridge, MA: HBS Press;61–88.

Chapter 5

Leadership Behaviors and Management Tools

"Management is doing things right; leadership is doing the right things."

PETER F. DRUCKER

Key Terms

Ambition: The use of available resources (intrinsic and extrinsic) and other effective strategies to promote professional and personal development.

Assertiveness: The quality of being proactive about new ideas, innovations, and change initiatives while maintaining respect for personal boundaries and the rights of others.

Benchmarking: Determining best practices by measuring one's performance against the best organizations in one's industry.

Brainstorming: A technique used to generate new ideas, in which the context is such that there are no "right" or "wrong" ideas.

Collaborating: Effectively participating with other professionals within the local or global community to achieve similar goals.

Context: The background information to an event; the integration of any number of external and internal variables, such as attitudes, belief systems, values, cultural bias, and symbols that make up a circumstance.

Contextual intelligence: The ability to recognize, assess, and assimilate several external and internal variables that make up any situation or environment.

Creativity: The willingness and ability to produce plausible ideas when asked or needed.

Critical thinking: The cognitive ability to make connections, integrate, and make practical application of different actions, opinions, and information.

Cultural sensitivity: The quality of promoting diversity by aligning diverse individuals and creating opportunities for diverse members to interact in non-discriminatory manner.

Discipline: The quality of demonstrating consistent and steady behavior.

Ethical behavior: Behavior characterized by reporting incompetent, unethical, and illegal practice objectively, factually, and according to current standards/procedures. Treating people equitably and fairly.

Hygiene factors: Variables that when absent contribute toward job dissatisfaction, such as status, job security, salary, and fringe benefits.

Initiative: Willingness to embark on a new venture.

Motivator factors: Variables that when present increase job satisfaction, such as challenging work, recognition, and responsibility.

Resilience: The ability to recover from and adjust to misfortune or change.

ifty billion dollars is spent annually on leadership development in the United States.[11] The value many Americans place on leadership is not without cause. There is a substantial body of evidence to suggest that leadership is important to organizational and individual success.[11] Attempts to delineate leadership have produced lengthy lists of behaviors, skills, and abilities. Athletic trainers should be aware of the leadership behaviors that contribute to organizational and individual effectiveness. A large part of leadership in athletic training involves using motivational techniques and management tools.

This chapter focuses on some of the specific leadership behaviors that the athletic trainer can implement in everyday practice. We will begin by discussing general health care leadership and evidence-based leadership. Next, we will discuss specific leadership behaviors that athletic trainers can implement. This is followed by a discussion of motivational theory and techniques that can be used by the athletic trainer. After motivation, we turn to a discussion of management tools that can be used by the athletic trainer to operate a more efficient athletic training room or clinic.

CRITICAL LEADERSHIP QUESTIONS

There are several important leadership behaviors perceived to be important for athletic training practice. Some of these behaviors are unique to athletic training and others are "generic"—that is, they transcend context and are not role- or title-dependent—and are beneficial in multiple settings and can be transferred between jobs, work settings, and social settings. Before delineating any specific leadership behaviors it will be helpful to perform a leadership awareness exercise. Based on your current level of understanding, take a moment to reflect on the following questions:

1. Who have I seen demonstrate leadership?
2. What specific actions did I observe in that person to make me think they were a leader?
3. How is leadership "success" often defined?
4. What leadership behaviors do I currently exhibit? and most importantly…
5. What is it about my becoming a better leader that will enhance the profession of athletic training?

It is important that everyone be able to answer these questions so that leadership development can be informed and intentional. Having a basic philosophical grasp of leadership and how it impacts the world around us is an important foundation to practical and useful integration of leadership behaviors and management tools.

Other questions important for leadership development include: is leadership an integrated cluster of tangible skills? Or, does leadership consist primarily of intangible abilities? The fact is, leadership consists of both tangible and intangible abilities. Some of the tangible (or observable) behaviors of leadership include strategic thinking, communication, initiative, and resilience. The intangible aspects of leadership consist of things like personality, interpersonal people skills, and attitude.

Intangible leadership skills are difficult to teach to another person; these skills are best developed internally after careful self-reflection. The tangible leadership skills are easier to teach to others. Therefore, the majority of leadership development has defaulted to teaching observable and measurable behaviors (or competencies). The next logical question then is, what are the leadership behaviors athletic trainers need to exhibit? The next section covers some of the general leadership competencies required of any health care professional. Finally, specific behaviors are identified for leadership within athletic training.

LEADERSHIP COMPETENCIES IN HEALTH CARE

Many leadership skills are similar between health care workers.[6] There is a growing body of evidence that suggests leadership skills may be transferable between industries and organizations.[5,12] In this sense there are generic leadership abilities that can be employed in almost any environment or setting.

The Pew Commission[9] identified 21 competencies of the competent health care professional. Many of the competencies identified are related to leadership. Those health care competencies are:

1. Embrace a personal ethic of social responsibility and service
2. Exhibit ethical behavior in all professional activities
3. Provide evidence-based, clinically competent care
4. Incorporate the multiple determinants of health in clinical care
5. Apply knowledge of the new sciences
6. Demonstrate critical thinking, reflection, and problem-solving skills
7. Understand the role of primary care
8. Rigorously practice preventive health care
9. Integrate population-based care and services into practice
10. Improve access to health care for those with unmet health needs
11. Practice relationship-centered care with individuals and families
12. Provide culturally sensitive care to a diverse society
13. Partner with communities in health care decisions
14. Use communication and information technology effectively and appropriately
15. Work in interdisciplinary teams
16. Ensure care that balances individual, professional, system and societal needs
17. Practice leadership
18. Take responsibility for quality of care and health outcomes at all levels
19. Contribute to continuous improvement of the health care system
20. Advocate for public policy that promotes and protects the health of the public
21. Continue to learn and help others learn

Interestingly, competency 17 "practice leadership" indicates that all health professionals, whether they seek administrative and managerial positions or not, should be exposed to experiences that improve their ability to communicate, negotiate, lead, and facilitate change.[9] The implications of this recommendation are that practicing leadership should not be restricted to those in formal positions of authority. Rather, it implies that communicating, negotiating, and facilitating change are the behaviors of leaders, regardless of position. Another aspect of leadership is the judicial application of evidence in decision making.

Leadership is an evidence-based professional activity.[3] Leadership decisions should not be made in a vacuum and should include any available evidence. **Evidence-based leadership** is a structured method for interpreting and applying evidence in the identification of appropriate actions and the innovative and creative implementation of decisions. Evidence in this construct includes past experiences and best-practices. Figure 5-1 is a graphic depiction of what "evidence" is available in an evidence-based leadership process. The available evidence includes knowledge of established leadership theory, the historical experiences of corporate and team decisions, knowledge of individual past decisions, outcomes of and reactions to those decisions, and context-specific knowledge. The next section will delineate some specific leadership behaviors important for athletic trainers. This is certainly not an exhaustive list, but serves as a sound starting point.

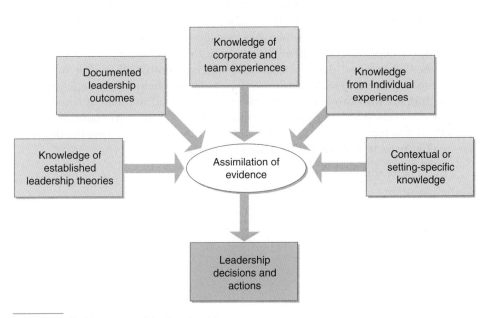

Factors for Evidence-based Leadership

FIGURE 5-1 Evidence used for leadership

LEADERSHIP BEHAVIORS IMPORTANT FOR ATHLETIC TRAINING

The existence of leadership ultimately is determined by behavior. Behaviors are those actions or reactions that a person demonstrates to others. Demonstrated behaviors are complex and are a result of several variables, including education, experience, socialization, values, and culture. Leaders tend to consistently demonstrate certain behaviors that are often credited for their effectiveness or success (however that might be defined). Forty-nine leadership behaviors have been identified as important for athletic training practice.[7] Athletic trainers who demonstrate these behaviors are likely to be perceived as leaders. A list of forty-nine leadership behaviors can be difficult to implement and even harder to assess. Therefore, to better understand and implement these leadership behaviors, they were organized into six broad leadership factors. The six leadership factors important for athletic training practice include the following:

1. Personal Qualities
2. Diagnosing context
3. People skills
4. Communication
5. Initiative
6. Strategic thinking

Table 5-1 is a list of the six leadership factors for athletic trainers. Under each factor is a list of specific behaviors associated with the factor.

Personal Qualities

Certain personal qualities are demonstrated in leadership. Personal qualities are greatly influenced by personality. Personality is developed early and may be well established by the time formal leadership development occurs. Because it is developed early on, personality is unlikely to be significantly affected by formal leadership development programs.[11] However, knowing which behaviors other athletic trainers perceive to be associated with a desirable personality can help inform self-reflection. Athletic trainers who can learn to effectively critique and implement some of the behaviors associated with the personality factor increase the perception of leadership others may have of them. Behaviors that contribute toward having the desirable personality characteristics of a leader include:

1. Ethical behavior
2. Responsibility
3. Personal discipline
4. Open-mindedness
5. Flexibility and adaptability to change or stress
6. Assertiveness
7. Creativity
8. Ambition

Of all the personal qualities, behaving ethically appears to be the most important.[7] **Ethical behavior** involves promoting ethical practice in the treatment of patients and in the pursuit of organizational goals and objectives. This behavior includes reporting incompetent, unethical, and illegal practice objectively, factually, and according to current standards/procedures, and treating people equitably and fairly. Additional aspects of ethics are discussed in chapter 14.

Ambition and assertiveness also are important aspects of personality that seem to be exhibited by leaders. **Ambition** is the use of available resources (intrinsic and extrinsic) and other effective strategies to promote professional and personal development. While ambition is deemed important, it is critical that it be tempered with ethical behavior. **Assertiveness** is being proactive about new ideas, innovations, and change initiatives while maintaining respect for personal boundaries and the rights of others. It is critical to remember that ambition or assertiveness themselves are not what is important. They are a small part of other personality characteristics and need to be integrated with them.

Another behavior associated with personality often perceived in leaders is open-mindedness. Being open-minded involves a willingness to consider new ways of

TABLE 5-1 Six Leadership Factors and Related Behaviors or Skills

Leadership Factor	Factor Definition	Specific Behaviors Exhibited in This Factor
Personal Qualities	Tendencies or behaviors that are primarily learned early in childhood development. Many of these characteristics are difficult to learn as part of a leadership development program, but can be reinforced or assessed later in leadership development.	Ethical behavior Thrives on responsibility Emotionally stable Disciplined Open mindedness Flexible or adaptive in times of change, crisis, or stress Assertive Creative/innovative leadership Ambitious
Diagnosing Context	The ability to assess and interpret contextual variables such as other people's biases, beliefs, and values and reconcile those with recognized cultural, religious, social, or political variables.	Dedicated Critical thinker Uses appropriate leadership style Socially responsible Leadership planner Contextual intelligence Change agent Resilience Willing to take appropriate risks
People Skills	The ability to align and influence people with different points of view and diverse backgrounds.	Consensus builder Cultural sensitivity Collaborator Protector Multicultural leadership Improves morale Nurtures professional relationships Delegates effectively
Communication	Concisely and articulately portrays meaning to others.	Written communication skill Empathetic Verbal communication skill Uses body language
Initiative	Willingness to begin or facilitate a new series of actions or embark on a new venture.	Intentional leadership Crisis management Applies known and attained knowledge Credible Identifies leaders Advocate Courageous
Strategic Thinking	Having a delineated plan of action that is based on the integration of relevant past experiences, present reality, and an anticipated future.	Future minded Organizational savvy Knowledgeable Ensures awareness of mission Influencer Controls risk

thinking or even abandoning former ways of thinking when evidence indicates that such a change is prudent. An open-minded disposition facilitates effective decision making by considering relevant evidence. Responsibility is another personality trait and involves two distinct aspects. The first is being responsible for actions, which is the ability to tactfully accept scrutiny and even criticism for personal actions and decisions that prove to be distracting. The second aspect involves thriving on responsibility, which is having a sense of duty to the profession and organization.

Exhibiting personal discipline is another key indicator of a leader's personality. **Discipline** is consistent and steady behavior. Being disciplined requires balancing consistency with flexibility and adaptability in crisis or stress. A temptation for many athletic trainers might be to maintain discipline and strict boundaries at the expense of being flexible or adaptable. However, longevity in athletic training requires adaptability.

One final behavior that lends itself to a desirable personality is creativity. **Creativity** is the willingness to produce plausible ideas when asked or needed. In other words, creativity is helping to generate or participate in brainstorming. **Brainstorming** is a technique used to generate new ideas or thoughts in a "safe" context where there are no "right" or "wrong" ideas.

Personality characteristics are only a small portion of what contributes to leadership. Many of the above behaviors, such as ambition, assertiveness, and creativity may be difficult to learn. Others, such as discipline, ethical behavior, and open-mindedness can be intentionally integrated into behavior, which may help to foster the perception of leadership. Another leadership factor is the ability to diagnose context. The next section will involve delineating the behaviors associated with diagnosing context.

Diagnosing Context

The context where the athletic trainer practices is dynamic. Health care in general is extremely dynamic and at times can be volatile. The **context** is the background of an event and involves a combination of any number of variables, such as attitudes, belief systems, values, cultural bias, and symbols. For example, there are often political, cultural, social, religious, and other factors present that define the context of any circumstance. Often in athletic training there is a mixture of physicians', parents', coaches', and athletes' values, biases, and beliefs. These variables, combined with organizational culture, historical precedent, and personal experiences, make each context unique. Being able to diagnose the context is an important leadership consideration for the athletic trainer.

The following list of behaviors lend themselves to being able to accurately diagnose context:

1. Contextual intelligence
2. Critical thinking
3. Use of appropriate leadership style
4. Resilience
5. Willingness to take appropriate risks

Contextual intelligence is the ability to recognize, assess, and assimilate several external and internal variables inherent in a given environment or circumstance. Simply stated, contextual intelligence is the ability to interpret and appropriately react to changing surroundings. Contextual intelligence is a skill that separates many leaders from non-leaders.

Critical thinking is an essential behavior of every professional and can be developed in formal athletic training education. Richard Paul is often cited as stating "critical thinking is thinking about your thinking, while you're thinking, in order to change your thinking."[10] The key idea about critical thinking is to make improvements in how you assess your options and organize your actions. A more pragmatic definition of **critical thinking** in light of leadership is the cognitive ability to make connections, integrate, and make practical application of different actions, opinions, and information.

Diagnosing context also involves demonstrating the appropriate use of leadership style. As noted in chapter 4, there are many leadership styles. The athletic trainer who knows which leadership style is appropriate is likely aware of the current context.

Other behaviors associated with diagnosing context include resilience and risk taking. **Resilience** is the ability to recover from and adjust to misfortune. It is also a personality characteristic, but is part of diagnosing context in that it demonstrates an ability to adapt to impending change. Willingness to take appropriate risks involves thought-out actions. It is the opposite of a cavalier attitude. Risk taking involves taking bold actions. Bold actions require precision and calculation, so that any foreseeable risk is minimized.

The next leadership factor involves those behaviors associated with relating to people. Obviously, leaders have to interact with people. Those athletic trainers who are comfortable with and around other people are likely to have other leadership attributes. The next section will include a brief discussion of important people skills for the athletic trainer to posses.

People Skills

A major component of any context is people. Therefore, contextual intelligence depends on the correct assessment of people. In fact, it is likely that leadership ability will be limited to the extent that one is comfortable interacting with others. People skills include the following specific behaviors:

1. Consensus building
2. Cultural sensitivity
3. Collaborating
4. Protecting others

Building consensus takes advantage of one's interpersonal skills to convince others to see the common good or a different point of view. This requires the ability to listen and communicate effectively, manage conflict, and diagnose context. **Cultural sensitivity** actively promotes diversity and aligns diverse individuals by creating opportunities for diverse members to interact in a non-discriminatory manner. Athletic trainers with people skills often create an atmosphere in their athletic training room that is inviting and conducive to the rich cultural and ethnic diversity in many athletic departments. **Collaborating** involves participating with other professionals within the local or global community in achieving similar goals. Finally, those with effective people skills protect others. Protecting in a leadership context means providing a secure and safe environment and doing what is possible or necessary to preserve that security. To develop authentic leadership the responsibility of protecting is important.

Effective people skills involve communicating. Communication is often cited as one of the most important roles or aspects of leadership. In the next section we will discuss the specific behaviors associated with communication. For a more detailed examination of communication, see chapter 2.

Communication

Rarely will anyone argue against the importance for a leader to communicate effectively. This does not mean every leader must always give great speeches, but they must be able to articulate their ideas clearly to others. Essentially effective communication is how well others understand what you are saying. Effective communicators use multiple techniques to get others to understand their message.

Communication is addressed extensively in chapter 2. Therefore, this section will only identify the specific behaviors of those leaders who communicate effectively. Three primary behaviors are:

1. Verbal communication
2. Written communication
3. Effective and appropriate use of body language

Skill in these three areas may dramatically enhance the perception of leadership by peers, subordinates, and supervisors. Likewise, poor written and verbal skills, accompanied with inappropriate use of body language, can seriously hinder leadership.

The next leadership factor involves initiative. Leaders simply must initiate action. The next section describes specific behaviors associated with initiative.

Initiative

Initiative is an individual's willingness to embark on a new venture. It also means the first in a series of events or steps. To initiate implies readiness and willingness to take an action, and may even include a calculated risk. Like the other factors, initiative is greater than the sum of it parts. The behaviors associated with initiative are:

1. Intentional leadership
2. Crisis management
3. Credibility

Intentional leadership is purposefully taking the actions necessary to become a better leader. It involves purposeful assessment and evaluation of one's own leadership performance and an acute awareness of one's own strengths and weaknesses. This assessment and awareness must result in new or changed actions. Practicing intentional leadership requires that knowledge gained from self-reflection be used as a framework from which to modify undesirable or unproductive behaviors. Intentional leaders must be open-minded, able to accept and synthesize feedback, and welcome the opportunity to develop themselves through interaction with others.

Athletic trainers with initiative handle crisis well on two fronts, internally and externally. "Internal crisis management" implies that the leader remains in control of his or her emotions. "External crisis management" implies that any response or action is deliberate and calm. In this context crisis management is not emergency response or preparedness (that aspect is covered extensively in chapter 13). Crisis management in the context of a leadership behavior is defined as effectively handling unforeseen crises, which includes limiting or correcting problems in a reasonable amount of time by using problem solving and dialogue. Athletic trainers who handle crisis effectively often provide effective strategies for conflict resolution soon after the crisis is identified.

The final aspect behind initiative is credibility. Nothing can potentially stifle a leader worse than a lack or loss of credibility. Being credible is critical to leading a successful initiative. Simply stated, credibility is gained by being believable, honest, trustworthy, and ethical in dealing with subordinates, peers, and supervisors. Everyone must believe you mean what you say and that you will do what you say. Without that level of believability, any initiative will falter right out of the gate.

In the next section we will discuss the final leadership factor important for an athletic trainer, strategic thinking. Strategic thinking is more than preparing a vision statement, identifying values, or a performing S.W.O.T. analysis (these aspects of strategic planning are outlined in detail in chapter 2). Strategic thinking involves specific actions based on awareness and intent.

Strategic Thinking

Strategic thinking is vastly different than strategic planning.[1,2,4,8] Strategic thinking involves having an intuitive awareness of the proverbial "big picture." Specifically, strategic thinking requires a holistic viewpoint that is based on the integration of the past, present, and future. Strategic thinking is demonstrated by anticipating certain outcomes and involves the following specific behaviors:

1. Future-minded
2. Use of influence
3. Organizational savvy

The future-minded athletic trainer has a forward-looking mentality and sense of direction and concern for where the organization should be in the future. To do this, the leader must manage several stimuli simultaneously. Because of the potential for so much stimuli, it is important to consult others and have a trusted group of people, with diverse backgrounds to help tailor or temper ideas. Ironically, awareness of history is an important aspect of being future-minded. History is important because the future cannot be correctly plotted if the starting point is not accurate. Furthermore, a future-minded leader needs to understand that the organization (and the individuals they lead) represent more that the sum total of their past. A future-minded athletic trainer is willing to embrace (and perhaps risk) that another individual's ability to contribute is not based solely on past successes or failures.

Appropriate use of influence is another behavior of strategic thinkers. The strategic aspect of influence involves knowing when, where, and how to use it. Appropriately using influence requires interpersonal skills to ethically and non-coercively affect the actions and decisions of others toward the future they envision.

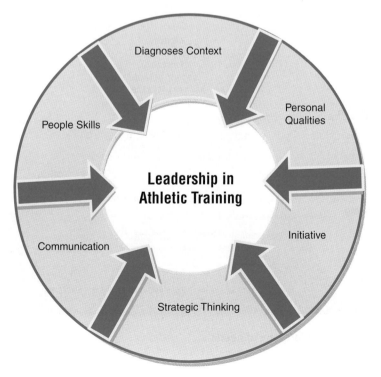

The last skill of the strategic thinker is organizational savvy. **Organizational savvy** requires profound understanding of the organization's infrastructure; its history; its future plans, policy and procedure; and its opportunities and threats.

Any one of these six factors will contribute toward leadership, but in isolation effectiveness is limited. To have the greatest impact as a leader all six factors need to be integrated. As stated at the beginning of this section, this is not a checklist that guarantees leadership. The athletic trainer at any level could use these factors and behaviors as part of a larger effort to improve on their current level of leadership.

MOTIVATIONAL THEORIES

Leadership necessitates motivating others. This is especially true in reference to human resources. The following is a brief review of some of the more common motivational theories and how you might apply them in athletic training.

Maslow's Hierarchy of Needs

Abraham Maslow (1908–1970) was a psychologist most noted for his theory of human motivation. Maslow believed that humans must have certain needs met in successive order. For example, need for water and food must be met before the need for security. The hierarchy of needs starts with physiological needs, then progresses to safety needs, then love/belonging, then esteem, and finally self-actualization. Figure 5-2 shows the pyramid of Maslow's hierarchy of needs, which identifies the five needs in sequential order. The needs identified at the bottom of the pyramid are the highest priority.

The athletic trainer can implement Maslow's theory by being attuned to the needs of those they influence (peers, athletes, or subordinates). For example, a

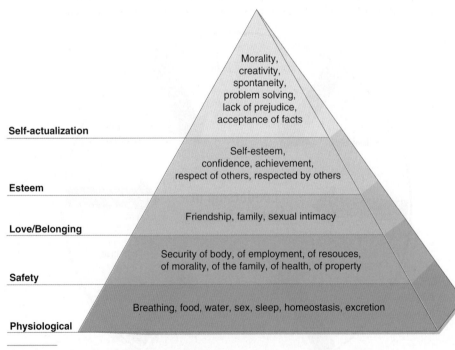

FIGURE 5-2 Maslow's hierarchy of needs

student athlete may have little money and be unable to pay rent or buy nutritious food, or even may be physically ill and not know how or where to seek help. That student athlete is going to respond and be motivated differently from others who have enough money, have a strong social network (i.e., family), are well fed, and are physically strong and healthy. The athletic trainer should have a referral network in place to support athletes whose basic needs are not met.

Herzberg's Hygiene Factors

Frederick Herzberg (1923–2000) was a psychologist who introduced the motivator-hygiene theory, which was popularized in business management. This theory states that there are two factors that contribute to job satisfaction and other factors that contribute to dissatisfaction. **Motivator factors** are things like challenging work, recognition, and responsibility. **Hygiene factors** are things like status, job security, salary, and fringe benefits. The presence of motivators give someone satisfaction in their work. Hygiene factors do not give satisfaction, but if they are absent they result in dissatisfaction.

For example, athletic training can be a highly satisfying career. There is often a high degree of responsibility and often the work is challenging. If hygiene factors, for example, salary and job security, are present, these motivator factors can help the athletic trainer achieve higher levels of performance as experience is gained. However, what frustrates many athletic trainers is often the salary and lack of job security. Therefore, in spite of challenging work and a high level of responsibility, the hygiene factors become an obstacle.

McGregor's Theory X & Y

Douglas McGregor (1906–1964) was a management professor at MIT. McGregor proposed that human motivation is based on either X or Y tendencies. Theory X is the assumption that subordinates are inherently lazy and will, if given the chance, avoid work. Therefore, managers who subscribe to theory X believe their workers need to be closely monitored and supervised. Belief in theory X has a profound effect on how a leader would choose to motivate.

Theory Y is the assumption that employees are self-motivated, desire greater responsibility, and exercise self-direction. In other words, theory Y managers tend to believe that if given the chance employees are creative and productive. Therefore, managers who subscribe to theory Y often delegate and share responsibility and can be more transformational leaders.

Athletic trainers hold to both theories. For example, motivating an athlete in rehab may require different techniques because one athlete exhibits theory X traits, whereas another exhibits theory Y traits. Furthermore, an athletic trainer may have a bias that all athletes exhibit theory X traits, which dictates how the athletic training room is managed, compared with a colleague who believes all athletes in general exhibit theory Y traits.

> ✎ *From the Field*
>
> *There are student athletes whose motivation to participate on a team is purely for social acceptance and not for the "love of the game" or passion to compete. In one particular circumstance, I remember discovering that an athlete only wanted to go on road trips for the per diem money. The athlete did not actually care if they competed; the motivation to be a part of the team and especially travel was driven by a financial need. Later it was discovered that he was saving the per diem money and using it to pay necessary expenses, such as rent and gasoline.*

CONTEMPORARY MANAGEMENT TOOLS

The above sections have all addressed leadership behaviors and motivational theories. The next section delineates tools at the leader's disposal to help facilitate an optimal environment, motivate, and track productivity of fellow workers.

360° Feedback

360° feedback has been called multi-source feedback and has become a very popular feedback and evaluation tool in health care. Used as a human resource tool for evaluating individual performance, this tool can also be very effective in evaluating programs, assessing outcomes, and assessing productivity and performance. Multi-source feedback can take extra time to complete, but it can provide valuable information. This multi-source approach also can focus in on specific aspects within an athletic training program needing attention.

360° feedback incorporates the feedback of several interested parties. Critical to the successful implantation of 360° feedback is anonymity. This is desirable because it may yield more honest results. Consider the head athletic trainer asking for a critical examination of how the athletic training room is operated during a staff meeting. As the assistant athletic trainer you may be hesitant to be honest, fearing repercussion. However, if a 360° feedback tool is used, the head athletic trainer asks for anonymous feedback from peer-level staff (maybe the head softball or track coach); subordinates (such as the assistant athletic trainer or athletic training students); patients (such as student-athletes); superiors (such as the athletic director or head team physician); and other stakeholders such as parents of athletes. These evaluations are then assessed by an unbiased third party and are compared to the head athletic trainer's own analysis. The evaluation and feedback is then given to the head athletic trainer and is used to make positive changes in the way the athletic training room operates. Another valuable aspect of 360° feedback is the opportunity to delineate and assess any existing gaps between the perceptions of the leader and other stakeholders.

Evaluation of the Strategic Plan and Leaders

Successfully integrating changes or innovations must be based on sound evaluation techniques and thorough assessment. In spite of all the effort, time, and resources put into program development, there are often unanticipated events and circumstances that are introduced which require flexibility. Fluidity in the plan requires a consistent evaluation process so that unforeseen circumstances or unmet objectives can be assessed. Therefore, programmatic evaluation is always necessary. During the evaluation process, weakness will be discovered and changes will be necessary. It is critical for the longevity of the program and credibility of the leader that these changes be made. A plan should never be implemented then left to fate. It is the evaluation process that allows us to alter the plan so that outcomes can be maximized.

Evaluation is more than checking to see if things are running smoothly or if things are on pace to be completed. Evaluation's core premise is the idea of taking what is working and helping it to work better. Evaluation transcends the "squeaky wheel gets the grease" syndrome. It is difficult for some people to realize that when things are working well they can, in fact, work better. Evaluation and benchmarking can help this realization. **Benchmarking** is determining best practices by measuring your performance against the best organizations in your industry. The evaluation and benchmarking process can document the need for change or improvement and serve as a vehicle to introduce innovation.

The continual evaluation of any program is significant to the longevity of that program. Evaluation is simply the process used to determine the worth or value of something. Any evaluation is better than no evaluation. Several types of programmatic evaluation can be used to assess the value and worth of a program relative to its stated objectives. Some of the evaluation tools include self-study reports, 360° feedback, and benchmarking.

Self Study

The self-study process is when an organization critically examines its program's structure and substance and results in a detailed written report. The self-study process is a critical aspect of the evaluation process. Self studies are used to rate a program's performance relative to stated objectives and goals and can be a valuable component of a S.W.O.T. analysis. The self study should also include a statement of purpose and provide clear evidence that an identifiable process actually took place and that information gathered has been used to make necessary changes.

CHAPTER SUMMARY

Leadership within athletic training requires assimilating several leadership behaviors, which can be organized into six general factors: personality characteristics, diagnosing context, people skills, communication, initiative, and strategic thinking. These factors should be integrated with management tools that increase effectiveness and organizational awareness. Management tools can be used to assess individuals and programs or to help motivate by articulating specific actions needed. Motivating others requires an understanding of the specific factors that might contribute to job satisfaction or dissatisfaction as well as awareness of someone's current need. The athletic trainer who is purposeful about leadership development will take the time to reflect critically on existing or absent leadership behaviors and will seek to understand what motivates others and learn which management tools can be used to facilitate desired outcomes.

▶ Leadership Application

You are a new assistant athletic trainer at State College. After a few days on the job, you were approached by a veteran assistant athletic trainer who informed you that the head athletic trainer and the educational program director have been competing to be the primary influencer in all athletic training–related decisions for years. After a few months you begin to notice that they both prefer that all decisions come through them. Furthermore, you realize that they rarely delegate tasks and each tries to "outdo" the other or have the last word. You begin to find yourself in casual discussions with the other assistants over this apparent interpersonal "drama" that is unfolding before your eyes. While your co-workers do not, you perceive this apparent tension as a real problem. One afternoon the head athletic trainer invites you to lunch and during lunch it is apparent that he is trying to lobby for your support over an upcoming staffing decision that is likely to be challenged by the program director at the next meeting. The decision involves hiring a new athletic trainer who will serve a dual appointment as a part-time faculty member and part-time assistant athletic trainer. What the head athletic trainer does not know is that the program director already spoke to you about the same issue. Based on what you have heard from both the head athletic trainer and program director, you are sure that the next meeting will involve an unnecessary confrontation.

Critical Thinking Questions

1. What interpersonal dynamics might be involved that would influence you to choose sides?
2. What leadership strategies can you employ to prevent becoming cynical about this apparent problem?
3. What skills might help navigate this complex environment, and why?
4. What leadership or management strategies can you employ to eliminate the apathy among your peers and motivate them to take action?

References

1. Abraham S. Stretching strategic thinking. *Strategy & Leadership* 2005;*33*(5):5–12.

2. Bonn I. Developing strategic thinking as a core competency. *Management Decision 2001;39*(1):63.

3. Field K. Evidence-based subject leadership. *Journal of In-service Education 2002;28*(3): 460–474.

4. Graetz F. Strategic thinking versus strategic planning: Towards understanding the complementarities. *Management Decision 2002;40*(5/6):456–462.

5. Groysberg B, McLean A, Nohria N. Are leaders portable? *Harvard Business Review 2006;* 92–100.

6. Hannam S. *Professional behaviors in athletic training.* Thorofare, NJ: Slack Inc.; 2000.

7. Kutz M. Importance of leadership competencies and content for athletic training education and practice: A Delphi technique and national survey [dissertation]. Boca Raton, FL: College of Business and Management, Lynn University; 2006.

8. Liedtka JM. Linking strategic thinking with strategic planning. *Strategy and Leadership 1998;26*(4):30–35.

9. O'Neil EH, Pew Health Professions Commission. *Recreating health professional practice for a new century.* San Francisco: Pew Health Professions Commission; December 1998.

10. Paul R, Binker A. *Critical thinking: What every person needs to survive in a rapidly changing world.* Rohnert Park: Sonoma State University, Center for Critical Thinking and Moral Critique; 1990.

11. Tubbs S, Schulz E. Exploring a taxonomy of global leadership competencies and meta-competencies. *The Journal of American Academy of Business 2006;8*(2):29–34.

12. Yntema T. The transferable skills of a manager. *Journal of the Academy of Management 1960;*8:79–86.

Chapter 6

Human Resources

"The human mind is our fundamental resource."

JOHN F. KENNEDY

CHAPTER RATIONALE

Role Delineation Study Components

Domain V: Organization and Administration

- Institutional and federal employment regulations (e.g., EEOC, ADA, Title IX)
- Human resource management

Educational Competencies

- Identify the principles of recruiting, selecting, and employing physicians and other medical and allied health care personnel in the deployment of athletic health care services.
- Identify common human-resource policy and federal legislation regarding employment such as The Americans With Disabilities Act, Wage and Hour, Family Medical Leave Act, Family Educational Rights Privacy Act, Fair Labor Standards Act, Affirmative Action, Sexual Aggression, and the Equal Opportunity Employment Commission.

Key Terms

Chronological resume: A resume that lists all education and work experience in chronological order (present to past) and is the "traditional" resume format preferred by many employers.

Core competency of an organization: The collective talent, experience, and creativity of the people within that organization that differentiates them from others.

Cover letter: A tool used to introduce oneself to potential employers and highlights important aspects of one's resume.

Functional resume: A resume designed around skills and experiences and that is used when there have been frequent job changes or long lay-offs between jobs.

Heroes or heroines: The people (alive or dead, real or imagined) who represent the ideals of the organization.

Human capital: The experience, education, and background that people bring to a job or role that contribute toward organizational success.

Knowledge workers: Specialized professionals who have a unique skill set.

Rituals: Those actions that fill social needs within an organization.

Symbols: The words or objects used to communicate ideas within an organization.

Values: Priorities held by the organization.

P eople are the greatest asset of any organization. Be it a large company, family-owned business, organization, hospital, clinic, or small department, people are central to organizational success. As implied in the opening quote, a person's experience, education, and background can be significant contributor's to positive growth and development of any enterprise. **Human capital** is what people bring and contribute to organizational success.[8] It is human capital that provides the knowledge, experience, creativity, and innovation required for an effective organization. Human capital creates the core competency of an organization.[8] The **core competency of an** *organization* is the collective talent, experience, and creativity of the people within that organization that differentiates them from others.[8]

Athletic training is no exception. The certified athletic trainers, athletic training students, and other members of the sports medicine team make an athletic training program distinctive. Discovering and maximizing human capital falls within the scope of human resources (HR). However, it is not the exclusive domain of HR. Effective leaders and managers often take a significant role in matters related to HR. Human resource activities include collaborating with others on strategic planning, employment and staffing, training and development, worker protection, and labor relations.[8] Effectively leading human resources includes creating policies and encouraging procedures that enhance and foster individuals and teams. Leading and managing those human resources becomes a critically important component to long-term success and must involve recruiting and retaining the right people for the right tasks.

As an athletic trainer, HR is likely to impact you in two ways. First, HR will impact you as an employee. Therefore, knowing how human resource managers and departments operate and their fundamental principles of operation can help in job searches, evaluations, and in assimilating more easily into a new organizational climate. Second, it is likely that at some point the opportunity to hire new staff, interview candidates, or sit on a search committee will present itself. Having basic knowledge of human resources will help you in any of these roles.

In this chapter we will outline the basic aspects of human resources. First, we will look at specific strategies that athletic trainers can use to find a job, including how to locate available jobs, build resumes, and interview for jobs. We will also discuss the elements of organizational culture in order to prepare job seekers to accurately evaluate employment opportunities. Next, we will turn to a brief discussion of human resource legislation and typical policies and procedures. Finally, we will examine employee retention issues, including training, development, and evaluations.

FINDING A JOB

Being aware of what employers go through trying to recruit qualified athletic trainers for their positions is important to understand. Finding a job that is a good fit for both the candidate and employer involves coordinating several activities. Those activities include understanding the job search and hiring timeline of the profession, preparing an adequate cover letter and resume, knowing how to make your resume visible to the right people, and understanding the art of interviewing.

Making your resume visible to the right people is a daunting task. It requires knowing the kind of job you are best suited for. Discovering this involves critical self-reflection as well as candid discussions with honest friends and trusted mentors. When deciding on the fit of a specific job, it is important to examine and perhaps rank several items. Prioritizing the following items is an important step in assessing the fit of certain jobs:

1. job security
2. opportunity for team work
3. opportunity for independent work
4. professional status
5. intellectual challenge
6. pleasant surroundings
7. ability to advance
8. financial rewards
9. challenging or stimulating co-workers

Ranking these items by importance will help determine which jobs are the most appropriate. Taking a job on the sole basis of it being the one that offers the highest salary or the best benefits is not a sound strategy. Making a selection based on interest, experiences, and overall fit is more likely to result in greater satisfaction.

For athletic trainers seeking jobs, an important question is, "What characteristics do employers most want to see in applicants?" Kahanov and Andrews[7] identified four factors, each with specific characteristics that employers look for when hiring athletic trainers. The four factors consisted of 1) personal characteristics; 2) educational experience; 3) professional experience; and 4) work-related attributes. Employers in different athletic training settings regarded certain factors as more important or less important depending on the setting. However, "personal characteristics" were rated as important by employers in all work settings. Athletic trainers seeking employment should consider these personal characteristics when searching and applying for jobs. Box 6-1 is a list of those specific characteristics employers look for in athletic trainers. Interestingly, eight of the personal characteristics identified by Kahanov and Andrews[7] are similar or identical to the characteristics identified by Yukl[12] for successful leaders.

BOX 6-1   Personal Characteristics That Employers of Athletic Trainers Look for in all Work Settings

1. Self-confidence*
2. Maturity
3. Interpersonal skills*
4. Assertiveness*
5. Enthusiasm/motivation
6. Technical skills
7. Ability to articulate goals*
8. Oral communication skills*
9. Leadership skills
10. Initiative*
11. Ambition*
12. Problem-solving skills*
13. Writing skills

---

* Indicate Yukl's characteristics of successful leadership

Resume Preparation

The resume is an important part of getting information about an applicant to potential employers. It is a common misunderstanding that the resume is used to secure a job. In fact, a resume is not intended to "get you a job." The resume has many functions, the first and foremost of which is to get the applicant an interview. Resumes are also helpful when used to supplement a job application by supplying potential employers with information that is not asked on an application.

Resumes should be a summary of pertinent information relevant to a desired job or position. Providing too much or not enough information can hinder an adequate review by potential employers. Traditionally, resumes provide a summary of formal education, work or professional experience, and other information relevant to a specific job. Within these three sections (i.e., education, experience, and other relevant information) there are several headings that can be used to highlight pertinent information. Box 6-2 contains a list of headings that have been used on resumes.

BOX 6-2 **Headings That Have Been Used in Athletic Training Resumes**
1. Objective
2. Education
3. Honors, scholarships, and/or awards
4. Professional experience
5. Work history or related experience
6. Licenses and certifications
7. Skills
8. Internships, volunteer work, and/or community service
9. Professional memberships
10. Publications and/or presentations
11. Military
12. Computer and/or technical skills
13. Conferences attended
14. Highlights or summary of qualifications
15. Hobbies & interests
16. Personal achievements
17. Professional development
18. References

Resumes can be prepared to be specific to individual jobs or more generic. It is recommended that applicants have several "versions" of a resume, tailoring each to specific job settings or roles. There are several types of resumes that can be created for job searches. The most common type is the **chronological resume**. A chronological resume lists all education and work experience in chronological order (present to past) and is the "traditional" resume format preferred by many employers. However, there are other viable formats. A second type of resume is the functional resume. A **functional resume** is designed around skills and experiences and is used when there have been frequent job changes or long lay-offs between jobs. An example of when to use a functional resume might be after returning to the workforce after a long stay at home to raise children. The functional resume is designed to highlight experience and skills. Finally, a combination format allows the candidate

John S. Doe
901 University Drive
Big Town, ST 55555
555-555-5555

EDUCATION
State University (Anywhere, USA)
Bachelor of Athletic Training (May 2009)
Suma Cum Laude

CERTIFICATES AND LICENSES
BOC Certified Athletic Trainer, 2009
State Licensed Athletic Trainer, 2009

ATHLETIC TRAINING EXPERIENCE
Athletic Training Student, State University (2005-2009)
- Spring 2009 Soccer
- Fall 2008 Football
- Fall -Winter 2007-2008 Women's Basketball
- Spring 2007 Softball
- Fall 2006 Track & Field
- Spring 2006 Student Observer

Sports Medicine Internship with Awesome Orthopedics, Inc. (Summer 2009)
- Organized sports physicals for three area high schools.
- Assisted Orthopedic surgeons with patient follow up care.
- Assisted in monitoring and supervising patient's rehabilitation protocols.

PROFESSIONAL MEMBERSHIPS
National Athletic Trainers' Association
American College of Sports Medicine
Student Member – State Athletic Trainers' Association

LEADERSHIP & VOLUNTEER ACTIVITIES
2007-2009, President Athletic Training Student Association
Spring 2008, Medical volunteer, Annual Mountain Climb 5K
Spring 2006, Volunteer for State-wide Special Olympics

Figure 6-1 Sample chronological resume

JOHN S. DOE, ATC

12344 ROAD STREET
ANY CITY, STATE 5555
PHONE/FAX
EMAIL

Education

M.S. (Athletic Training)   University of XYZ   date – date
B.A. (Athletic Training)   ABC University   date – date

Summary of Qualifications

- Authored more than two-dozen articles and scholarly papers on sports medicine topics
- Considered by peers to be a "change agent" and innovative thinker
- Excellent written and oral communication skills
- Understands and works well within team dynamics
- Experienced presenter and public speaker
- Very proficient with various types of technology

Leadership & Management History

- Created and implemented entrepreneurial initiatives
- Managed day-to-day operations of a non-profit organization
- Planned and supervised international humanitarian relief teams
- Directed an educational program and served on several committees and sub-committees
- Supervised full-time staff, mentor peer-faculty, oversee student workers and volunteers
- Initiated new programs and services for regional hospitals
- Supervised and managed up to seven different department simultaneously
- Facilitated and directed staff meetings
- Demonstrated ability to create a dynamic working environment with peers, subordinates and supervisors

Professional Experience

St. John's Medical Center   Head Athletic Trainer   date – date
Advanced Rehabilitation Center   Head Athletic Trainer   date – date
University of XYZ   Graduate Assistant   date – date

Licenses, Certifications, & Memberships

State License (#AT1234)
BOC Certified (# 123456789)
Member, National Athletic Trainers' Association

Figure 6-2 Sample functional resume

to list experience in chronological order, but also uses space for listing skills and abilities. (Figures 6-1 and 6-2 are samples of chronological and functional resumes.)

When employers critique resumes, they are typically looking for several things:

1. The ability to communicate concisely
2. Markers of intelligence (demonstrated through a strong educational background)
3. Special skills or experiences
4. Self-knowledge (the ability to highlight strengths and recognize weaknesses)
5. Leadership experience
6. Creativity and innovation

It is common practice to include "action words" throughout the resume. Examples of action words are included on Box 6-3. Action words are used to convey that a behavior has been demonstrated, which implies competence. Box 6-4 is a list of tips to consult when designing a resume.

BOX 6-3 Action Words Used in Resumes	
Achieved	Generated
Administered	Implemented
Analyzed	Improved
Attained	Led
Budgeted	Maintained
Collaborated	Managed
Communicated	Organized
Created	Passed
Delegated	Provided
Developed	Reviewed
Edited	Succeeded
Executed	Supervised
Facilitated	

Cover Letters

Another important aspect of the resume is the cover letter. The **cover letter** is used to introduce yourself and to serves as a map to your resume. Used correctly, a cover letter will guide the reader to the important aspects of the resume and serve as an echo or perhaps even a brief explanation of what is summarized on the resume. Cover letters typically follow a certain format. In the greeting, introduce yourself by stating your name, and how you came to know about the available position. If you are going to "name drop," now is the time. For example, "Mr. Smith (who is a famous person or someone known to the reader) referred me to this position." After the introduction, identify briefly why you believe you are the best candidate for this job. Now is the time to echo some of the items you want to highlight from your resume. For example: "As you will note on my resume, I am suited for this position because…" This strategy will take the reader directly to your resume and helps the reader make a connection between your experience and their job requirement. The

> **BOX 6-4   Basic Resume Tips**
>
> 1. Be honest, do not lie or exaggerate.
> 2. Center, bold, and enlarge your name at the top.
> 3. Contact information should be easy to locate (preferably close to your name).
> 4. Keep the sections lined up and consistent.
> 5. Do not use odd or fancy fonts (use Times New Roman or Arial).
> 6. Keep font size at 11–12 points, except for your name and headings.
> 7. Try to avoid two-page resumes for entry-level positions.
> 8. If you have a two-page resume, be sure to fill the second page at least halfway.
> 9. Most professional organizations frown on graphics, borders, or boldly colored paper.
> 10. Leave out personal data, photos, and unrelated hobbies.
> 11. Use consistent formatting (i.e., if you abbreviate dates and states, abbreviate throughout; if you spell them out, spell out throughout).
> 12. Proofread!
> 13. Have a friend or colleague proofread it!

next section should conclude the cover letter and reiterate how excited you are about the opportunity. Figure 6-3 is a cover letter template.

Interviewing

Ideally, a resume generates enough interest to warrant an interview. Typically, interviews occur in two stages, a phone interview and a face-to-face interview. The best advice for phone interviews is to be prepared. Practice the phone interview and be sure to be in a quiet room where risk of interruption is low. A land-line phone is preferable; cellular phones are convenient and usually more accessible, but the risks of a bad connection, dropped calls, or static are high. If the phone interview is with a committee, be sure to address specific individuals. Keep a legal pad near by to write down questions or thoughts that arise during the phone interview. Again, the goal of the phone interview is to set up a face-to-face interview, so be concise and brief when asking or answering questions. Do not mumble, ramble, chew gum, or interrupt when on a phone interview.

Face-to-face interviews can be stressful, but if prepared for properly can produce a great outcome. The face-to-face interview is what can secure or lose the job. The resume, cover letter, and phone interview were all designed to get you face to face with a potential employer. Once in a face-to-face interview, remember that someone thinks you deserve to be there. It is still competitive, but half the work is already done. The next step is to present yourself well. Attire, preparation, and confidence are now your best allies.

When choosing interview attire, be conservative and well groomed. For men, that means a dark suit, regular tie (not too bold), dress shoes, and white shirt. For women, that means a traditional pants suit, mild perfume and make-up, closed toe and heel shoes, and a conservative neckline.

Preparing for an interview includes researching the organization. Research should be thorough enough to provide questions about an organization's operations or procedures. It is not enough to know only the company name, location, and founder. Visit the websites of the organization (including their HR page), local chamber of commerce, and some local business; these should provide enough information about the organization and community to give you a solid background and sensible

Your Street Address
City, State Zip Code
Telephone Number
Email Address

Month, Day, Year

Mr./Ms./Dr. First Name Last Name
Title
Name of Organization
Street or P. O. Box Address
City, State Zip Code

Dear Mr./Ms./Dr. Last Name:

Opening paragraph: State why you are writing; how you learned of the organization or position, and basic information about yourself.

2nd paragraph: Tell why you are interested in the employer or type of work the employer does. Demonstrate that you know enough about the employer or position to relate your background to the employer or position. Mention specific qualifications which make you a good fit for the employer's needs (refer to your resume). This is an opportunity to explain in more detail relevant items in your resume. Refer to the fact that your resume is enclosed. Mention other enclosures if such are required to apply for a position.

3rd paragraph: Indicate that you would like the opportunity to interview for a position. State what you will do to follow up, such as telephone the employer within two weeks. State that you would be glad to provide the employer with any additional information needed. Thank the employer for her/his consideration.

Sincerely,

(Your handwritten signature)

Your name typed

Enclosure(s) (refers to resume, etc.)

Figure 6-3 Template cover letter

BOX 6-5   Common and Illegal Interview Questions

COMMON INTERVIEW QUESTIONS

1. What is the most challenging injury or patient you have ever worked with?
2. What are your career goals?
3. Tell me about yourself?
4. How did you decide to apply for a position with us?
5. What are your strengths?
6. What are you weaknesses?
7. Why did you leave your last job?
8. What types of activities do you find to be rewarding and why?
9. What types of activities do you find to be frustrating and why?
10. Tell how you handled the last disagreement you had with a peer or supervisor?
11. In what ways have your college experiences prepared you for this job?
12. Are your best contributions made as part of a team or individual?

SOME ILLEGAL INTERVIEW QUESTIONS

1. Are you a United States citizen?
2. What was the date of your last physical exam?
3. What is your birthday?
4. What are your childcare arrangements?
5. Where do you go to church?
6. How much do you weigh?
7. Where were you/your parents born?
8. How old are you?
9. Do you plan to have a family?
10. How many children do you have?
11. What clubs or social organizations are you a member of?

---

questions. The goal is to get a snapshot of the community and begin to assimilate how the organization fits into the community. Next, know your resume! Be thoroughly familiar with the information submitted to the potential employer. It is also a sound practice to take extra resumes; during the course of an interview additional resumes may be required.

During an interview you can expect questions that relate to your resume and industry-specific tasks or knowledge. For an athletic trainer, that means questions about educational experiences, level of proficiency pertaining to specific competencies, and leadership and teamwork related questions. As an interviewee it is important to be aware of illegal or improper interview questions. Questions that ask about age, race, religious affiliation, alleged arrests, medical history, disability, martial status, pregnancy, or childbearing plans are illegal. If asked an illegal question, it is appropriate to state that you would rather not answer or state that the issue has no bearing on the ability to perform the job. Box 6-5 is a list of questions that some employers might ask as well as a list of some illegal questions.

The sequence of an interview typically follows a uniform format. However, some interviews involve meals or may even take a couple of days. In most cases the sequence tends to follow a particular order. That order is the interviewer(s) give a brief explanation of the company and the position. This is followed by review of the interviewee's background and experience and their strengths and weaknesses. The interviewee is given an opportunity to explain how he or she believes they can contribute to organizational or team goals. Usually there is time allotted for the interviewee to ask questions. When given the opportunity to ask questions, be sure to have some prepared. Always have a few backup questions ready, often times the original question is answered during the course of the interview, so be prepared with additional questions. Sometimes compensation packages are discussed, other times they are not. Do not be presumptuous; wait for the interviewer to bring up that issue. The interviewer knows compensation is on your mind. Typically there are closing remarks at this point be sure to thank everyone present for their time. A day or two after the interview is over, follow up with a thank-you card, thanking the interviewer for their time and for providing the opportunity to interview.

Understanding Organizational Culture

All athletic trainers should make an effort to assess the organizational culture of potential employers. Organizational culture is important because it can help define boundaries, establish identities, facilitate stability and comfort, and help regulate attitudes and behaviors. Furthermore, organizational culture plays a role in determining the areas in which the organization is able to learn easily and those areas in which the organization is likely to resist change.[2] Often the leadership style and strategies that will be used by your supervisors or that you might be expected to use largely depend on the organizational culture. Organizational culture is the personality of the organization and stems from organization's beliefs, knowledge, attitudes, and customs; it is the framework and assumptions deemed true by the organization's employees.

The foundation of organizational culture is determined by the presence of four elements: symbols, heroes and heroines, rituals, and values.[11] **Symbols** are the words or objects used to communicate ideas within an organization. For example, the use (or lack of use) of technical jargon can establish a certain culture. Written or unwritten performance expectations can also be powerful symbols. **Heroes or heroines** are the people (alive or dead, real or imagined) that represent the ideals of the organization. For example, awarding the Sayers "Bud" Miller Award to a distinguished athletic training educator or the Dick Butkus award to an outstanding linebacker indicates those individuals may be heroes within the organization and the behaviors and attitudes they represent are desirable traits. **Rituals** are those actions that fill social needs within an organization. An example might be casual Friday or opening each staff meeting a certain way. Finally, **values** are the priorities held by the organization and are an important part of organizational culture. Failure to embrace an organization's values can lead to a frustrating career, if not termination.

Whereas organizational structure is easier to delineate (i.e., organizational charts and hierarchy), organizational culture is less tangible and can be difficult to measure. Often any symbols, beliefs, attitudes, and rituals of organizations are implied (as opposed to stated explicitly). Because they are not explicitly stated does not make them any less important. Caccia-Bava[3] identified four types of organizational culture.

1. **Developmental**. Typically, developmental cultures are flexible and have an external focus. The external focus is typically on gaining a competitive advantage by being aware of what others are doing. Developmental cultures are often adaptable, focus on growth, provide adequate resources, are willing to take necessary risks taking, resist formal hierarchy, and are governed by ideology.

2. **Group**. Typically, group cultures are flexible and have an internal focus. Internally the focus seems to be on systems and clear lines of communication. Group cultures are often cohesive, have a high morale, develop human resources, are

very supportive and clan oriented, and are governed by affiliation and sense of belonging.

3. **Rational**. Typically, rational cultures are predictable (vs. flexible) and have an external focus. Rational cultures set a high priority on strategic planning and goal setting, operate efficiently (based on expected outcomes and polices and procedures), value competence, and are governed by contract (i.e., transactional).

4. **Hierarchical**. Typically, hierarchical cultures are predictable and have an internal focus. Hierarchical cultures value stability, and place a premium on control and the internal environment. Information is a powerful tool and is disseminated cautiously. There is often a value placed in conservative and cautious thinking. Hierarchical cultures gain compliance by promoting rules and regulations and are similar to a bureaucracy.

HUMAN RESOURCE MANAGEMENT

Human resource management is based on the value of human capital and creating and maintaining good labor relations. Today, human resource management (HRM) is not only about making sure employee's interests are represented, but HRM also has grown to encapsulate improving employee performance. Human resource management (or personnel management) has become a major area of focus within organizational development and business administration. It has evolved into entire schools and academic programs devoted to educating professionals to deal exclusively with human resources. HRM includes several dimensions, including employee recruitment and selection, employee motivation, performance appraisal, salary and benefits, talent management, and policies and procedures. Polices and procedures have a far-reaching scope and include items such as grievances, time-sheets, pay scales, job descriptions, and promotion policies. Basically, anything that involves an employee and his or her work environment falls under the domain of human resources.

Viewing people as a valuable resource was not always a popular school of thought. However, today it is a common belief that a principal component to long term, sustained success is to invest in the people within the organization. Unfortunately, many leaders and managers still hold to Theory X assumptions (i.e., that people are inherently lazy and will do anything to avoid work) and fear that "perks" such as breaks, flex hours, decent wages, providing needed training, and an ergonomic workplace might undermine their authority or create lazy employees. Human resource managers need to encourage leaders and managers to recognize that investing in employees sustains positive returns.

Pfeffer[9] identified seven characteristics of effective human resources. These characteristics should be at the heart of all personnel-related decisions and serve as the values for the human resource profession. These seven characteristics when implemented have been shown to increase employee performance:[9]

1. Emphasizing employment security – this involves making sure employees feel as if their job is secure and stable even during turbulent times.

2. Using self-managed teams – this involves placing people on teams with enough authority to accomplish their tasks and objectives.

3. Decentralizing decision making – this involves delegating the necessary decision-making authority to appropriate teams or members.

4. Hiring selectively – this involves recruiting a large applicant pool and choosing relevant and rigorous selection criteria.

5. Reducing barriers and distinctions between individuals – this involves removing symbols or classifications that foster barriers between employees or teams and promoting diversity.

6. Providing all necessary training – this involves providing ongoing training and required continuing education to all employers at or above industry standards.

7. Linking compensation to performance – this involves offering competitive salary and benefits as well as rewards based on performance.

In addition to these characteristics, human resource managers need to build a specific personnel strategy based on their unique organizational culture and goals. This involves creating and fostering a philosophy where everyone values employees similarly. Good human resource representatives convey to others the value people bring to an organization. This includes establishing and recommending highly selective hiring and interviewing procedures. Once the right people are hired it is important to ensure that they stay. This includes protecting jobs, promoting from within, creating grass-roots training and promotion policies, offering development opportunities (both personal and organizational), providing structured and safe modes of feedback, and fostering equality and diversity. While these ideals seem lofty, it is HRM that champions many of these causes.

In spite of all these lofty ideals it is still the recruitment and selection of employees that human resources is known for. Truly selecting the right personnel makes all the other aspects of HRM easier.

Searching for and Selecting Personnel

One of the major responsibilities of HRM is recruiting and selecting personnel. Selecting personnel requires a substantial amount of time and energy. Athletic training is a knowledge-based profession, meaning it requires what Peter Drucker referred to as a "knowledge-worker." **Knowledge-workers** are specialized professionals who have a unique skill set. It is possible that many human resource managers lack the background in athletic training (i.e., knowledge of the BOC's *Role Delineation Study* or the NATA Educational Competencies) to make informed personnel decisions. Therefore, some HR directors may depend on athletic trainers when it comes to recruiting qualified personnel who are able to contribute to athletic training and organizational goals. Athletic trainers should take initiative to educate human resource managers on the unique aspects of athletic training, including federal and state regulations. It is also recommended that athletic trainers and those familiar with the profession be included in athletic training-related hiring decisions. Figure 6-4 is a sequence map for recruiting and selecting athletic training personnel.

Getting a New Athletic Training Position Approved

One of the first aspects of recruiting involves a needs analysis. Requesting a new athletic training position must be supported with sound rationale. Before any position can be approved a need should be documented. There are times when the need is obvious, but often justification is required to get administration to set aside the required resources necessary. One tool that an athletic trainer in a traditional athletic training setting can use to document a need for additional personnel is the *Recommendations and Guidelines for Appropriate Medical Coverage of Intercollegiate Athletics*. This is a document published by NATA and can help delineate personnel needs. Another approach to determining a need for additional personnel is benchmarking. Benchmarking involves comparing the size and activities of your staff to a similar institution or an institution who you desire to mimic. Finally, personnel can be justified by assessing work load of current employees or cost-benefit ratios for hiring.

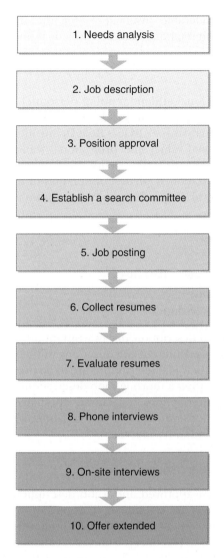

Figure 6-4 Process of searching for and selecting qualified athletic trainers

There are several tools available for assessing employee work loads or cost-benefit ratios.

Another aspect of a needs analysis involves determining the type of employee needed. In general when determining personnel needs consider the following:

1. Stakeholder expectations of a new employee.
2. Duties or responsibilities that will be required.
3. Skills and abilities required for those responsibility, and which skills are a "must have" and which skills are preferred.
4. Specific qualifications (i.e., experience, credentials, and education) that might be necessary.

Resources for a new position consist of more than the money for a salary. Bringing in new personnel requires infrastructure to support additional personnel such as adequate work space (i.e., office space), computer and technology resources, benefits, and training expenses. Then there are the expenses involved in recruiting and reviewing candidates. This includes advertising positions, travel and hotels for candidates, and food, all of which can significantly impact a budget. Therefore, a needs analysis can offer considerable justification for the immediate and on-going expenses of recruiting and retaining qualified athletic trainers.

Job Descriptions

Once the need for additional athletic training personnel has been documented a job description needs to be generated. Job descriptions should be based on objective information from a job analysis (i.e., BOC's Role Delineation Study) and should take into account organizational values and professional standards and competencies. Preparing a job description typically occurs simultaneously to seeking approval. Depending on the organization, a job description may or may not be required to be submitted prior to approval. Regardless, a job description needs to clearly articulate the following information:

1. Name and title of position
2. Reporting structure
3. Position rationale (usually a narrative)
4. Minimum qualifications
5. List of responsibilities or duties

Figure 6-5 is a sample job description for an assistant athletic trainer that includes each of the above sections. Different organizations will have their own preferences or even template of how their job descriptions are to be presented. However, regardless of job title or work setting a thorough job description should include the above information. Clear job descriptions can curtail workplace confusion and help to delineate roles and functions, which can foster collaboration, teamwork, and understanding between peers and with supervisors.

Vacancy Notices/Advertising

After a position has been approved and a job description prepared, it is time to advertise the job to prospective candidates. This portion of the job search includes preparing the job announcement and posting the position where it will be seen by as many potential employees as possible. Job announcements are similar to job descriptions, but serve a different purpose. The purpose of the job announcement is to recruit candidates and market the organization (or position), whereas a job description is intended to delineate responsibilities, lines of authority, and functions. Adequate job announcements should include all the following information:

1. Name and title of the position – similar to a job description, list the name of the employer and full title of the available position.
2. Description of the position – similar to a job description provide a brief narrative of the requirements of the position.
3. Minimum qualifications – list each of the criteria required to be eligible as a candidate.
4. Employer information – provide a brief synopsis of the organization or department as well as location and any salient facts about the employer. You may also want to consider providing access or links to community opportunities (i.e., chamber of commerce, local school districts, places of worship, etc.)
5. Contact information – provide detailed information on who to contact should there be any questions.
6. Application procedures – provide specific instructions on what is required for a complete application, who to send application materials to, and deadlines for submissions.

Employer: XYZ University
Job Title: Assistant Athletic Trainer

Reports To: Head Athletic Trainer.

Basic Duties: The assistant athletic trainer will be responsible to supervise two varsity sports, assigned by the head athletic trainer and assist in the day-to-day operations of the athletic training room. It is expected that the assistant athletic trainer have excellent interpersonal communication skills. Other duties will include, advising athletes on the proper use of equipment. Planning and implementing comprehensive athletic injury and illness prevention programs. Developing training programs and routines designed to improve athletic performance. Travel with athletic teams is expected. Instructing coaches, athletes, parents, medical personnel, and community members in the care and prevention of athletic injuries is also expected. Head athletic trainer will also consult with coaches in order to select appropriate protective equipment.

Minimum Qualifications: BOC-certified; state license or eligible, bachelor's degree in athletic training or related filed, master's degree preferred; Current first aid and CPR certification.

Knowledge, Skills and Abilities: As defined in the Board of Certification (BOC) role delineation study:

- Injury prevention
- Recognition, evaluation and assessment of injuries
- Immediate care
- Treatment, rehabilitation and reconditioning
- Organization and administration
- Professional development and responsibility

Figure 6-5 Sample job description

7. Special instructions – provide any special requirements, such as instructions for applicants with a disability.
8. Federal or state required disclaimers or notices – provide equal opportunity or affirmative action statement.

Figure 6-6 is a sample position notice similar to what might be posted on the NATA career center web site.

After the position notice is completed it is important to decide when and where to post it. Many athletic training jobs are posted on the NATA career center website. However, there is a fee associated with posting on this and other professional forums. Other options for advertising an athletic training position include organization, state or district web sites. Local or regional outlets such as newspapers or trade magazines are also an option, but these have limited drawing power due to limited

Position: Graduate Assistant Athletic Trainer/Intern
Category: College-Part-time/Graduate Assistant/Intern

Description:
XYZ University is seeking 1 position for a graduate assistant athletic trainer. XYZ University is a NCAA Division I school that offers healthcare to student-athletes on 12 intercollegiate sports teams. Primary responsibilities include, but are not limited to: serving as an assistant athletic trainer to football, practice and event coverage, travel, communication with supervising ATCs, Team Physicians, and coaches, and the prevention, rehabilitation, and care of athletic injuries. The position also requires applicant to maintain accurate and current medical records, supervision of student athletic trainers as well as any other duties assigned by the Head Athletic Trainer. The position is 22 months in length and would start June 1st.

Qualifications:
Requirements: State Licensure or Eligible, BOC Certified. Current CPR/AED certification, Bachelor's Degree in Athletic Training.

Location:
XYZ University
Sports Medicine
5555 Main Street
Anywhere, State 55555-555
Phone: 555-555-5555
Fax: 555-555-5555

Contact:
Mr. Athletic trainer
Email: ATC@XYX.edu

Application Procedure:
Please send a resume' and 3 references to Mr. Athletic trainer at XYZ University
Apply-By Date: position is open until filled
Starting Date: June 1, 2008

Figure 6-6 Sample position notice

TABLE 6-1 List of Places to Search for Athletic Training Jobs

Name of Organization	Contact Information
NATA Career Center	http://www.nata.org(membership required)
State or NATA District	Sites vary (for a list of district and state associations, visit http://www.nata.org)
Career City	http://www.truecareers.com
Career Path	http://www.careerpath.com
Career Web	http://www.careerweb.com
Career Builder	http://www.careerbuilder.com
USA Jobs	http://www.usajobs.opm.gov
Monster	http://www.monster.com
Chronicle of Higher Education	http://chronicle.com/jobs
NCAA News (the Market)	http://ncaa.thetask.com/market/jobs/browse.php
HigherEdJobs	http://higheredjobs.com

circulation. Table 6-1 is a list of internet sites that athletic trainers commonly search for available positions.

The recruiting process does not end once the position has been posted. Human resources and search committees must vigilantly review and critique applications, check references, set up and conduct phone interviews, and ultimately interview candidates. These activities can be very time consuming. Reducing a large applicant pool down to the three to five most qualified candidates is reasonably easy. However, deciding the top or even top two candidates from a pool of five is much more difficult. Coming to consensus as a search committee can be challenging. It is helpful for a search committee to have prepared in advance a list of qualifications and expectations for all candidates once formal reviews begin.

Human Resources Polices and Legislation

Human resources is responsible for writing and maintaining the policies and procedures that pertain to all employees throughout an organization. A policy is the formal statement needed to ensure a behavior or activity within an organization occurs. When used effectively, policies help focus attention and resources on actions that promote the organization's vision and values. Procedures are the operational processes required to implement an organization's policies. Procedures (or operating practices) can be formal or informal, specific to a department or applicable across the entire organization. Polices tend to address the "what" and "why" of operations and procedures typically address the "how," "when," and perhaps the "who" of carrying out those policies. Furthermore, polices tend to be more concrete and change less frequently than procedures. Lastly, polices are usually broad in application whereas a procedure is more detailed and specific. For example, it may be policy that every employee's performance must be evaluated annually. Specific procedures may be delineated that outline how and over what competencies each evaluation is to be completed, which may vary by department.

There is a social and ethical responsibility associated with writing polices and procedures, which includes not violating an individual's sense of community, implementing governmental requirements, not presuming moral obligations, and keeping the best interest of all parties without violating anyone's rights. Box 6-6 is a sample of some human resource policies. Also, it is important that polices be created that address legislation. For example, policies should address employees with disabilities, minimum wage, leave, and harassment.

> ### BOX 6-6 List of Sample Polices Often Written by Human Resources Managers
>
> 1. Absenteeism and Tardiness
> 2. Access to Personnel Records
> 3. Application for Internal Job Opportunities
> 4. Attendance Policies
> 5. Bereavement Leave
> 6. Benefits Roundup
> 7. Dress Code
> 8. Candidate Evaluation Form
> 9. Code of Ethics
> 10. Drug Testing/Screening Policy Development
> 11. Fair Labor Standards Act (FLSA)
> 12. Family and Medical Leave Act (FMLA)
> 13. Harassment Investigation Steps
> 14. Health Insurance Portability & Accountability Act (HIPAA)
> 15. I-9 Form: Employment Eligibility for Employers
> 16. Job Descriptions
> 17. No Smoking Policy
> 18. Maternity/Paternity/Adoption Leave
> 19. Open Door Policies
> 20. Personal Days
> 21. Personnel File Policy
> 22. Personnel File Access Policy
> 23. Professional Training/Continuing Education
> 24. Sexual Harassment Complaint: How to Address
> 25. Sick Leave

The Americans With Disabilities Act

The Americans with Disabilities Act of 1990 (ADA) was enacted to ensure that disabled persons would have equal access. The ADA is a civil rights law that prohibits, under certain circumstances, discrimination based on disability. Disability is defined as "a physical or mental impairment that substantially limits a major life activity." Human resources must have polices established that comply with ADA regulations. The ADA addresses four areas of compliance and miscellaneous issues.

1. Employment – prohibits denying disabled persons based on their disability employment or the rights and privileges of any employee once employed.
2. Public services – ensures that all public services (i.e., all governmental agencies or office, be they local, state, or federal) are accessible and that public transportation is accessible to all disabled persons.
3. Public accommodations – ensures that no individual is discriminated against on the basis of disability with regards to the full and equal enjoyment of the goods, services, facilities, or accommodations of any place of public accommodation. "Public accommodations" include most places of lodging (i.e., hotels), recreation, transportation, education, and dining, along with stores, care providers, and others.
4. Telecommunications – ensured that those who are deaf, hard of hearing, and/or speech-impaired have functionally equivalent services to telecommunications.

Family Medical Leave Act

The Family and Medical Leave Act of 1993 (FMLA) ensures that an employee can take unpaid leave due to a serious health condition that makes the employee unable to perform his or her job or to care for a sick family member or to care for a new child (by birth, adoption or foster care). FMLA ensures that all workers are able to take extended leaves without fear of being terminated from their jobs or from being forced into a lower job upon their return. Basically, employees are entitled up to 12 weeks of unpaid leave. An employer is not obligated to grant this extended leave until 12 months of employment have accrued.

Fair Labor Standards Act

The Fair Labor Standards Act of 1938 (FLSA) The FLSA established a national minimum wage, guaranteed time and a half for overtime in certain jobs, and prohibited child labor. The premise of the FLSA is fair compensation. However, most professional careers (such as athletic training) are exempt for this act. There are many exemptions an employer can claim that will not require them to satisfy minimum wage, overtime, or record-keeping requirements. The most notable exception is the "white collar" exemption. The exemption is applicable to professional, administrative, and executive employees. Athletic trainers are exempt from this Act and employers of athletic trainers are not required to pay minimum wage nor are they required to pay overtime. However, athletic trainers can approach employers or state legislators about these issues if there are unfair practices, which can be evaluated on a case-by-case basis.

Affirmative Action

Affirmative action refers to enacting policies and procedures intended to provide minorities with additional access to education or employment. Affirmative action occurs whenever an organization devotes resources to making sure that people are not discriminated against on the basis of their gender or their ethnic group.[4] Ultimately affirmative action is about increasing diversity. Opponents of affirmative action argue that it is another form of discrimination, by citing that a qualified applicant is denied entry to higher education or employment because they belong to a majority group. Obviously there is much controversy over affirmative action policies; human resources should have a prepared statement concerning affirmative action practices.

Sexual Harassment

Sexual harassment should be a concern for athletic trainers.[10] The Equal Employment Opportunity Commission (EEOC)[5] has defined sexual harassment as "unwelcome sexual advances, requests for sexual favors, and other verbal or physical conduct of a sexual nature." Sexual harassment policies should be disseminated to all employees and not just to those is supervisory positions.[10] Athletic trainers should be aware of the sexual harassment policy within their organization or department. Athletic trainers should work closely with HR to see that their athletic training rooms or clinical settings comply with sexual harassment laws.[10]

Equal Opportunity Employment

Equal Opportunity Employment (EOE) was created to prohibit federal contractors from discriminating against employees on the basis of race, sex, creed, religion, color, or national origin. Equal opportunity is very similar to affirmative action. They differ in that EOE seeks to ensure that discrimination will not be tolerated once it is detected, whereas, affirmative action, is proactive and seeks to actively recruit minorities.

Employee Retention and Promotion

Another aspect of HR is the retention of employees. Retention includes such things as evaluating, motivating, improving morale, and training and development. "Improving employee retention can result in a number of positive outcomes for an organization. Productivity and quality of work should be higher because experienced employees know their jobs well and require less training and development."[1] HR managers should be adept at assessing the morale of employees and keeping them motivated. By keeping morale high, retention efforts are much easier.

However, skilled employees are presumably going to be in high demand and despite all efforts there are still those who leave for "greener pastures." Employee turnover is not always because of organizational factors, there are a myriad of personal reasons for turnover, which the HR manager has no control over. For example, an employee may leave because they have to care for a sick family member; cost of living is too high in one locale, or issues with children. No one can foresee every reason, but there are strategies to reduce employee turnover.

High employee turnover has a negative impact of performance and lowers morale.[1] Nearly 50% of employees who plan to leave their current job do so because they perceive their skills and abilities are not being utilized, compared to 25% who plan to leave because salary is too low.[6] The implication of this is that utilizing an employee's skills is a greater factor in retaining that employee than paying them a larger salary. There are strategies for increasing retention, which include:

1. Careful employee selection – make sure there is a good match, not only of professional competency and KSAs, but also of values and vision.

2. Encourage and foster use of expertise – many employees have similar competencies, but each has different interests and passions that shape how they use or define those competencies. Create an environment that allows employees to put their expertise into action.

3. Offer professional training and development – be sure to offer employees a chance to learn and grow. Offering opportunities for personal development (in addition to professional development) is equally as important.

4. Offer attainable chances for promotion – make sure opportunities and expectations for promotion are clearly delineated.

5. Adequate compensation – salary, benefits, and time off must be competitive with similar size organizations in a specific locale. This includes offering benefits and vacations that consider employee's families and dependents.

6. An early opportunity to contribute – provide employees with opportunities to share ideas, innovate, and contribute creatively. Take the ideas generated by employees seriously!

7. Foster friendships – provide opportunities for employees to socialize with each other.

8. Recognize success – be sure to thank employees (publicly and privately) for a job well done, for new ideas, or for anything that contributes to the success of the organization's, department's, or team's goals or for upholding core values.

9. Conduct exit interviews – no matter how great an organization, employees will leave. Some have good reasons to leave others do not, both hurt. Regardless of the reason an employee leaves, be sure to conduct an exit interview.

Training and Development

Training and development takes on many forms. Early training and development will foster employee buy-in and sense of ownership. The most common forms of early training and development are employee orientations and in-services. Other types of training include times for specialized development and continuing education. An important aspect of professional responsibility for the athletic trainer is to stay abreast of new knowledge and relevant legislation.

Training and development can be invaluable to promoting an organization's mission, vision, and values and for creating a viable and stable work force. Orientations are usually an athletic trainer's first real encounter with the organization's or department's culture. A well-planned orientation serves to motivate employees and get them off on the proverbial "right foot." Orientations serve as the time to review pertinent policies and familiarize employees, co-workers, and other supervisors on the facility and existing or new procedures.

In-services or competency development is another form of training and development. Competency development can also help to serve personal and professional development needs. For example, during a performance evaluation competency or proficiency in a specific athletic training skill is noted by an employer or perceived by the employee to be weak, such as post-op shoulder rehab. Therefore, the employee is sent to a conference or seminar on that specific topic in order to improve core knowledge or review relevant skills. Continuing education can be used in the same vein. Continuing education is an important aspect of professional responsibility and development and will be addressed in more detail in a later chapter. Regardless of whether the opportunity is an orientation, in-service or seminar, human resources should provide opportunities for athletic trainers to gain new knowledge that is relevant to their personal and career goals.

Employee Evaluations

Another important aspect of employee retention and promotion are evaluations. Evaluating employees occurs throughout the employee's life-cycle within an organization. Performance evaluations typically occur on an annual basis and are based on the employee's job responsibilities or professional job analysis, such as the Board of Certification's Role Delineation Study for athletic trainers. Evaluations are designed to provide constructive feedback as to whether an employee is doing their job and to what level they are performing. Typically, employee performance is ranked based on some matrix or rubric that gives a point total. That number is then used to justify any merit raise or increase in benefits and is used to set goals for the upcoming year. Early in an employee's tenure, reviews may be more frequent. An example is that some employees must clear a probationary period (typically 90 days) before they are allowed to collect health benefits or other perks.

Performance evaluations, if used creatively, can be used as a tool to increase organizational effectiveness as well. Evaluations should be approached by both parties (i.e., the evaluator[s] and the employee) as a chance to learn something. Performance evaluations should be relevant, free of bias, and based on objective and quantifiable facts. However, it is important to include some level of subjective information. The performance evaluation should not be the first time an employee hears or realizes he or she is performing poorly or well. It is merely the time when things are formally recognized and recorded. Evaluations should provide a positive experience for the employee and result in an opportunity to improve. A well thought-out evaluation considers the future plans of the organization or department. Finally, performance evaluations should be organized and conducted in a formal environment.

A well-planned evaluation begins well before the formal evaluation and should include input form multiple sources. A very valuable technique is having perform-

Leadership Application

As the first and only athletic trainer at a small university with limited funding, it becomes obvious that there is a need for an additional athletic trainer. Coaches are complaining about the available coverage. Furthermore, traveling with teams is restricted because when one team is away another has a home event or practice. In your opinion the needs of the coaches and athletes are not being adequately met. Furthermore, you are feeling pressure to continually put in additional time to cover all the events. The athletic director is sympathetic, but claims his hands are "tied." When questioned about it, his response always seems to be one of two responses. One, you knew the workload would be high when you were hired or, the overtime you are asked to do is more than compensated for because you are allowed the summer months (June and July) off.

Critical Thinking Questions

1. What could have been done differently during the interview and hiring process to let you know more about the job expectations?
2. What type of organizational culture might you guess this university is?
3. What are some strategies you might implement to help the coaches and athletes understand your dilemma?
4. How might you justify to the administration the need for additional athletic trainers?

ance appraised from four different perspectives. Some might call this or similar versions 360-degree feedback. The four perspectives are intended to yield appraisals from everyone "surrounding the employee" (i.e., 360°). The first perspective is the employees. Employees should be given the chance to evaluate themselves independent from their supervisor and given a chance to justify their self-appraisal. The second perspective is based on the appraisal and feedback of their supervisor. Obviously, the supervisor provides input into the evaluation process and should justify comments and ratings on specific performance events that can be cited and not conjecture or hearsay. The last two perspectives should be anonymous and serve as guidance to the supervisor's evaluation. It should also be allowed to be reviewed in its entirety by the employee being evaluated. The last two perspectives are a peer-based review and subordinate or patient review. A peer or peers can be asked to submit an anonymous critique of a co-worker. The format of the peer-review is more subjective and not as detailed as a self or supervisor's review and should not carry much weight in the overall evaluation process. However, it is valuable source of information. Finally, subordinates or patients can also be asked to evaluate an employee. Again, these last two perspectives are anonymous and primarily subjective.

Ultimately, the evaluation process should benefit the employee by giving specific and measurable objectives for the upcoming year. It should also be a time of reflection and a time to implement needed change for the employee, the supervisor, and perhaps the organization. Some of the information gathered form annual reviews can be very useful to strategic planning. A well-planned and executed performance evaluation can boost morale and ultimately aid in employee retention.

CHAPTER SUMMARY

Human resources is a central aspect of any organization or department. Athletic trainers will often be required to perform many HR-based functions. Knowing how to approach HR and what to expect of HR will help the transition into new jobs and help facilitate long-term employment. Understanding the job search timeline, what is required, and how to prepare complete and accurate application information can go a long way in making the job search and selection process pleasant and exciting.

References

1. Arnold E. (2005). Managing human resources to improve employee retention. *The Health Care Manage 24*(2):132–140.

2. Berthoin A, Dierkes, M. Hahner, K. (1997). Business perception of contextual changes: sources and impediments to organizational learning. *Business and Society 36*(4):387–407.

3. Caccia-Bava M, Guimaraes T, Harrington S. (2006). Hospital organization culture, capacity to innovate and success in technology adoption. *Journal of Health Organization and Management 20*(3):194–217.

4. Crosby FJ, Iyer A, Sincharoen S. (2006). Understanding affirmative action. *Annual Review of Psychology 57*:585–611.

5. Equal Employment Opportunity Commission. (1980). *Title VII guidelines on sexual harassment.* Washington, DC: U.S. Government Printing Office 189–191.

6. Gering J, Conner J. (2002). A strategic approach to employee retention. *Journal of The Healthcare Financial Management Association 56*(11):40–44.

7. Kahanov L, Andrews L. (2001). A survey of athletic training employers' hiring criteria. *Journal of Athletic Training 36*(4):408–412.

8. Mathis R, Jackson J. (2008). *Human resource management.* Mason, OH: Thompson.

9. Pfeffer J. (1998). *The human equation: Building profits by putting people first.* Boston: Harvard Business School.

10. Velasquez BJ. (1998). Sexual harassment: A concern for the athletic trainer. *JAT 33*(2):171–176.

11. Waters VL. (2004). Cultivate corporate culture and diversity. *Nursing Management 35*(1):36–38.

12. Yukl GA. (2002). Leadership in organizations. Englewood Cliffs, NJ: Prentice-Hall.

Information, Fiscal, and Risk Management

Chapter 7

Managing Technology

"The first rule of any technology … is that automation applied to an efficient operation will magnify the efficiency."

BILL GATES

Key Terms

Asynchronous: Not occurring at the same time; in this case, in reference to electronic communications.

Bandwidth: The rate or speed of data transfer; often used synonymously with data transfer rate.

Central processing unit (CPU): The part of a computer that includes the circuits controlling the processing and execution of instructions.

Computer network: Two or more computers connected together using a telecommunication or wireless system for communicating and sharing resources.

Computer technology: The application of computers for manipulation and management of information or data.

Computer virus: A program introduced from an external source that replicates within a computer's system and can render it useless and can destroy data files.

Cyberspace: The virtual world accessible via the Internet.

Data mining: The process of examining a large pool of information and summarizing it into more useful information.

Download: The transfer of data from an external source unit (i.e., server, network, internet, or software program) to a personal unit (i.e., personal computer).

Firewall: A software program that inspects and regulates the traffic into a network and either allows files to pass through or restricts access based on predefined rules.

The Health Insurance Portability and Accountability Act (HIPAA): A law enacted by the U.S. Congress in 1996 that ensures health care coverage for employees who change or lose their jobs and ensures confidentiality and that minimum technical standards of those records are met as they are transferred.

Innovation: Implementation of a brand new idea or a different application of an existing product or idea.

Intranet: A private computer network used to foster communication and data sharing within an organization.

Netiquette: Network etiquette; acceptable behaviors for electronic communications.

Random access memory (RAM): The physical memory used to store data while a computer is operating. More RAM will normally contribute to a faster PC.

Spam: unsolicited junk e-mail or other electronically transmitted propaganda.

Technology: The beneficial application of scientific advances or discoveries.

Universal serial bus (USB): A computer port that is compatible with many devices.

Upload: The transfer of data from a smaller unit (i.e., PC) to a larger unit (i.e., server or network).

---

*A*thletic trainers use technology every day. **Technology** *is the beneficial application of scientific advances or discoveries. Therefore, anything people make can be considered technology. However, the concept of technology usually is applied in the context of putting new knowledge to a practical use. For example, in athletic training this includes the application of the electromagnetic spectrum as therapeutic modalities. Technology is revolutionizing the way health professionals manage information and medical resources.[3] Using technology appropriately is an essential competency for all health care professionals in today's health care context.* **Computer technology** *is the application of computers for manipulation and management of information or data. If used to its full potential, incorporating technology into athletic training leadership roles and management functions greatly enhances the efficiency and impact of athletic trainers.*

In this chapter we will consider uses for technology followed by uses for computers, along with the implications of hardware and software. Our treatment of software will cover commercialized injury tracking programs, which have special significance to athletic training. Next, we will discuss computer networks and how they can enhance the athletic trainer's function within an organization, department, or as part of a team. Finally, we will examine information management, considering electronic documentation.

USES AND NEED OF TECHNOLOGY

Change is facilitated by advances in technology.[1] Arguably nothing has caused more societal change than innovations in technology. As technology is introduced, it is expected that the delivery of health care will keep up with technological advancements. **Innovation** is the implementation of a brand new idea or a different application of an existing product or idea. The concept of technology in athletic training should go beyond computer literacy and include experimenting with new uses for existing data storage and retrieval devices and taking full advantage of different communication systems. Athletic trainers need to be technologically savvy. Technology is changing and advancing so quickly that it requires an intentional effort to recognize how it can best be used to facilitate the values and goals of an organization and promote the profession.

In today's global context, technological literacy has been equated to being bilingual.[1] Technology is rapidly becoming a major component of knowledge acquisition and dissemination. In other words, technology is becoming a central vehicle to education. To maximize the impact of technology, the athletic trainer needs to implement innovation, rational thinking, and business savvy. Although not all are covered in this text, there are many applications for technology, including medical record keeping, database searches, data collection and analysis, e-mail, smart modalities, web-casting, *e*-learning, and pod-casting. These applications of technology can influence athletic training.

COMPUTER TECHNOLOGY

The personal computer (PC) was first introduced with the advent of microprocessors in the early 1970s. Early on, PCs were costly and were a luxury with an uncertain future. Today the PC is essential for conducting day-to-day business in any organization. Computers are an important tool and athletic trainers need to understand the scope of its uses. Computers are used for multiple applications, such as generating records, storing files, word processing, communicating, data mining, tracking inventory, creating graphics, marketing, and educating and training. **Data mining** is the process of examining a large pool of information from a diversity of sources and summarizing it into more useful information. In short, data mining is involves sorting through large amounts of information and picking out what is relevant.

Before purchasing a computer, it is important to be aware of technology needs. Computers come with a variety of customizations and a needs analysis should be conducted before purchasing a computer. A basic needs analysis for purchasing a computer includes answering the following questions:

1. What will the computer be used for?
2. How often will the computer be accessed?
3. Who will have access to the computer?
4. Where will the computer be located?
5. How much information will be stored on the computer?
6. Who will provide technical support for the computer?

Answering these questions will help determine how to manage security issues, assess space allocation of hardware, and decide which software to purchase.

Security

Security is a major issue with the use of computers. Using computers to their full potential typically requires having access to the Internet and therefore be linked to cyberspace. **Cyberspace** is the virtual area beyond one's personal computer that can be accessed by anyone. This poses a serious security risk. Furthermore, when entering patient data into a computer program (either to downloaded software on a specific PC or uploading it to a web-based Internet site), there is significant risk that the data may be intercepted. Keeping patient data and organizational communications secure must be a major priority for the athletic trainer.

Keeping data secure and computers functioning efficiently involves a few practical steps. Incorporating passwords onto each computer is a critical aspect to security. Make sure that every computer is password protected. This will ensure that only those people with the password can access the data files on that specific computer. It is good idea to change passwords regularly, which also helps in another aspect of security, managing computer access. Passwords should be easy to remember and difficult to guess. It is unwise to use personal information such as pets', spouses', or children's names, Social Security numbers, or birth dates as passwords. Passwords should be case sensitive and include numbers and letters. After implementing passwords, physical access needs to be managed.

Managing computer access involves keeping common computers in an area of high visibility, but in a secure space. For example, computers used to input patient data, injury information, or treatment logs should be kept in the athletic training room where they can be locked when an athletic trainer is not present. Keeping computers in the athletic training room will also help to ensure only staff and athletic training students have access. This will allow use on the computer to be monitored, curtailing inappropriate use or access.

Computers used to input injury and patient data should not be accessible to the general population and unless it is someone's personal computer should not be used by others for personal reasons, such as e-mailing, surfing the Internet, or gaming. If possible, having one specific computer designated solely for data entry and injury tracking is preferable. This allows for staff member's computers to remain private.

Other security risks involving computers include viruses and hackers. Ways to protect computers form outside hackers or Spam include anti-virus software and **firewalls**. Anti-virus software can be purchased or downloaded onto specific computers. Ant-ivirus software routinely scans files to identify and eliminate **computer viruses**. A computer virus is a "bug" (i.e., program) introduced from an external source that replicates within a system and can render a computer useless and often can destroy data files. A firewall inspects and regulates the traffic into a network and either allows files to pass through or restricts access based on predefined rules. Frequently firewalls are used to intercept Spam. **Spam** is unsolicited junk e-mail or other electronically transmitted propaganda. Taking the necessary precautions to protect the medical and organizational information stored on computers by using passwords and firewalls and monitoring access are critical steps to gaining the trust of patients and using technology responsibly.

Hardware

Computer hardware consists of the physical equipment of the computer, such as the **central processing unit** (CPU), digital circuitry, the monitor, speakers, keyboard, and output devices such as printers and scanners. The CPU is the part of a computer that includes the circuits controlling the processing and execution of instructions. The efficiency of a computer's CPU is based on available RAM. **Random access memory (RAM)** is the physical memory used to store data while a computer is operating, so the computer does not have to take the time to access the hard drive to find the file(s) it requires. More RAM will normally contribute to a faster PC. Other devices that may influence hardware or software uses include:

1. **Universal serial bus (USB)**, which is a connection port on a computer that is universally compatible with many devices, such as, printers, speakers, or scanners.
2. Video and sound cards.
3. Some type of removable media writer (or drives) such as CD/CD-ROM drive, CD writer, DVD/DVD-ROM drive, DVD writer, floppy disk, or tape drive (used for backup).
4. Network card used for DSL/cable Internet, and/or connecting to other computers.

A USB thumb drive (flash drive or jump drive) is an external storage device that fits into the USB port on a computer. Thumb drives are capable of storing large data files and are easily transferable between PCs (Fig. 7-1). It is important to determine if the software that is desired can be used in conjunction with the available hardware (i.e., sound or video cards). For example, if the desired software (i.e., injury management program) or external devices (i.e., printer or scanner) requires too much RAM, does not have a suitable video card, or does not have a USB port, the current computer may not be able to support the needs of the athletic trainer.

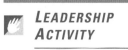

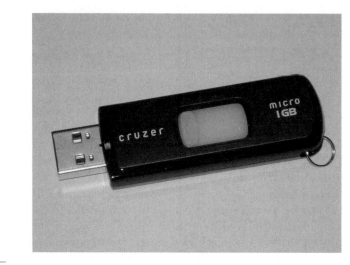

FIGURE 7-1 Thumb (or flash) drive for a USB port.

Software

Software, sometimes called programs, is an application that can be **downloaded** or **uploaded** onto computers that permits the computer to perform specific tasks. Downloading is the installation of external software or file into a computer. Downloading is typically from a larger unit or server to a smaller unit (i.e., PC). Uploading is the transfer of data from a smaller unit (i.e., PC) to a larger unit (i.e., server or network). Examples of software include operating systems such as Microsoft Windows® or Mac OS®. Software also includes applications such as a word processor, spreadsheets, databases, or web browsers. Important things to consider when purchasing software are:

1. expense
2. technical support
3. training to use the software
4. how often the software requires an upgrade.

Software should be selected that has a wide appeal. For example, selecting software that is highly specialized or unique can have a negative influence on ease of employee transitions or hiring if in-depth technical training is required.

Sports Injury Tracking Software

There are several commercially available software programs for tracking and monitoring injuries. Many of these injury tracking programs are either hosted on an external website where a membership or access fee is required and data is uploaded to the host, or it can be purchased as downloadable software and installed on specific PCs. Many of these programs are very versatile and offer the athletic trainer options to create team or individual injury reports, compare injury trends across seasons, years, or teams, quantify treatment efficiency, and an overall easier way to manage records.

There are pros and cons to using computer-based injury tracking programs. Some of the drawbacks include time-intensive data entry. It often requires a significant amount of time at the initial onset to code in all the necessary patient or team information. Other risks of using injury-tracking software are common to computers. There are risks of network failures or viruses contaminating or destroying records. There is also risk of document exposure. Athletic trainers must be vigilant to keep

---

✎ From the Field

As faculty member in a small university Athletic Training Education Program (ATEP), I worked closely with the head athletic trainer in the clinical context. As I spent more time in the athletic training room, I discovered that we needed to better integrate technology into education. Part of the decision to remedy this included purchasing standard injury-tracking software.

Upon trying to implement this software, several road blocks occurred. First, there were licensing issues, which needed to be settled by our IT department. Settling the licensing issue required several days of meetings and e-mails. Questions needed to be answered, such as, how many computers need a license, are they network or non-network computers, if network can all computers campus-wide have access to the software, how do we safeguard the data once coded or entered, if students have access are there state or federal regulations that govern the data and its access and dissemination? Once these issues were satisfactorily resolved, a requisition for a "public" use computer in the athletic training room (an individual campus policy) needed to be filed. Up to this point, the only computer in the athletic training room was the one in the head athletic trainer's office. Once we received approval to have a special computer for AT students only, we had to determine range of use. For example, to save money and because we intended to only use it for data entry, the IT department wanted to give us a very old computer. However, the "old" computer was not able to support the "newer" software. After successfully arguing for a new computer (which required several more weeks of meetings and emails), the new injury tracking software is now working and students are learning to enter data and query results successfully.

Not long after this, our head athletic trainer resigned to pursue other interests. The new head athletic trainer arrived and soon discovered that he did not like the injury tracking software we recently installed. He quickly uninstalled the new software, citing that he did not like it, did not know how to use it, and the format and data entry screens made no sense to him. This action confused the athletic training students who were just getting familiar and comfortable with that software.

The head athletic trainer proceeded to requisition new injury tracking software. The request for new software did not get approved (on the grounds the AD just bought new software for the same reason). In response, the head athletic trainer commissioned a friend who was somewhat of a competent computer programmer to create an injury tracking program that he liked and was unique to his style. After a few weeks the new software arrived and all the students were retrained on this new software. After a few weeks with the new software, a similar situation occurred, and this "new" head athletic trainer left the university for a different position. This left the university, students, and staff with specialized software and no technical support.

---

data and medical records confidential. This includes monitoring printed documents or reports. Be sure to retrieve printed documents with any kind of patient information or names from the printer immediately, especially if using a public or network printer.

Another drawback is the perception that these programs may not always seem time effective. Many athletic trainers record injury data or SOAP notes on paper or a pre-made form and place it in a physical file to be retrieved and referenced later. Taking the time to enter the data after it has been collected on the paper form may seem to be recording the same injury data twice. However, paper-only systems are not conducive to generating the many reports that are extremely beneficial to the athletic trainer.

In light of these drawbacks, there are some significant advantages to using computer-based injury-tracking software. The main benefit is generating useful reports. Most injury-tracking software includes features that allow the athletic trainer to create reports and sort or filter data to specific conditions. For example, a common feature in many applications is the option to easily generate customized reports. Reports can be used to identify statistics of certain athletes, specific injuries, or teams. Injury or illness trends can be identified, which ultimately can help shape prevention and risk management plans. This type of software can also track referrals, which can be used to calculate revenue generated to outside providers. Many of these programs can be integrated with a personal digital assistant (PDA) or laptop so data can be entered from remote locations. Some common injury-tracking software available includes:

1. Sportsware™
2. Simtrak®
3. Safety Software® (OSHALOG® 300)
4. injuryTRACKER (Presagia, Corp.)
5. Assistantcoach.net

The programs listed above only represent a selected sample of what is available. Each has its own features that may appeal to different athletic trainers based on specific needs or context. Before purchasing this type of software, know what information and reports you need to produce. Some of these programs listed are designed (or customizable) specifically for athletic trainers, others are designed for occupational settings. Some can be purchased and downloaded from the Internet and others are hosted on websites or servers. Part of managing well includes being a wise consumer. Before purchasing injury tracking software get feedback from other athletic trainers on the products you are considering (Figures 7-2 and 7-3).

NETWORKS

A **computer network** is at least two computers connected together using a telecommunication or wireless system for the purpose of communicating and sharing resources.[2] A computer connected to an external device (i.e., a printer) may also represent a computer network. There are several types of networks as well as several kinds of servers. Servers, as the name implies, allows connections to other network users. For example, mail servers facilitate the sharing of information via e-mail. The most common type of network is a Local Area Network (LAN). LAN is limited to a relatively small spatial area such as a room or a single building. Networks are important in athletic training so that communication (i.e., e-mail), data output (i.e., printing), intranet, and other essential tasks can occur. The use of networks also allows teams a cost-effective means to share equipment. For example, having one network printer to which everyone can print may be more cost effective than purchasing desktop printers for every employee.

Electronic Communications

Networks are an important tool in communications. Without networks, functions such as printing, e-mailing, and web-browsing could not occur. These functions are an important piece of modern global communication and are an important aspect of organizational communications.

Intranet

The **intranet** is an organization's private "Internet." It requires network connectivity and is almost identical to the internet with the expectation that it is confined to a single network. Intranet is a powerful communication tool and information sharing

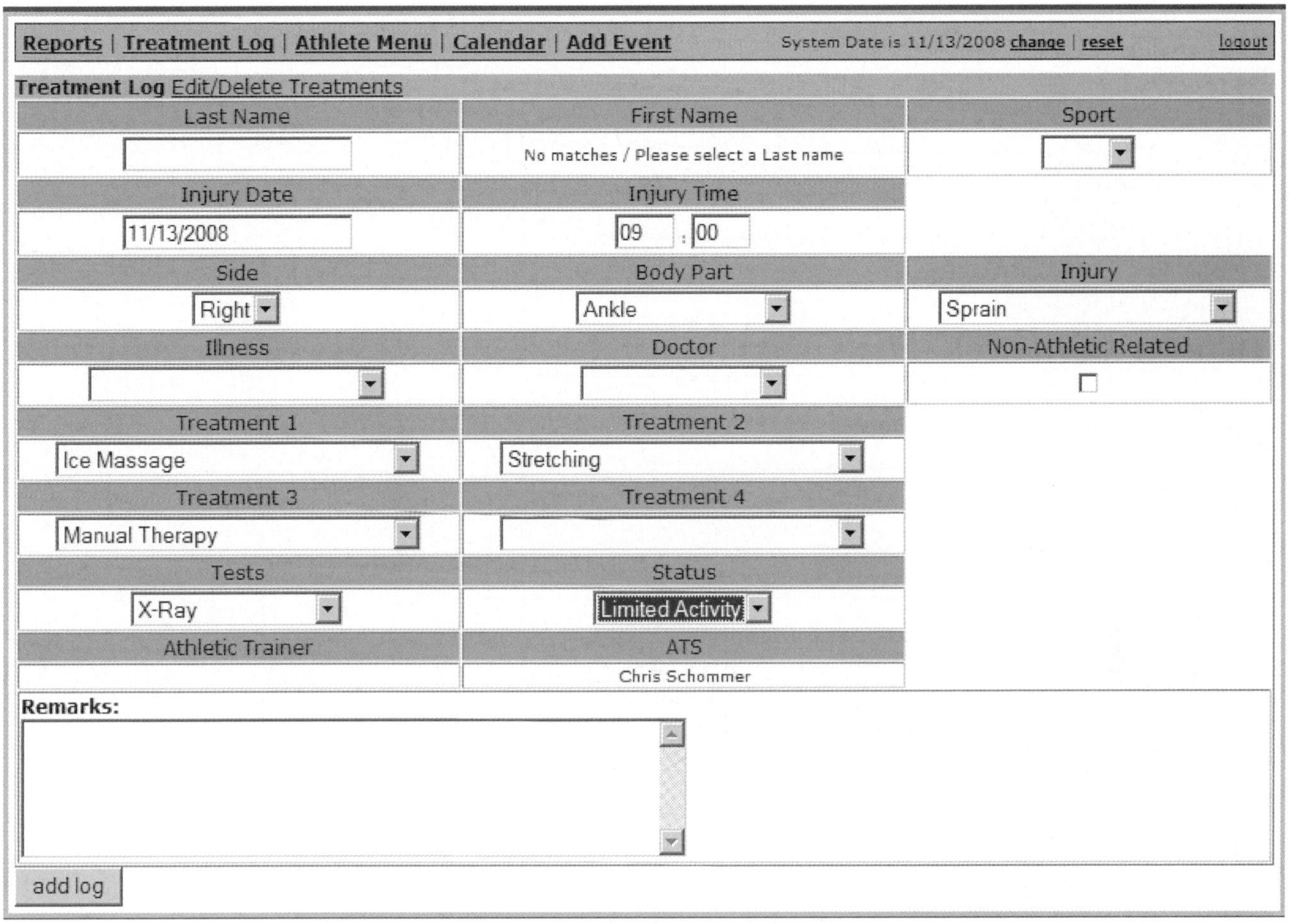

FIGURE 7-2 **Injury report entry form.** Courtesy of Shamrock Net Design, http://www.shamrocknd.com.

system. For example, Ford Motor Company has more than 175,000 employees in 950 global locations, each having access to the company's intranet. This gives employees up-to-date information about benefits, demographics, salary history, general company news, and human resources forms. Many organizations that employ athletic trainers, such as hospitals or universities, also make use of intranet services. The athletic trainer can use their intranet to maximize time, for communication within the organization, to access policies and procedures, forms and documents for record keeping and data gathering, as well as generating and submitting internal reports.

E-mail Netiquette

Electronic mail (e-mail) is a great way to maintain individual, organizational, and global communication. Obviously, leaders need to use e-mail appropriately, if used appropriately it can be an excellent tool for communicating. However, e-mail should not be used as a replacement of face-to-face conversation. A large portion of face-to-face or verbal communications involves the use of body language, gestures, and tone of voice, which can be lost in an e-mail. Care should be taken to craft an e-mail message that is not misconstrued or misunderstood.

Netiquette (network etiquette) is a term applied to the proper and correct use of e-mail and is a set of rules for behaving properly online (Box 7-1).[5] Being mindful that the people you are e-mailing are actual people, will also foster netiquette. For example, typing an e-mail in ALL CAPS signifies shouting or raising your voice.

| Reports | Treatment Log | Athlete Menu | Calendar | Add Event | System Date is 11/13/2008 change | reset | logout |

Current Data Reports

First Name	
Last Name	
Sport	MSC ▾
Athletic Trainer	▾
Date From	
Date to	
RLB	Left ▾
Body Part	Ankle ▾
Injury	Sprain ▾
Non-Athletic Related	☐
Treatment 1	Ice Pack ▾
Treatment 2	Stretching ▾
Treatment 3	Manual Therapy ▾
Illness	▾
Tests	X-Ray ▾
Status	Limited Activity ▾
Doctor	
Remarks	
	Search

FIGURE 7-3 Daily treatment log. Courtesy of Shamrock Net Design, http://www.shamrocknd.com.

Newsgroups and list-serves are examples of other network communication formats that have unique rules. For example, posting to a list-serve (such as the athletic training educators list-serve) has specific rules to posting topics and has an administrator to help impose those rules. One example, of netiquette for list-serve participants is to not resurrect old topics that have been closed, especially if nothing new

---

BOX 7-1 Basic Netiquette Tips

- Use the subject line, do not leave it blank.
- Replying to pertinent recipients only; if there is a large distribution list with an e-mail, do not automatically "reply to all."
- Business e-mail accounts should rarely be used for personal correspondence.
- Be aware that many e-mail accounts are set up for official company communications and are often monitored.
- Abbreviations (i.e., text messaging format) should only be used in personal communications.
- E-mails in all capital letters signify yelling at the recipient.
- Do not send large data files or attachments that require a lot of memory.

can be contributed. Furthermore, it is important to stick within the topic being discussed, if a new issue arises, start another post or thread to address the new issue.

The core rules of netiquette are[5]:

1. Remember the human: if you would not say it directly to the person's face, do not write it.
2. Adhere to the same standards of behavior that you follow in real life. Because you cannot physically see the other person, does not mean they are less human or less worthy of respect.
3. Know where you are in cyberspace, each domain has its own set of netiquette rules. Do not just enter into a domain chat, post, or thread without knowing the purpose and intent of the hosts.
4. Respect other people's time and **bandwidth** (rate or speed of data transfer), do not send large attachments, forwards, and files unless they are requested.
5. Be forgiving of other people's mistakes.

ELECTRONIC INFORMATION MANAGEMENT

Information management (IM) has been described as getting the right information to the right person at the right place at the right time. Information management is a valve phenomenon, meaning there is input and output. Managing the incoming information (input) as well as the outgoing data (output) requires time and purposeful managing. Figure 7-4 is a schematic representation of information that goes through an athletic trainer before sufficient outcomes can be implemented.

Information management is rapidly becoming an issue of technology. However, managing some information can still be done with hard-copy, pen and paper methods. For example, smaller athletic training programs with limited resources and space may still prefer to do their bookkeeping and inventory with a handwritten ledger. Several reasons for this exist including fear of losing information, lack of resources, lack of technical knowledge, or fear of becoming over dependent on computers. In athletic training, it might not be uncommon to still keep daily treatment logs on a sign in sheet where the athletic trainer reports the injury and treatment on a check-sheet system, which may be coded into a computer at a later or more convenient time.

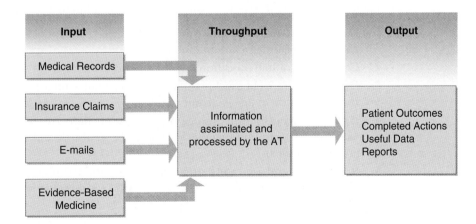

FIGURE 7-4 Information management in athletic training.

However, competent health care professionals will integrate and utilize technology in daily operations and patient care or risk becoming obsolete. Furthermore, there are several athletic training stakeholders (i.e., physician offices, clinical sites, insurance companies, etc.) who use technology in their day-to-day operations. In order to maintain the relationships, it is important to use technology that is equitable to athletic training's stakeholder groups. Pen-and-paper injury documentation, evaluations, treatment logs, progress (SOAP) notes, and reports perhaps meet minimum standards of care, but may not be adequate in our technology-rich health care industry.

In spite of all the actual and perceived benefits of electronic documentation, there are also emerging issues that need to be addressed. With the advent of a technology-savvy culture comes new risks. In recent years the increase of identity theft has been cause for alarm concerning management of records, especially those records that are digital. For example, use of an individual's Social Security number (SSN) as an identifier has been widely used in health care. New forms of identification and adherence to HIPAA regulations can help limit identity theft and make transitions to electronic records more manageable. HIPAA is the **Health Insurance Portability and Accountability Act** enacted by the U.S. Congress in 1996. This act ensures health care coverage for employees who change or lose their jobs and ensures confidentiality and that minimum technical standards of those records are met as they are transferred.

Other aspects of electronic data include retrieving information. Evidence-based medicine is one practice that has benefited from the proliferation of technology and electronic communication. For example, paper journals, that once could only be accessed form libraries (or if you had a subscription) are now far more accessible. The accessibility to scientific, peer-reviewed data makes quality of care and evidence-based practice easier to implement. Furthermore, the dissemination of knowledge, acquiring continuing education, and formation of **asynchronous** groups via technology makes professional responsibilities easier as well. Asynchronous communications are those that do not occur at the same time. This enables team members to not have to adjust schedules to accommodate everyone.

Transitioning to Digital Records

Digital or electronic record keeping is the process of storing, for retrieval purposes, medical or program administration documents. Digital records allow for ease of production, sharing, and transmission. However, transitioning from a pen-and-paper system to paperless is an involved process. Moving to a paperless system can be very challenging. The American Health Information Management Association (AHIMA) has identified several steps to ensure a smooth transition to a paperless office:

1. Ensure buy-in from all employees on the merits of a paperless (all electronic) record keeping and documentation.
2. Consider a gradual transition.
3. Develop a comprehensive plan of actions and milestones for each step involved in the transition to an electronic system.
4. During the transition, consider developing an index or matrix that describes where and how to find specific documents (e.g., history and physical exam forms and SOAP notes).
5. Research federal, state, and organizational standards and regulations (including HIPAA, Accreditation standards (e.g., CARF), and regulations regarding retention of records and electronic signatures).
6. Consider confidentiality issues (HIPAA compliance, access, transferring data, i.e., can it be attached as an e-mail)

Once records and forms are digital and no longer also kept on paper, managing that system requires a unique perspective and dedication. Managing electronic records requires decision making and planning throughout the entire life cycle of the electronic record—from planning, creation, processing, distribution, maintenance, storage, and retrieval to its ultimate end (i.e., archival or destruction).

Managing Patient Information

Using technology becomes important for managing patient information because of the sheer volume and complex nature of documentation, filing, and reporting. Effective use of technology in managing information can help to satisfy legal requirements, professional standards, insurance requirements, and helps facilitate information sharing between professional colleagues concerning common patients. These records can be requested by third-party payers in order to evaluate a claim, can be used in legal proceedings to determine if standards of care were satisfied, or to help fellow health care professional's clinical decision making, if called upon to consult on patient care. Computer technology, e-mail, intranet, and the Internet can be great resources for athletic trainers in regards to information management.

Electronic Documents

Technology is a tool used to generate multiple reports to assist the athletic trainer in disseminating information.[4] Such reports include injury rates and statistics, medical histories, rehabilitation reports, physical exam results, treatment logs/records, and progress notes. Each of these (and other) reports can be generated with computers and made easier by using athletic injury software. Furthermore, disseminating reports can also be done electronically, which can facilitate groups that might not ordinarily be able to meet face-to-face or increase number of group interactions. For example, electronic reports can be generated and disseminated from remote locations, when a meeting is not possible or for a group that normally only can meet once a month, can now have asynchronous weekly meetings via e-mails, discussion threads, or newsgroups.

Furthermore, these types of systems can supplement hard-copy interoffice memorandums (and other hard-copy reports), which limits two-way interaction. Use of electronic media to deliver reports or memos, creates an opportunity for enhanced communication.[1] For example, a hard copy memo distributed via interoffice mail to 20 employees does not afford the recipient a chance to respond or rebut. However, electronic distribution of a memo facilitates communication, by allowing opportunity for recipients to respond (anonymously if desired), which fosters two-way communication.

THE FRONTIER

Paperless administration and record keeping is now a real possibility. With the capabilities of digital photos and communications, archiving, and retrieval, the future of record keeping is here. For example, digital photos, such as x-rays are being sent from the imaging center directly to the team physician or athletic trainer as an e-mail attachment. The future of technology in relation to managing records and patient data is unlimited. New technology is being developed and updated daily to make record keeping and managing information easier and more convenient.

With innovations and advances in technology athletic training is likely undergo additional changes and even experience greater visibility. This increased visibility needs to be intentionally monitored to ensure that athletic training is being portrayed properly. Web pages, blogs (i.e., web logs), and other Internet-mediated formats, such as http://www.facebook.com and http://www.myspace.com can be beneficial or damaging. It is imperative that athletic trainers and students remain professional and always consider the ramifications that postings might have on their professional image, job searches, and the profession's reputation.

CHAPTER SUMMARY

The use and inclusion of technology by the athletic trainer is essential for a productive and relevant work setting. Computer technology and the PC have made record keeping, data and report generation, electronic filing, communication, and other management duties streamlined and time efficient. Considering specific programmatic needs when purchasing computer hardware and software is essential to get the most out of the technology. Technological innovations such as networks, servers, intranet, Internet, and e-mail have made communication within the local and global health care context extremely reliable. This enhanced ability to communicate ideas and information has allowed managers and leaders greater access and influence with subordinates and peers. Electronic information management, such as electronic documents and paperless record keeping systems has allowed organizations to implement sustainable practices as well as streamline their effectiveness and share information more easily. However, these benefits are not without their drawbacks. Because of increased technology, the health care industry is at greater risk for identity theft and breaches in confidentiality, which must be well managed by the athletic trainer.

▶ Leadership Application

Bill is the new director of athletic training services at Athletic Training Resources, Inc., a busy sports medicine clinic in a large metropolitan city. He arrives to find that the record keeping and injury-tracking programs are not utilized to their full effectiveness. In fact, they are only used by the secretary to input patient billing information. Bill is not familiar with the current software, but quickly familiarizes himself with it and within a few days is very proficient at using it. Now that he is familiar and comfortable with the software, he implements a new policy requiring all records and injury data from now on be kept electronically. Initially, the staff is excited about this transition. However, after a week of trying to code in new data and transfer old records to an electronic format, the staff revolts. The staff cites that the job is too big to do, and that, while the software is easy enough to use, it is just too time consuming and inconvenient.

Critical Thinking Questions

1. Why do you think the staff is initially excited about the transition? How can access to this data benefit the organization?
2. Why do you think the staff is revolting, is there truth to their complaints?
3. What leadership skills can help Bill solve this problem?
4. What strategies can Bill implement to change the staff's opinions?

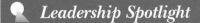

Leadership Spotlight

MALISSA MARTIN

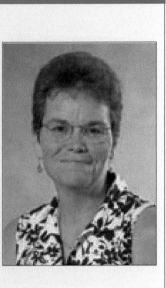

EDUCATION:

Post Graduate Certification in Alcohol/Drug Studies, University of South Carolina

EdD, Curriculum and Instruction, University of South Carolina, 1995

MEd Education/Health, University of South Carolina, 1987

BS, Health Education (Concentration in Athletic Training), Indiana State University, 1982

CURRENT JOB:

Professor and Director, Athletic Training Education Program, College of Mount St. Joseph, Cincinnati, OH

FIRST ATHLETIC TRAINING JOB:

Athletic Trainer for Women's Sports, University of South Carolina

PROFESSIONAL INTERESTS/RESEARCH FOCUS:

Health Issues in Female Athletes; Pedagogy

ATHLETIC TRAINING–RELATED AWARDS/HONORS:

- 2008 Educator of the Year, Greater Lakes Athletic Trainer's Association
- 2007 Historical Women in Athletic Training, Greater Lakes Athletic Trainer's Association
- 2005 Most Distinguished Athletic Trainer, National Athletic Trainer's Association
- 2002 Outstanding Athletic Training Educator and Administrator, Southeast Athletic Trainer's Association
- 1998 National Athletic Trainer's Service Award, 1998

Q & A

What first inspired you to enter the athletic training profession?

Originally I was under the assumption that athletic trainers were individuals who conditioned and trained athletes. After sitting through my first AT class at Indiana State University, I quickly discovered that ATs were health care providers. Since I was majoring in health education and I enjoyed the medical field and sports, athletic training became a natural fit for me.

How would you define leadership in athletic training?

I observe leadership as being a servant. I believe leaders serve others and assist others in getting where they want to in life. A true leader inspires others to make the most of a situation and guides others in making quality decisions. They play a major role in the growth and development of organizations and individuals by listening and recognizing that everyone has a voice and, more importantly, there is no I in TEAM! Leaders do not always follow the path of popularity. Great leaders carve their own path, have courage to think outside of the box, and transform their thoughts into actions. They have vision and can see the big picture and consider multiple viewpoints.

What is the best advice you ever received from another athletic trainer?

The best advice I received from an ATC is to spread your own wings and carve your own path.

What has been the most enjoyable aspect of athletic training?

My most enjoyable moments and what keeps me in clinical or teaching practice is the time I spend with students in and outside of the classroom. The day I no longer enjoy this interaction and engagement is the day I will retire from the profession.

What has been the least enjoyable aspect or your biggest challenge in athletic training?

The biggest challenge I think for me and others is the basic need for communication. I believe most frustrations can be resolved through communication with parties involved. I have a difficult time with colleagues who do not follow CAATE rules in relationship to clinical requirements for students.

What advice would you give a first year athletic training student?

A first year ATS should always be a sponge—but an active sponge. Get engaged, be active, but know your limitations. Learn or review at least one skill or concept each and every day. The opportunities for a freshman ATS are endless.

What advice would you give a brand new BOC-certified athletic trainer who is deciding between taking that first professional job or entering graduate school to pursue a master's degree in athletic training, and why?

With the current state of the economy and the rising cost of higher education, I believe this decision is based largely upon the financial and personal status of the individual. I always encourage ATs to attend graduate school; however, most of the time the students do not pursue a masters in AT, rather they chose education, health, or exercise physiology. I do believe that, in the long run, if an ATC does not eventually attain a master's degree, he or she will not move up the ladder in employment pursuits.

What other interests outside of athletic training have you pursued?

Other than administration and the business side of AT, I have not pursued other interests.

Where do you think (or hope) athletic training will be in the next 10 years?

I hope athletic trainers will be fully recognized by the average person on the street as the number one health care provider for physically active individuals. I hope that sports announcers will properly address us as athletic trainers and *not* trainers. I hope that more students pursuing athletic training degrees stay in athletic training and pursue employment in athletic training.

References

1. Goldsmith M, Greenberg C, Robertson A, Hu-Chan M. (2003). *Global leadership: The next generation.* Upper Saddle River, NJ: Prentice Hall.
2. Groth D, Skandier T. (2005). *Network +.* Hoboken, NJ: Sybex, Inc.
3. Pew Health Profession's Commission. (1998). *Recreating health professional practice for a new century.* Accessed February 26, 2007 at http://www.futurehealth.ucsf.edu/pdf_files/recreate.pdf
4. Rankin J. (1997). Technology and sports health care administration. *Athletic Therapy Today* 2(5):14–16.
5. Shae, V. (1997). *The core rules of netiquette.* San Francisco, CA: Albion Books. Accessed February 27, 2007 at http://www.albion.com/netiquette/corerules.html

Chapter 8

Record Keeping

"… nowadays there is so little useless information."

OSCAR WILDE

CHAPTER RATIONALE

Role Delineation Study Components

Domain V: Organization and Administration

- Institutional guidelines for referring patients to health care services
- Institutional informed consent policies and procedures
- Documentation protocols

Educational Competencies

- Explain the typical administrative policies and procedures that govern first aid and emergency care, such as those pertaining to parents/guardians, informed consent, media relations, incident reports, and appropriate record keeping.
- Develop a comprehensive patient file management system that uses both paper and electronic media.
- Identify the components of a medical record (permission to treat, emergency information, treatment documentation, and release of medical information) and the common medical record-keeping techniques and strategies, and the strengths and weaknesses of each approach.
- Use appropriate terminology and medical documentation to record injuries and illnesses (e.g., patient encounters, history, progress notes, discharge summary, physician letters, treatment encounters).
- Identify the current injury/illness surveillance and reporting systems such as, but not limited to, NEISS, National Athletic Head and Neck Injury Registry, and NCAA.

Key Terms

Administering: Giving medications in a dose that is to be consumed within 24 hours.

Dispensing: Giving medications in a dose that is to be consumed in a period of time greater than 24 hours.

Evidence-based practice: The integration of individual clinical expertise with the best available external clinical evidence from systematic research.

Explicit knowledge: Knowledge that has been or can be articulated, codified, and stored in media and that is easily transmitted to others.

Information: Data that has been sorted, analyzed, and displayed and typically has been communicated through text, figures, or tables.

Input: The information or data received from an external source.

Knowledge management: Any number of practices that identify, create, represent, and distribute knowledge for reuse, awareness, and learning.

Output: Data or information that has been converted into a usable form.

Privacy: The right to protection against unreasonable and unwarranted interference with the patient's solitude.

Referral: A written recommendation from one health care provider for a patient to receive medical care from another health care provider.

Tacit knowledge: The knowledge, typically based on personal experiences, that individuals may or may not be aware of and that, therefore, is difficult to disseminate and share.

ealth care is information intensive. Athletic trainers are required to track, organize, and record enormous amounts of information. The information that an athletic trainer needs to keep track of comes from several places. Information is generated from athletes, coaches, parents, patients, administrators, physicians, professional agencies and organizations, from evaluations, and from research. Organizing and making sense of this information requires accurate and reliable record keeping as well as a high level of critical thinking ability.

Accurate record keeping has implications for several aspects of athletic training, including technology, legal and ethical behaviors, and evidence-based practice. Because information is so abundant, has multiple sources, and because of its wide implications, organizing information for assimilation, assessment, and retrieval becomes a central task of the athletic trainer.

Managing information becomes an important element of longevity and success. Information consists of input and output. **Input** *is the information or data received from an external source. Examples of input include information gained from any number of athletic training practices including observation, special tests, questions, or clinical experience.* **Output** *is what the input is converted into once it has been documented. For example, output can be evidence-based medicine sheets, injury statistics, case studies, or research data. Output is used to facilitate actions or make informed decisions. The work of documenting (i.e., making input into output) is almost entirely a management task. Information is always being generated, and in health care, information is becoming less and less trivial. Therefore, record keeping for the sake of documentation has become a critical management skill for athletic trainers.*

In this chapter we will discuss the importance of knowledge management as well as challenges associated with managing different types of knowledge. The importance of confidentiality will be discussed, followed by a brief description of evidence-based practice. Then we will cover the medical record and what belongs in it. Finally, we will make note of some common errors in medical records and how to handle them.

KNOWLEDGE MANAGEMENT

Knowledge is an indispensable asset to athletic trainers. Athletic trainers are knowledge workers who must manage their knowledge wisely. A knowledge worker is one who works primarily with information or one who develops and uses knowledge in the workplace. Knowledge work typically is a non-repetitive, non-routine, activity that requires a large amount of critical thinking and decision making.[9] As knowledge workers, athletic trainers must have access to information and data that is accurate and reliable. The onus of providing the knowledge worker with correct, accurate, and reliable information falls to the organization. The onus of making sure the information is usable falls to the knowledge worker. Therefore, both parties need to engage in knowledge management. **Knowledge management** is any number of practices that identify, create, represent, and distribute knowledge for reuse, awareness, and learning. Fundamentally, knowledge management is the process of organizing and analyzing information to make it understandable and applicable to problem solving or decision making.[1] The knowledge-based work of athletic trainers requires support in the following areas:

1. Storing clinical data
2. Retrieving clinical data
3. Translating data into information
4. Linking data and information to domain specific knowledge (i.e., competencies)
5. Assimilating clinical data.[9]

The appropriate application of leadership skills is essential to knowledge management. Leadership that can facilitate the judicious use of information and therefore, knowledge management, includes the following skills:

1. Skilled communicator: to disseminate information appropriately
2. Ethical: to use information appropriately
3. Collaborator: to involve others in the use of information
4. Knowledgeable: to use information in the correct context
5. Future-minded: to apply information toward vision and goals
6. Critical thinker: to critique and assimilate information for use
7. Open-minded: to use information in new or creative ways

It is important that leaders understand how data, information, and knowledge support their operations. Leaders must ask critical questions about where knowledge exists, how information flows, what data is collected and where is it collected, and who is involved in the process.[1]

Types of Knowledge

Information is data that has been sorted, analyzed, and displayed and typically has been communicated through text, figures, or tables.[2] Knowledge requires transforming information into something usable or applicable.[2] Transforming data (records) into information and information into usable knowledge can be a difficult task.

Knowledge is either tacit or explicit. **Tacit knowledge** is the knowledge, typically based on experiences, that people carry around in their minds; they may or may not be aware of this knowledge and therefore it is difficult to disseminate and share. The transfer of tacit knowledge usually is very time intensive and requires trust and relationship. **Explicit knowledge** is knowledge that has been or can be articulated, codified, is stored in media and is more easily transmitted to others. Examples of explicit knowledge include texts, journal articles, documents, and procedures. Skyrme[7] described four ways these two types of knowledge can interact or be disseminated:

1. Tacit-to-tacit: where individuals acquire new knowledge directly from others. Examples might include lecturing or mentoring.
2. Tacit-to-explicit: the articulation of knowledge into tangible form through dialogue or other media (i.e., writing). Examples might include writing an article summary or a critique.
3. Explicit-to-explicit: combining different forms of explicit knowledge, such as in documents or databases. Examples might include compiling injury data.
4. Explicit-to-tacit: learning by doing, where individuals internalize knowledge from documents into their own body of experience. Examples might include a clinical experience or internship.

Athletic training preparation takes advantage of all four kinds of knowledge transfer.

Leadership and Knowledge Management

As with other leadership responsibilities, knowledge management has specific challenges. These leadership responsibilities include controlling volume, security, quality, and accessibility of information.[1]

Controlling the Volume of Information

The volume of information that the athletic trainer needs to manage can be intimidating. Athletic trainers are often required to maintain treatment records, insurance claims, physical evaluation forms, rehabilitation programs and protocols, SOAP notes, inventory, purchasing and receiving records, employee or staff evaluations, waivers, and much more. Managing and organizing all this information requires effective knowledge management practices. One way to control the volume of information is to have a systematic method of storing and retrieving what is important. This can take several forms, from a file-based system to an electronic storage system. The first step in this process is to prioritize the information. Once prioritized, define frequency of use; in other words, define how often this information needs to be retrieved. Information requiring frequent retrieval should be kept in a convenient location, but it is most important to create a system where information can be found easily, even if it is rarely needed. Once a system is created to manage the volume, controlling security and access become central factors.

Controlling the Security and Accessibility of Information

Keeping information secure and confidential can be a challenge. Obviously, there are legal and ethical ramifications behind security and confidentiality of information. Pragmatically, keeping information secure also helps in later retrieval and the decision-making process. Because of the nature of many athletic training rooms (open-door policies and near 24-hour service) and the relationship many athletic trainers enjoy with students, patients, peers, and superiors, ensuring that documents and other patient-related information is kept confidential presents unique challenges to athletic trainers. Using technology, educating others, and adhering to professional and ethical standards can help keep information secure.

Patients have a right to privacy of the medical record. **Privacy** is the right to protection against unreasonable and unwarranted interference with the patient's solitude.[9] Privacy is understood in health care as the protection against 1) using a patient's name or image for its own advantage; 2) intrusion by the institution into the patient's affairs; 3) disseminating facts that place the patient in a negative light; and 4) public disclosure of private facts. Every athletic trainer in every setting should take patient privacy and confidential record keeping seriously.

What is often misunderstood is that, as a primary source of information, the medical record is the property of the institution. Therefore, the institution must maintain it. The patient has a right to the copy of the entire medical record, but only a copy. The same is true even if records are subpoenaed. The institution need only supply a verified and true copy of the original record. Therefore, direct access is limited to the institution, but the institution must provide a reasonable way for patients and others to obtain legal copies of medical records.

It is best to restrict patient information to only those who "need to know." Those who need to know are the patient and direct providers, (i.e., the physician, nurses, therapists, and technicians). At times, administrators or researchers may need to see medical records for analysis, staffing implications, or to review quality of care. There are others who also may "need to know," but it is wise to always secure the patient's permission in writing regardless of why or by whom a record needs to be reviewed.

Controlling the Quality of Information

It is essential that the data and information collected be of adequate quality. Ensuring quality is difficult. All information needs to be valid and reliable and should be able to be converted into usable output to help make meaningful decisions. Valid information supplies data about what is actually being asked. Valid information is accurate. Reliable information supplies data that is consistent. Reliable information is trustworthy and the source is objective and unbiased. Data and information that are poor in quality can ultimately hinder or sabotage the decision-making process. Careful safeguards should be established to ensure that any information collected is from a notable and reputable source, is objective, and current.

THE IMPORTANCE OF DOCUMENTATION

Information and records that are valid and reliable can be used to:

1. secure reimbursement
2. aid in communication
3. facilitate informed decisions
4. adjust clinical practice
5. facilitate better patient outcomes

Furthermore, keeping accurate records can help reduce liability by demonstrating certain actions did or did not take place. Keeping accurate records also serves a very pragmatic role, remembering what was done.

Regardless of setting, the athletic trainer's work life can be very hectic. Often the details of what treatments, what injuries, what modalities, what exercises, or what messages are forgotten. Keeping documentation can help the athletic trainer remember exactly what happened.

Documents take on many forms and often evolve quickly. Many different settings and roles require different kinds of documentation, logs, or records. Typical forms in athletic training include (but are certainly not limited to) the following:

1. Daily treatment logs
2. S.O.A.P. notes
3. Injury evaluations
4. Performance evaluations
5. Waivers and consent forms
6. Insurance sheets
7. Health history forms

Much of the paper work listed above is an important part of the medical record.

The Medical Record

The medical record is the sum of all patient information ranging from health history to all treatments and interventions. The medical record is often kept in a folder, frequently organized by sections. Box 8-1 is a list of documents often kept in a medical record. The following section is a brief description of some of documents that may be kept in a patient's medical record.

> ### BOX 8-1 Paperwork Often Kept in a Medical Record
>
> 1. Insurance information
> 2. Pertinent personal information
> 3. Emergency contact information
> 4. Health history
> 5. Physical exam
> 6. Injury forms
> 7. SOAP or progress notes
> 8. Informed consents
> 9. Waivers
> 10. Discharge notes

Insurance Documents

Insurance information is often the first thing asked for when visiting most health care facilities. This information is important to the provider because it demonstrates there is a payment plan in place and ensures the provider that at least a portion of the expenses will be paid by a third party. Often there is a questionnaire asking insurance-related questions as well as a photocopy of the patient's insurance card. It is important to collect the policy and group number of the insurance plan as well as information on the insured (or policy holder).

Personal Documentation

Personal information is also often part of the medical record. Personal information may be a part of other forms (such as the medical history) or may be a separate form. Personal information must be pertinent. Under no circumstances should personal information be used to discriminate. Examples of pertinent information include height, weight, eye and hair color, gender, occupation, date of birth, and home address. Personal information may also include emergency contact information. Emergency contact information should include the name, address, and phone number of someone the patient has designated ahead of time to contact in case of an emergency. Emergency information might also include a list of allergies or current medications, as well as a quick reference to insurance information.

Health History

A health history is also a very important piece of the medical record. The health history includes a list of all past medical conditions. A health history needs to include personal history, such as previous surgeries, fractures, injuries, illnesses, allergies, and concussions. A health history also needs to include a detailed family history. A family history can help to uncover any inherited conditions and usually includes at least biological parents and grandparents. If a patient is adopted and does not have access to his or her biological parent's medical histories, it is important that the patient is aware that inherited conditions may exist. In such cases, the athletic trainer and the patient have to make do with the information available.

Physical Examinations and Progress Notes

The pre-participation physical examination (PPE) is also included in the medical record. The PPE serves as the clearance to participate and identifies any pre-existing conditions that might disqualify or modify the patient from participating.

Injury forms are also kept in the medical record. Injury forms that document each specific injury. Typically injury evaluations follow H.O.P.S. (i.e., History, Observation, Palpation, Special Tests) or S.O.A.P. format. Injury forms should include the name of the evaluator, the injury date as well as the date the injury was reported (if not the same), as well as differential diagnosis, referral or treatment plans, and a place for a signature and date of evaluator.

SOAP (i.e., Subjective, Objective, Assessment, Plan) notes or progress notes are also an important part of the medical record. Often these are kept after the initial injury form has been filed and are used on a regular basis to keep information on the initial injury up to date. However, SOAP note format may also be used for the initial evaluation. The information gained from a SOAP note includes what the athlete reports to be feeling, objective measurements (i.e., ROM, girth), a differential diagnosis, and the plan of action, which often includes treatment plan, rehab plans, or referral plans. The SOAP note should be concise using common medical language and terminology so that it can be read and quickly understood by any member of the health care team. For samples of the common forms used, see the appendices at the end of the book.

Waivers

Waivers and informed consents are also kept in the medical record. Informed consent is for legal purposes and clearly articulates any risks associated with participation in an activity and is an acknowledgement by the participant that he or she was made aware of the risks either verbally or in writing or both. Waivers can include several different releases. For example, waivers are often included that release a related party from liability. Figure 8-1 is a sample of an assumption of risk waiver. Figure 8-2 is a consent form. General liability and equipment (e.g., football helmet) are common waivers. A release of medical information is also typically part of the medical record. Figure 8-3 is a sample medical information release.

Documenting Medications

The medical record is also a place to list information concerning the medications being taken by patients. All prescriptions should be handled within the patient, physician, and pharmacist triad. Other than recording the medications patients are taking, most athletic trainers should not need to be involved with handling, dispensing, or recommending medications.

However, some athletic trainers in collegiate settings have additional roles concerning medications.[3] At times the collegiate athletic trainer is asked to administer or keep records of athlete's medications. While not an ideal situation, it does occur and the athletic trainer must be well versed in specific state licensure laws, practice acts, and federal mandates concerning the handling and dispensing of medications.

Obviously, there are legal ramifications with administrating or dispensing of medications, both over-the-counter (OTC) or prescriptions. There are many state and federal regulations that mandate how and under what conditions medications can be handled and by whom.[3] It is illegal in every state for athletic trainers to dispense medications (prescriptions and OTC). **Dispensing** medications is defined as a dose that is to be consumed in a period of time greater than 24 hours. However, there is variability between states as to whether a licensed athletic trainer can administer medications. **Administering** medications is defined as a dose that is to be consumed within 24 hours. Not every state allows licensed athletic trainers to administer medications. It is prudent to consult individual state practice acts before attempting to administer any type of medication. Note that consumption time and not package

Assumption of Risk From

I am aware that playing, practicing, training, and/or other involvement in any sport can be a dangerous activity involving MANY RISKS OF INJURY, including, but not limited to the potential for catastrophic injury. I understand that the dangers and risks of playing, practicing, or training in any athletic activity include, but are not limited to, death, serious neck and spinal injuries which may result in complete or partial paralysis or brain damage, serious injury to virtually all bones, joints, ligaments, muscles, tendons, and other aspects of the musculoskeletal system, and serious injury or impairment to other aspects of my body, general health and wellbeing.

Because of the aforementioned dangers of participating in any athletic activity, I recognize the importance of following all instructions of the coaching staff, strength and conditioning staff, and/or Athletic Training Staff. Furthermore, I understand that the possibility of injury, including catastrophic injury, does exist even though proper rules and techniques are followed. I also understand that there are risks involved with traveling in connection with intercollegiate athletics.

In consideration of (insert name of university) permitting me to participate in intercollegiate athletics and other activities and travel related to my sport, I hereby voluntarily assume all risks associated with participation and agree to hold harmless, indemnify, and irrevocably and unconditionally release (name of university), and their officers, agents, and employees from any and all liability, any medical expenses not covered by the (name of university), and any and all claims, causes of action or demands of any kind and nature whatsoever which may arise by or in connection with my participation in any activities related to intercollegiate athletics.

The terms hereof shall serve as release and assumption of risk for my heirs, estate, executor, administrator, assignees, and all members of my family.

I fully understand that this authorization shall be effective and valid for one year (52 weeks) after the termination of my playing and/or academic career at (name of University).

_____   _____

Student-Athlete Signature   Date

_____   _____

Parent's Signature required if Student-Athlete is under 19   Date

FIGURE 8-1 Assumption of risk form

University
Consent Form

Athlete's Name (print) _____

Please read the following consent forms carefully. If you are under 18 years of age, your parents must also sign. The basic content of each is:

A. **Shared Responsibility for Sport Safety:** Acknowledges that there are certain inherent risks involved in participating in intercollegiate athletics and that you are willing to assume responsibility for such risks.

B. **Release of Information:** Allows those listed to release information concerning your injuries to the media.

C. **Release of Information:** Allows those listed to release information concerning your injuries to your parents or guardians.

D. **Release of Information:** Allows those listed to release any and all information concerning you, including records and other items listed, to professional teams, agents, scouts, etc.

E. **Medical Consent:** Allows those listed to treat any injury or illness you receive while at XYZ University.

F. **Responsibilities:** Acknowledges that you have read and understand the responsibilities of being a XYZ University student-athlete. If you should choose to refuse to sign any of these, please write "Refused to sign", date, and your signature.

Shared Responsibility for Sport Safety - Part A
Participation of sport requires an acceptance of risk of injury. Student-athletes rightfully assume that those who are responsible for the conduct of sport have taken reasonable precaution to minimize such risk and that their peers participating in the sport will not intentionally inflict injury upon them. Our athletic trainers and physicians will periodically analyze injury patterns to refine rules and make safety decisions. However, to legislate safety via a rule book and equipment standards, while often necessary, seldom is effective by itself; and to rely on officials to endorse compliance with the rule books is as insufficient as to rely on warning labels to produce compliance with safety guidelines. "Compliance" means respect on everyone's part for the intent and purpose of a rule or guideline.

I have read the above shared responsibility statement. I understand that there are certain inherent risks involved in participating in intercollegiate athletics. I acknowledge the fact that these risks exist and I am willing to assume responsibility for such risks while participating at XYZ University
Signature:_____ Date:_____

Release of Information - Part B
This is to authorize XYZ University athletic trainers, team physicians, athletic coaches, and administrators to release to the XYZ University Sports Information Department and the media at any time, all medical information on my son/daughter/myself including but not limited to any information concerning illness or injury relative to my past, present, or future participation in athletics at XYZ University.
Signature:_____ Date:_____

Release of Information - Part C
This is to authorize XYZ University athletic trainers, team physicians, athletic coaches, and administrators to release medical information on my son/daughter/myself, to my parents or guardians, any information concerning illness or injury relative to my past, present, or future participation in athletics at XYZ University.
Signature:_____ Date:_____

FIGURE 8-2 (*Continued*)

Release of Information - Part D

I hereby give my consent for the team physicians, athletic trainers or other medical personnel of XYZ University to release such information regarding my medical history, record of injury or surgery, record of serious illness and rehabilitation results as may be requested by the scout or representative of any professional or amateur athletic organization seeking such information.

I understand that a record will be kept of all individuals requesting such information and the date of the request. This information is normally confidential and, as provided in this release, will not be otherwise released by the parties in charge of the information.

Signature:_____ Date:_____

Medical Consent - Part E

I hereby grant permission to XYZ University team physicians and/or their consulting physicians to render my son/daughter/myself any treatment and medical or surgical care that they decm reasonably necessary to the health and well being of the student-athlete. I also hereby authorize the athletic trainers at XYZ University who are under the direction and guidance of the XYZ University team physicians, to render to my son/daughter/myself any preventative, first aid, rehabilitative or emergency treatment that they deem reasonably necessary to the health and well being of the student athlete.

Also, when necessary for executing such case, I grant permission for hospitalization at an accredited hospital.

Signature:_____ Date:_____

Responsibilities - Part F

I furthermore…

A. Understand that it is my responsibility to report all injuries and illness to my staff team athletic trainer as soon as possible.

B. Understand that I am expected to report promptly as scheduled for treatment and/or rehab;

C. Understand that I will continue to receive treatment/rehab until released by my staff team athletic trainer.

D. Understand that XYZ University cannot be held responsible for any previous medical condition(s) I might have.

Signature:_____ Date:_____

My signature release remains valid until revoked by me in writing.

FIGURE 8-2 Consent form

size differentiates dispensing from administering. In other words, it is important to realize that giving a "handful" of single dose packets of any medication constitutes a dispensed dose and is illegal for athletic trainers to do.

There are also federal regulations that mandate how medications must be stored, how they are labeled, and how records are kept. Labeling requirements for all administered medications must include directions for use as well as the patient's full

---

Authorization to Release Medical Information

Full Name:_____

Permanent Address:_____

Home Phone:_____ Cell Phone:_____ DOB:___/___/____

I hereby authorize (name of university) Athletic Training and (another organization) to inspect or secure copies of case history records, laboratory reports, imaging results and any other data covering this and/or previous confinements and/or disabilities. A photocopy of this authorization shall be deemed as effective and valid as the original. This authorization will automatically expire one year from the date signed. This authorization will be updated according to the academic year, not the calendar year. I understand that I may revoke this consent at any time except to the extent that action has been taken in reliance thereon.

_____   _____

Student-Athlete Signature   Date

_____   _____

Parent's Signature required if Student-Athlete is under 19   Date

---

FIGURE 8-3 Release of medical records

name. Furthermore, all records concerning medications must include inventory, reconciliations, and drug usage logs.

Athletic trainers who work in settings where prescription medications are stored and administered need to consult their state's practice act, obtain legal counsel, work closely with their team physician and pharmacist, and have strictly enforced written policies and procedures on the handling and recording of all medications.

Making Referrals

The medical record is also a place to note any referrals made. **Referrals** are written recommendations from one health care provider to receive medical care from another health care provider. Most athletic trainers note the initial referral in the plan of a SOAP note. There are also formal recommendation forms that can be used. For example, athletic trainers should refer all illnesses or injuries that require care beyond their scope of practice. Referral forms vary by organization and it may be that the health care provider receiving the referral has a special form that they use. Figure 8-4 is a sample referral form used to refer a university athlete to the university medical center. Some examples of what might constitute needing a referral include manipulations; diagnostic imaging (i.e., x-rays or MRIs); need for prescription or over-the-counter (OTC) medications; and medical emergencies. For example, many athletic trainers in collegiate settings refer athletes to the university medical center or school nurse for general medical condition such a fever, cold, virus, or bacterial infections. For specific referral guidelines, the best practice is to consult organizational policy and procedure.

Common Errors in Documentation

Errors in documentation are likely to happen. No amount of care or thought can totally eliminate every error. Many facilities have policies and procedures in place for handling mistaken entries or errors. A typical rule of thumb to use when an error is made in an entry is to write the phrase "mistaken entry" next to the error. Never erase or cover up an error entirely. The original note along with the error needs to be able to be read. This will help to preserve the caregiver's credibility and keeps entire notes or documents from becoming suspect. Another way to handle mistake is to simply draw a single line through the error, initial it, and write the correct statement beside it.

If an error is discovered in the coding or billing process such as an incorrect diagnostic (ICD-9) or treatment code (CPT), the best course of action is to notify the third-party payer, usually in writing, of the error as soon as possible. Often if the diagnostic code does not match the treatment code the insurance company catches the error and denies payment for the treatment. Other common issues with coding usually include illegible hand writing, using old coding procedures, or transposing numbers or forgetting commas or periods. Another common mistake is made when trying to "squeeze in" additional information after the fact, e.g., trying to squeeze in a new or additional sentence between lines or in the margins. Avoid this altogether and simply add the information you wish to add at the end of note.

INJURY SURVEILLANCE AND REPORTING

There are several agencies that have created searchable databases that document and track injuries. This information can be used to track demographics or injury patters and trends. Injury trends can be queried by sport, gender, age, or date. This information can be helpful when creating emergency action plans, performing a risk assessment, needs assessment, or just to get a background on injury patterns for a certain demographic. This information can also be used to generate research. Two

ATHLETIC TRAINING UNIVERSITY
Student-Athlete Referral / Consultation Form

Name _____ SS# _____

Sport _____ Date of Birth _____

Date of Injury _____ Date of Referral _____

Injured Body Part- ☐ Right ☐ Left _____

History / Reason for Referral:

Referred To:

☐ ABC Orthopedics   ☐ Student Health Services
☐ Dr. Jim Smith, DO   ☐ Local Hospital
☐ Dr. Joe Smith, MD // Family Health Center   ☐ Dr. John Smith
☐ East State Dental (Dr. Jones, DDS) ☐ Specialty Brace & Limb
☐ Dr. Sue Smith (Optometrist)   ☐ Sports Bracing Assoc.
☐ Regional MRI   ☐ Pharmacy

☐ Other _____

Referred By: _____
     Name   Title

☐ **Sport Related Injury / Illness:**
  a) The student-athlete's primary insurance information is attached.
  b) The ATU and its athletics department is the **SECONDARY** insurance carrier for this referral.
  c) All claims and charges should be submitted directly to the student-athlete's primary insurance company.
  d) Remaining or unpaid charges should then be submitted, with an *itemized statement, HCFA or UB92, & an EOB from the primary insurance company* to:

  ATU
  Attn: Athletic Insurance Coordinator
  AT Sports Center, Room 133
  PO Box 123456
  Anywhere, ST 55555-5555
  (555) 555-5555 // fax- (555) 555-5555

☐ **Non-Sport Related Injury / Illness:**
  Injury / Illness is **NOT** the direct result of intercollegiate athletic participation at the ATU. Submit all
  charges directly to the aforementioned student-athlete and/or his/her primary insurance company.
  The ATU CANNOT, per NCAA regulations, remit payment for these charges.

_____   _____
Athletic Trainer Signature   Date

I, the undersigned, consent to the use or disclosure of my protected health information by the ATU Athletic Training Department and/or the aforementioned medical and/or allied health personnel for the purpose of diagnosing or providing treatment to me, obtaining payment for my health care bills or to conduct health care operations for the ATU Athletic Training Department and/or other medical entities.

I understand that I have the right to revoke this authorization, in writing, at any time, by sending such written notification to the ATU Athletic Training Department and/or the aforementioned medical and/or allied health entities. I understand that a revocation is not effective to the extent that the ATU Athletic Training Department and/or the aforementioned medical and/or allied health entities have relied on the use or disclosure of the protected health information.

_____   _____
Student-Athlete Signature   Date

White Copy: Provider Copy
Yellow Copy: Athletic Training Room Files
Pink Copy: Student-Athlete's Files

FIGURE 8-4 Sample referral form

common injury tracking (or surveillance) programs include the National Electronic Injury Surveillance System and the National Collegiate Athletic Association.

National Electronic Injury Surveillance System (NEISS) is a national probability sample of hospitals in the United States. Injury information is collected from each NEISS hospital for every emergency visit involving an injury associated with consumer products.[5] The NEISS database can be accessed via the Internet and allows certain estimates to be retrieved. Note that the search includes limiters such as, age range of the patient, dates of the injuries, diagnosis, body part, and area the injury occurred. For example, when using the NEISS, results can be limited to frequency of ankle injuries that occurred during sport or recreation for boys ages 6 to 18 years.

The *National Collegiate Athletic Association Injury Surveillance System* (ISS) was created to provide current and reliable data on injury trends in intercollegiate athletics.[4] The injury data are collected yearly from a sample of NCAA member institutions. The NCAA Committee on Competitive Safeguards and Medical Aspects of Sports then reviews the data. The committee's goal is to reduce injury rates through suggested changes in rules, protective equipment, or coaching techniques based on data provided by the ISS. For example, by using the ISS you can determine that during the 2004–05 wrestling season 73% of all injuries occurred during practice and 27% occurred during matches. Interestingly, the trend is almost reversed for ice hockey, where over 68% of injuries occurred during games. This information can be critical when rehearsing and planning for emergency situations as well as when managing human resources. You can access the ISS via the Internet at the NCAA's website.

Other injury registries include the *National Athletic Head and Neck Injury Registry*, *National Football Head and Neck Injury Registry*. There are international registries as well, such as the *Injury Surveillance On-line* in Canada, and the *Queensland Injury Surveillance Unit* in Australia. Because of the useful data tracking injuries can provide, maintaining these registries is an important professional responsibility for athletic trainers.

LEADERSHIP ACTIVITY

Schedule a meeting with your ACI (as a small group or individually) to discuss evidence-based medicine. Start the meeting by agreeing to work together on developing a strategy that you can use on a regular basis to evaluate whether treatment protocols are meeting current evidence-based practice recommendations. Once that process is established, develop a policy that will help implement evidence-based standards for common treatments or interventions done in the athletic training room or by athletic trainers. Also develop a policy that effectively deals with common treatments that might not achieve evidence-based standards. If your ACI is not able to meet with you, create a fictional strategy and resulting policies you might use in a clinic or athletic training of which you are the director.

EVIDENCE-BASED PRACTICE

Effective knowledge management is a key to implementing an evidence-based practice. **Evidence-based practice** is the integration of individual clinical expertise with the best available external clinical evidence from systematic research.[6] As information and knowledge increases, advances in clinical practices must follow.[2] Therefore, the effective leader will implement strategies to gather and assimilate valuable knowledge in an expedient manner. Building knowledge through surveying data and scanning the scholarly literature, then applying that knowledge in a clinical context is necessary to advance athletic training and critical for positive patient outcomes.

Evidence-based practice requires assimilating clinical judgment and systematic research.[8] Clinical decisions are based on multiple sources, i.e., experience, sound advice, scholarly research. Therefore, critical thinking and contextual intelligence are important skills for evidence-based practitioners.

Critics of evidence-based practice, often cite that evidence, when considered in isolation, is used to create a "cookie-cutter" approach to clinical practice. Therefore, multiple forms of evidence, including random controlled trials, meta-analysis, non-experimental research, case studies, qualitative research, and personal experience should be considered and integrated when making clinical decisions. Box 8-2 shows a list of scholarly journals often used by athletic trainers for clinical information.

> **BOX 8-2** **Popular Scholarly Journals Used by Athletic Trainers**
>
> 1. American Journal of Physical Medicine & Rehabilitation
> 2. American Journal of Sports Medicine
> 3. Athletic Therapy Today
> 4. Clinical Journal of Sports Medicine
> 5. Clinics in Sports Medicine
> 6. Exercise and Sports Science Reviews
> 7. International Journal of Sports Medicine
> 8. Journal of Athletic Training
> 9. Journal of Biomechanics
> 10. Journal of Orthopaedic & Sports Physical Therapy
> 11. Journal of Sports Rehabilitation
> 12. Journal of Strength and Conditioning Research
> 13. Medicine Science in Sports and Exercise
> 14. Physical Therapy
> 15. Physician and Sports Medicine
> 16. Sports Medicine
> 17. Sports Medicine and Arthroscopy Review

 Leadership Application

As an athletic training student you are assigned to an ACI whose primary responsibility is football. It is Saturday evening and the day's game is over and everyone is cleaning up the athletic training room for the weekend. The team physician has already left for the evening. The last of the football players are starting to leave when the starting quarterback stops in and complains to your supervising ACI of a headache. Your ACI gives you the keys to the medicine cabinet and asks you to grab six sample-size packets of ibuprofen. You did not ask, but you suspect the ACI intends to give him all six packets to tide him over till Monday, when he can come back and see the team physician.

Critical Thinking Questions

1. What are some concerns you may have or specific questions you might ask your ACI about this request?
2. Are there any legal or ethical considerations in this scenario, how would you find out if there are any?
3. Assume now that the team physician asked the ACI to grab the same medication from the cabinet, and you were simply an observer. What might you be asked to document?

CHAPTER SUMMARY

Knowledge management is an important responsibility for athletic trainers. Organizing and disseminating tacit and explicit knowledge is a task that can be both rewarding and challenging. As a knowledge worker, athletic trainers need to be leaders when it comes to knowledge management by applying and implementing knowledge in several contexts, especially in the clinical context. One way to put information to use is through evidence-based practice. Evidence-based practice makes use of systematic research and clinical judgment to formulate a clinical plan of action for patients.

The medical record and documentation of injuries is a major managerial role athletic trainers must play. This managerial task is the responsibility of all athletic trainers regardless of their role or function within the organization. Knowing the proper medical terminology, state and federal regulatory policies on record keeping, injury-tracking registries, and how to address errors in documentation can help turn information into usable knowledge and provide foundations for effective emergency planning and preparation.

References

1. Association of State and Territorial Health Officials. (2005). *Examples of knowledge management in public health practice.* Washington, DC: ASTHO.

2. Dawes M, Davies P, Gray A, Mant J, Seers K, Snowball R. (2005). *Evidence-based practice: A primer for health care professionals.* Edinburgh, Scotland: Elsevier.

3. Kahanov L, Furst D, Johnson S, Roberts J. (2003). Adherence to drug-dispensation and drug-administration laws and guidelines in collegiate athletic training rooms. *JAT 38*(3):252–258.

4. NCAA (n.d.). NCAA ISS retrieved May 18, 2007 from http://www1.ncaa.org/membership/ed_outreach/health-safety/iss/index.html

5. NEISS (n.d.) Retrieved May 18, 2007 from http://www.cpsc.gov/library/neiss.html

6. Sackett, D, Rosenberg, W, Gray, J, Haynes, R, & Richardson, W. (1996). Evidence based medicine: what it is and what it isn't. *BMJ 12*(7023):71–72.

7. Skyrme D. (1997). From information management to knowledge management: Are you prepared? *OnLine Information Proceedings 1997.* Learned Information Europe. Retrieved May 8, 2007 from http://www.skyrme.com/pubs/on97full.htm

8. Steves R, Hootman J. (2004). Evidence-based medicine: What is it and how does it apply to athletic training? *JAT 39*(1):83–87.

9. Yoder-Wise P. (2003). *Leading and managing in nursing.* St. Louis, MO: Mosby.

Chapter 9

Fiscal Management

"In all realms of life it takes courage to stretch your limits, express your power, and fulfill your potential.. it's no different in the financial realm."

SUZE ORMAN

CHAPTER RATIONALE

Role Delineation Study Components

Domain V: Organization and Administration

- Knowledge of institutional budgeting and procurement process
- Knowledge of storage and inventory procedures

Educational Competencies

- Develop operational and capital budgets based on a supply inventory and needs assessment.
- Explain the components of the budgeting process, including purchasing, requisition, bidding, and inventory.

Key Terms

Bid sheet: A list of needed supplies and equipment for the upcoming year that is sent to multiple vendors. Each vendor then estimates the cost of all or some of the supplies and returns a proposal for the total cost of the supplies to the athletic trainer for consideration.

Budget freeze: Suspension or stoppage of spending.

Capital budget: Money that is set aside and disbursed for expensive equipment that is intended to last for more than one budget cycle.

Formula budget: A budget model that uses a ratio of full-time employees to students as a means to determine total disbursement of funds.

For-profit organization: A legal corporate entity that distributes any profit to shareholders and investors.

Inventory: All of the goods and materials available for use by an athletic training program.

Line-item budget: A budget model that distributes a fixed amount of funds for each function within a program.

Lump sum budget: A budget model that distributes funds in a single amount for the entire budget cycle without delineating specific expenditures.

Not-for-profit organizations: A legal corporate entity that reinvests any profits back into the organization.

Performance budget: A budget model similar to program based, but money is allocated based on athletic training functions (i.e., record keeping, inventory, etc.).

Pooled bidding: Bidding in which several organizations join their resources so that a larger order can be placed, in an attempt receive a reduced price on certain items.

Program budget: A budget model in which funds are distributed based on services provided to patients; i.e., based on organizational goals and objectives.

Purchase order (PO): The securing of permission (or pre-approval) for a payment to a vendor.

Return on investment (ROI): A measure of the total benefit or outcome of an expenditure.

Supply chain management: An approach that involves organizing details of all activities involved in forming supply and service agreements, obtaining supplies and services, and paying for supplies and services.

Vendor: A sellers or distributor of athletic training supplies and equipment.

Zero-based budget: A budget model that does not take into consideration previous spending patterns. Therefore, each expense must be justified annually.

T*he athletic trainer has a large financial responsibility when it comes to managing and leading an athletic training program. Financial management can be a source of strength and credibility for a leader or it can be a tremendous weakness. Allocating and assigning money typically falls to athletic trainers in leadership roles.*

How well financial resources are managed often plays a disproportionate role in perceived leadership effectiveness. In other words, mismanaging money can ruin the reputation of an otherwise brilliant leader. On the other hand, poor leaders can overcome many weaknesses with savvy financial management. Athletic trainers in most settings must deal with several aspects of finances. Allocating resources, budgeting, purchasing, and managing supplies and inventory are major duties of many athletic trainers.

In this chapter we will outline the financial responsibilities of athletic trainers. We will start by examining the health care financial trends in the United States and follow that with how athletic trainers manage their supply chain. Next we will discuss the different types of budgets used by athletic trainers and how athletic trainers can implement a budget. After that we will discuss managing inventory, purchasing, and controlling costs.

HEALTH CARE COSTS IN THE UNITED STATES

Most health care organizations are experiencing all-time highs in expenses. These rising expenses contribute to a higher cost of health care in the United States. It is estimated that approximately 20% of the gross national product (GDP) will be spent on health care by 2015.[1]

Health care costs in the United States are covered by four sources: the government (i.e., Medicare and Medicaid), which covers about 45%; private insurance, which covers about 33%; out-of-pocket expenses, which covers about 16%; and private donors cover the remainder.[9] To help put this in perspective, consider that in 2006, a popular athletic training employer reported over 3 billion dollars in net operating revenue, 47% of which was from Medicare patients.

TYPES OF CORPORATIONS AND FISCAL MANAGEMENT

Corporations are either **not-for-profit** or **for-profit**. Profit is the amount of money left over after all the expenses are paid (profit = revenue − expenses). For-profit organizations distribute their profit to shareholders and investors. Not-for-profit

> ### From the Field
>
> *I have had the opportunity to work with both for-profit and non-profit athletic training and reha-*
> *bilitation facilities. Each of these experiences was educational and had different budgetary phi-*
> *losophies. Both required me to generate revenue for the organization. However, the emphasis*
> *and consequences were dramatically different. In the for-profit system, the amount of revenue I*
> *generated was a significant factor in determining my annual as well as my personal budget. If my*
> *revenue generation met or exceeded a certain expectation, I was rewarded with a bonus. The*
> *more revenue generated, the greater my bonus. Furthermore, if revenue met or exceeded projec-*
> *tions, my operating budget (for supplies and equipment) was increased. However, if revenue was*
> *lower than expected, there was a much lower personal bonus and funds were redirected to pro-*
> *grams or departments that generated more revenue.*
>
> *On the other hand, when working for non-profits, revenue was not directly tied to my operating*
> *budget. Revenue was also extremely important, but there were other values placed on the ath-*
> *letic training services than just revenue generation. For example, revenue expectations were less*
> *(compared to other referral based programs), but that was justified because athletic training*
> *had a much higher public relations presence in the community. In fact in the non-profit arena, my*
> *budget for supplies was shared by the community. I was contracted to a certain high school for*
> *athletic training and the supplies and equipment budget were shared between my employer and*
> *the school. I presume the portion of the supply budget that came from my employer was justified*
> *as a public relations or marketing expense.*

organizations must reinvest their profits back into the organization. Athletic training professionals work in both types of corporations.

Many athletic training departments are part of not-for-profit organizations, such as high schools, colleges and universities, and most hospitals. This should not be interpreted to mean that profit is not expected or that generating revenue is not essential to survival. It is just that the profit needs to be reinvested into the organizations instead of to a board or shareholders. In other words, not-for-profit organizations are under equal pressure by stakeholders to operate at a profit. Likewise, there is a growing number of athletic trainers who work for organizations that are for profit. For-profit organizations that might employ athletic trainers include private rehabilitation clinics, private physicians' offices, and fitness or wellness clubs. There is also a growing number of athletic trainers who are entrepreneurs and own their own athletic training facility.

It is important for athletic trainers to realize that regardless of their organization's profit status, it is important the athletic trainer contribute to the bottom line. If expenses remain greater than revenue, the organization will experience loss. Even if the athletic trainer does not bring in direct revenue, it is important for him or her to contribute to the organization's financial status by managing the supply chain, budgeting, managing inventory, and controlling costs.

SUPPLY CHAIN MANAGEMENT

It is important to point out that athletic training is a service and certain supplies and equipment are needed to perform this service. Part of managing fiscal resources effectively includes **supply chain management** (SCM). Supply chain management incorporates organizing details of all activities involved in forming supply and service agreements, including obtaining supplies and services, and paying for supplies and services. Thorough SCM includes coordinating and collaborating with suppliers, intermediaries, third-party service providers, and customers.

Supply chain management can be an involved process, which requires advance planning. It involves much more than just selecting and ordering supplies, logging inventory (receivables), and noting low stock. It also includes monitoring why and how inventory was used, who used it, and if it was used as originally intended. This information is then used to inform future purchases and budget planning. Supply chain management typically addresses the following issues:

1. **Distribution of services**: This includes managing the number and location of service areas. For example, an athletic trainer may have to operate out of a clinical setting in the morning and an athletic training room in the afternoon. Managing the logistics of two locations requires advance planning. These logistics may also include different stakeholder values. In the previous "From the Field," the athletic trainer had to manage the expectations of the clinical director in the morning and the expectations of the athletic director and coaches in the afternoon. At times, there may be conflicts between what each person expects of the athletic trainer or in what services the athletic trainer is expected to supply. The financial implications include when, where, and how the athletic trainer is able to produce a profit. With different stakeholders and venues, the issues of how supplies are dispensed and how and where revenue is collected become a consideration.

   A second example may include managing a department that operates multiple facilities. For example, the head athletic trainer at a large university may have several athletic training rooms to operate. There is one central budget, but managing purchasing, inventory, distribution of supplies between the different athletic training rooms requires advance planning and coordination.

2. **Distribution strategy**: This includes organizing centralized versus decentralized, direct shipment, and third-party logistics. For example, an industrial or occupational athletic trainer who has multiple sites to manage and multiple sites for which to order supplies and arrange services. Having a distribution strategy involves asking questions such as, are the same services provided to each location and what supplies are needed at each location for the services being supplied? Do all supplies need to come from one supplier and do they go to a centralized location or directly to a specific site where the service is provided?

3. **Information**: Requires integrating systems and processes through the supply chain to share valuable information, such as inventory. For example, athletic trainers can use treatment or usage records to determine the most commonly used equipment or modalities. They use that information to determine purchasing patterns, strategies, supply or equipment needs, training and development opportunities for staff, and to change strategies or performance indicators for the department.

4. **Inventory management**: Requires the management of inventory, work-in-process, and finished goods. This means that the athletic trainer keeps track of inventory respective to the services provided. For example, tracking inventory so that everyone is aware that there are only four elastic bandages left will alert you to fact that you may need to order more bandages soon. However, the premise of inventory management from a supply chain perspective also requires knowing why and how those ace bandages were used (not just that stock is low). This will serve to better inform future purchases and help in strategic planning.

BUDGETING

A budget is a planning and controlling tool used specifically to state anticipated outcomes and is expressed in monetary terms.[4,9] A budget is a means to express expected income and intended expenses. The value of a budget extends beyond records of revenue and expenses. Budgeting combines several different management functions such as, strategic planning, coordinating, and controlling.[9] The budget is a tool that facilitates programmatic assessment and assists in supplying rational for using resources more effectively and efficiently.

Types of Budgets

Although many types of budgets exist, most athletic trainers will use one of the following six types of budgets: lump sum, formula, line-item, program, performance, or zero-based. Each of these types of budgets has advantages and disadvantages. In the sections that follow each of the types of budgets is described.

Lump Sum

Typically, lump sum budgeting involves the allocation of a "lump sum" of money to the athletic training department. **Lump sum budgets** often have a high-level of flexibility and control by the athletic training department. The athletic training department can allocate any portion of their "lump sum" as it sees fit, as such there is little accountability and spending is often not related to stated goals. For example, the athletic department of a high school allocates $5,000 to the athletic training department on an annual basis. The head athletic trainer, in conjunction with any staff, then decides how and where to spend that money. As along as purchases are reasonably justified by the athletic training staff, very few restrictions are enforced. Often the only restriction is not to exceed the allocated lump sum.

The benefit of lump sum budgets is that there is a high degree of autonomy for the athletic trainer. Often the athletic trainer makes the sole decision on what is to be purchased and how resources are spent. However, the drawbacks to lump sum budgeting include, purchases may have a poor relationship to larger organizational goals, and a higher risk of misappropriated spending.

Formula Budget

Formula-based funding is used primarily in schools. The advantage of formula-based budgeting is that it is one way to ensure that administrators do not engage in disproportionate spending with respect to certain schools.[3] When being funded through the **formula budget**, the budget allocation is typically tied to a numeric value such as full-time-equivalencies (FTEs), i.e., number of FTEs of registered students multiplied by a fixed dollar amount yields the budget amount. For example, if there are two athletic trainers and 100 student athletes, each athletic trainer accrues $25 of cost per student and a student athlete is budgeted $50 the resulting budget is $5,000 ([25×2] × 100 = 5,000). When a formula budget is used it is typically used in a school or university setting where number of FTEs and students can be estimated accurately.

Formula budgeting has some disadvantages. The most obvious drawback is the uncertainty of variables. For example, the number of student athletes or staff members may change suddenly. Often these numbers change and can change at the last minute leading to uncertainty in budget forecasting. Therefore, timing is a critical factor in formula budgeting because the number of FTEs is often not known until the last minute, which does not allow for much advanced planning. Other drawbacks include the fact that most schools have special-need students (or staff) that require more than the allotted amount. This fact makes it is impossible to allocate 100% of a budget via an equal formula. Therefore, what often happens is that 75% of funds are allocated by the number of students. The remaining 25% is reserved for schools with a higher number of students with quantifiable special educational needs.

Line-Item Budget

The **line-item budget** includes all income and expense associated with the department's planned spending. The line-item budget is a more traditional method of developing a budget and often uses the previous year's budget as a base and additional spending requires justification.

A line-item budget provides data of how much athletic training will spend on every item it uses that year (or financial cycle). The rationale for a line-item budget is that there is a time and place for everything. Within a line-item budget, there are broad categories with several sub-categories. For example, there may be a category for professional development expenses. Within "professional development" there may be sub-categories for travel, membership dues, books and journal subscriptions, and continuing education expenses. The sub-categories are often broken down further. For example, "professional development-travel" line may have additional lines for airfare, lodging, meal per diems, taxi/shuttles, mileage, and tolls.

Line-item budgets are fairly easy to prepare and provide a picture of exactly what is spent and where. Therefore, the primary goal of most line-item budgets is to provide spending safeguards by controlling what a department spends and delineating who is accountable for the expenditures. Table 9-1 is a sample form of a typical line-item budget.

The advantages of line-item budgets include ease of preparation and detail. Furthermore, this is an excellent planning vehicle as a means of comparing performance from one fiscal period to another fiscal period. The drawbacks include the propensity for perpetuating a line that is no longer necessary or is losing relevance. Another tendency may be to allocate too many items to the "miscellaneous line."[8]

Program and Performance Budgets

By its nature, a **program budget** focuses on the services provided to patients. Ideally, program-based budgets change the perception of the resource requester from self or departmental to services provided, thus creating organizational or service orientation as opposed to "get and spend whatever I can." Therefore, the program budget more readily relates to organizational goals and objectives. The program budget development is very similar to the line-item budget. Each program appears separately (as a line) and is broken out in categories. For example, within athletic training there are often several services (i.e., programs) that exist. Those services might include injury prevention, rehabilitation, and emergency care. Each "program" then has a budgeted amount, which is broken down by specific items within the

TABLE 9-1 Line-Item Budget

Line Item	Code	FY 2008	FY 2009	Difference	% Change
Professional Development	**AT007**	$2,000	$2,500	$500	+25%
Travel	**AT007-1**	400	1650	1250	+75%
Airfare	*AT007-1a*	*(100)*	*(800)*	*700*	
Mileage	*AT007-1b*	*(100)*	*(300)*	*200*	
Lodging	*AT007-1c*	*(100)*	*(500)*	*400*	
Tolls	*AT007-1d*	*(100)*	*(50)*	*−50*	
Conference registrations	**AT007-2**	500	400	−100	−20%
In-state	*AT007-2a*	*(150)*	*(150)*	*NA*	
Out-of-state	*AT007-2b*	*(350)*	*(250)*	*−100*	
Books & Journals	**AT007-3**	100	100	100	**NA**
Membership dues	**AT007-4**	500	350	−150	−30%

TABLE 9-2 Program-Based Budget

Line Item	FY 2007	FY 2008	Difference	% Change
Athletic Training Department	$2,000.00	$2,000.00	–	–
Injury Prevention	$1,000.00	$1,000.00	–	–
Tape	*$750.00*	*$650.00*		*−13%*
Lace-up ankle braces	*$250.00*	*$350.00*		*40%*
Rehabilitation	$500.00	$500.00	–	–
Surgical tubing	*$250.00*	*$250.00*		
Foam rolls	*$50.00*	*$50.00*		
Ankle weights	*$200.00*	*$200.00*		
Emergency Care	$500.00	$500.00	–	–
Spine Board	*$500.00*	*$500.00*		

program. Injury prevention services may require funds to purchase tape and braces; rehabilitation services may require funds to purchase exercise equipment (capital equipment) and non-capital equipment such as exercise tubing, foam rollers, and ankle weights. Table 9-2 is a sample form of a typical program-based budget.

The advantage of the program budget is that resources are allocated based on specific program goals and therefore force the athletic trainer to prioritize or place delineated values on certain programs; this is useful in establishing priorities relative to the organization or department. A disadvantage associated with the program budget is that it forces staff to rethink and analyze themselves and their value along program lines in contrast to the comfort zone associated with previous budgeting methods. In other words, people can become defensive when required to analyze, report, and justify how they spend their money and time.[8]

Similar to a program budget is a **performance budget**. Performance budgets share similar characteristics with program budgets, but performance budgets focus primarily on different athletic training functions. Performance budgets focus on tasks rather than programs. Among the items displayed within a performance budget are administrative tasks (i.e., record keeping, inventory processing); patient education (i.e., brochures, handouts, in-services); and rehabilitation tasks (i.e., therapeutic exercises, modalities, reconditioning). Expenses for each of these activities are calculated to determine the annual budget. Obviously, performance budgeting can get quite extensive after each of the tasks an athletic trainer performs is delineated. The strength of a performance budget is that it provides for the monitoring of staff members and for developing unit costs. The primary disadvantage associated with performance budgets is the emphasis on quantity, not quality, of the activity being monitored.[8]

Zero-Based Budget

Zero-based budgets require that a "clean slate" be the starting point of budget development each year. Zero-based budgeting shifts the emphasis from comparing present performance to the past. Therefore, the emphasis is shifted toward future projections and away from comparisons of past spending patterns. The zero-based budget justifies its expenditures at the time the budget is created. Zero-based budgets are typically embraced by managers because, in effect, they can start over each year and not be influenced by previous budgets. Zero-based budgets typically allocate dollars to specific categories. For example, if you have a $5,000 annual budget, you might budget $2,000 for tape, $500 to first-aid supplies, $2,000 to modalities, and $500 to office supplies. You now have zero dollars left to later spend. If you decide you want $200 more for first aid supplies then you will need to pull $200 from one of those other categories. Failure to plan ahead with zero-based budgeting can get athletic trainers in trouble, because inventory in other categories often suffers. However, zero-based budgeting is a simple and effective way to track expenditures. Zero-based budgeting is a very useful tool for management because every dollar must be accounted for, in relationship to its assigned category.

With zero-based budgeting is it easier to keep value-added items in the budgeting process. Once the most valued activities are identified, then the associated costs are estimated and planned. Accompanying zero-based budgeting is the concept of "decision packages," a method used to examine each proposed program and rank its merits in relation to organizational or departmental goals and objectives. Advantages of zero-based budgeting include its focus on identifying programs that will advance departmental goals for the future. Most zero-based budgeting advocates maintain that the method promotes innovation, effectiveness, and efficiency.[2] The downside of zero-based budgeting is its time-consuming nature. Starting at "zero" implies that all aspects of athletic training will undergo examination and justification each year, regardless of past success or tradition.

Capital Budget

Capital budgeting, also called an investment appraisal, is the planning process used to determine investments in more expensive, longer-lasting equipment. Capital budgeting includes planning for the purchase of new equipment, replacing equipment, building new facilities, or offering new services. To be considered "capital equipment," the item typically has a life span of greater than one year and meets a minimum cost level determined by the organization. In most athletic training settings, minimum capital equipment costs range between $500 to $1,000.

Capital budgets are usually their own entity and are not on the same record as the annual budget. Many capital budgets are projected out over a span of several years, typically three, four, or five years in to the future.[5] Capital budgets are subject to many variables and as such often change from year to year. Urgency and need typically take priority over practicality. Equipment to be purchased may rise or fall on the priority list based on several factors. These factors include depreciation or obsolescence of current equipment, cost of training required to use the equipment, necessity, and competitive advantage associated with owning the equipment.

Implementing a Budget

Budgeting is a cyclical process and in spite of some efforts to the contrary is difficult to separate completely from the previous year's spending patterns. Preparing the budget requires advanced planning and time. Liebler and McConnell[4] outlined three phases of the budgeting process. Each organization or department that houses athletic training will have different policies and procedures pertaining to specific details of how the budget is to be prepared and the timelines for preparation, but the following steps can serve as a guide to many health care organizations. The major phases to implementing a budget include initial preparation, review and approval, and implementation.

Initial Preparation

The initial preparation phase is the most involved and requires several action steps. The first step is to assess the previous year's budget, equipment use, and maintenance logs. Assessing these items provides trend data for the current budget as well as information on depreciation of equipment that can help provide useful data for needed equipment purchases or upgrades (which can also inform capital budget planning). While not always consulted, it is advantageous to involve individuals who will be directly affected by the budget and those who regularly operate the purchased equipment. It also can help if budget planners ask for suggestions about needed equipment, needed replacements, supplies, and if there are any special resources available of which they might not be aware.

Another aspect of initial preparation includes noting trends in spending patterns, prioritizing budget items, and stating special initiatives for the upcoming year that requires resources.[4] Identifying these needs is not a one-time occurrence. Analyzing the needs of the athletic training department is part of the ongoing "cyclical process" of budgeting. Once spending trends, equipment data, and needs are analyzed and identified, the budget is prepared and submitted to appropriate staff and perhaps certain administrators for an informal review and final suggestions before the proposed budget is submitted for final review and approval.

Review and Approval

Once the proposed budget is submitted, the second phase of review and approval begins. Review and approval process includes the competing, bargaining, and compromising in the allocations of resources between departments.[4] Often departments compete with each other for limited resources. Sometimes departments need to request resources for similar items, items that if organized might be able to be shared. It is also possible that another department has the requested equipment already. The review and approval phase can help curtail any unwarranted competition or double purchases.

This phase is best performed independent of those of who developed the proposed budget. Often up until this point in the budgeting process the proposed budget is a "wish list" that includes every possible item that could be used in the following year. During this phase the proposed budget is scrutinized and items are eliminated from the budget by those who have responsibility to allocate resources. However, these decisions cannot be made completely independent of knowledge about the requesting department or program. Therefore, it is the athletic trainer's duty to provide justification concerning the items requested on the budget. Often it is possible to reallocate or divert funds from other programs or departments to purchase equipment that will make an immediate impact or that has multiple uses. Making sure that those individuals who are ultimately responsible for allocating resources and approving the budget are familiar with and understand the scope of practice and roles of athletic trainers is an important aspect of this phase of the budgeting process. Once a budget is reviewed and approved, it needs to be implemented.

Executing an Approved Budget

The final phase is budget execution. This is simply when the allocated resources are spent on the items that have been approved. However, this is typically an ongoing process, resources may or may not be available or released all at once. It is likely that a portion of the approved resources will be released then periodically released on a designated timeline until the approved amount has been released. There are several reasons to release funds in increments. Primarily it serves to monitor revenues, but it can also be done to ensure resources are being spent judiciously as well as to reduce the risk for misappropriation.

Once a budget has been approved, there is the chance of a **budget freeze**. A budget freeze occurs when administrators stop releasing funds. Funds are typically "frozen" because revenue has decreased or is not meeting expectations. In athletic training a budget freeze usually effects travel money, short-term supplies, overtime,

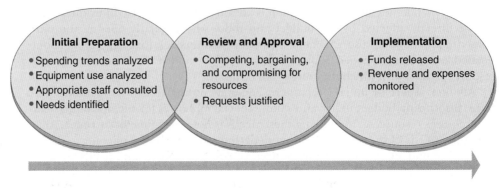

FIGURE 9-1 Chain-of-events map that delineates the budgeting process

and personnel hires. Once revenue catches up or expenses come down, the freeze can be lifted. Figure 9-1 is a chain-of-events map that outlines the budgeting process.

After a budget is executed, purchasing begins. As purchased equipment and supplies arrive, it becomes necessary to manage the growing inventory. In the next section we will discuss inventory management.

INVENTORY MANAGEMENT

Inventory includes all of the materials, equipment, or supplies that are immediately available for use by the athletic training program. Sound inventory management includes measuring **return on investment** (ROI). ROI is measuring or finding out the total benefit or outcome of expenditures. The traditional athletic training room is unique in that inventory is usually not converted into revenue. Therefore, the benefit of the inventory is proportional to the value it adds to the athletic trainer's performance or clinical outcomes.

When budgets are small, certain pieces of equipment become a luxury and not a necessity; in other words, they have a low ROI. For example, an expensive piece of equipment such as a fluidotherapy, laser, ultrasound, or electrical stimulation may not be as much of an overall benefit to the athletic program in a small rural high school than first aid supplies or preventative braces or tape might be. Therefore, the athletic trainer has to assess value of expensive equipment that may only get used periodically against supplies that are used every day or that are necessary to have on hand in case of a medical emergency.

Inventory management is a cyclical process involving several steps. These steps include communicating with vendors, purchasing, receiving and stocking, dispensing, and recording.

Communicating With Vendors

Communicating with **vendors** can take many forms. Some athletic trainers maintain a relationship with vendors purely through e-mail and Internet-based or catalog ordering; others visit vendors at conferences and exhibits; still others know a specific vendor by name and have a long-standing relationship with that specific vendor. On the other hand, there are athletic trainers who use multiple vendors for various supplies and equipment. Regardless of how the relationship is maintained, athletic trainers need to have a method for selecting and ordering equipment and supplies.

Purchasing

A very important aspect of managing inventory is knowing when to replace inventory and then having those supplies available the second they are needed.[7] Therefore, buying requires advanced planning. Deciding how much inventory to stock is also an important aspect of managing inventory. For example, answering the question of how much tape to have on hand is an important question. Should the athletic training department order all the tape needed for an entire year all at once, order it season by season, or by semester? If all the tape is purchased at once, what happens if it runs out sooner than expected, which is a risk if more is on hand and easily accessible?

Some organizations or vendors may require a purchase order (PO). A **purchase order** is an easy way to purchase supplies or equipment from an outside vendor. Essentially, a PO is the securing of permission (or pre-approval) for a payment to a vendor, which allows the athletic trainer to purchase supplies without spending money out-of-pocket.

Wise purchasing practices include the following considerations:[6]

1. Do not over purchase. Buying too much at once increases the risk of using it unnecessarily and wastes financial resources, which could be used more judiciously on higher priority supplies.

2. Purchase smaller amounts of hazardous or materials with expiration dates. Buying items that will expire in smaller amounts decreases the risk of having to throw it out if it goes unused for a longer then expected period of time.

3. Reduce the number of items purchased that are used for the same purposes. By reducing the number of items purchased that have redundant value can free up resources for other equipment or supplies.

4. Consider the available storage. Buying equipment or supplies in an amount that exceeds the available storage space increases the risk of lost or misplaced supplies.

Perhaps the most common method used for purchasing equipment in athletic training is the bid sheet.

Bid Sheets

Bid sheets are a popular method for controlling costs that allows for ordering a large bulk of items at one time. To create a bid sheet the athletic trainer compiles a master list of all needed equipment and supplies. A bid sheet includes the details of each item such as item price, number of items needed, item or order numbers, and total price (Table 9-3). The use of bid sheets allows a variety of different vendors to compete with each other. For example, the athletic trainer compiles the master list and sends it out to several different vendors. The vendors then return the bid with a sale price for either all of the items or some of the items on the submitted list. Then the athletic trainer decides from which vendor to purchase their supplies and equipment based on total cost and convenience. Depending on the vendor, this method allows athletic trainers to select the least expensive items from several vendors, ensuring a lower cost for the needed equipment. For example, vendor X sells tape for $46 a case, while vendor Y sells it for $43 per case, but vendor X also sells gauze pads for $3 per box, while Y sells them for $6 per box. After comparing each vendor's bid the athletic trainer can purchase tape from vendor Y and gauze pads from vendor X. However, some vendors place conditions on their bid and prices are only valid if all the items are purchased from a single vendor. Furthermore, vendors may not carry the same items that you are requesting and therefore, may not bid the item or may automatically include a substitution. The athletic trainer needs to be careful

LEADERSHIP ACTIVITY

Collect three different sports medicine vendor's supply catalogs (or visit their websites). Once you have at least three sources, create a mock bid sheet (with the appropriate columns, i.e., item number, item cost, quantity, total cost) of the supplies that are needed to stock an athletic trainer's medical kit. Compare the total cost of stocking a kit between each vendor, then calculate shipping and taxes for the total order. This may require contacting a sales representative from the vendor. Be sure to tell them you are a student and that this is a class project; they should be very willing to help because you are a future customer. Finally, take all three item lists and select the least expensive item from each of the vendors and create a fourth item sheet that is a composite of the least expensive items from each vendor. Compare your composite list's grand total to the least expensive list from a single vendor.

TABLE 9-3 Bid Sheet Excerpt

Item #	Item Description	Quantity	Unit Price	Price
33260	Toe aligning splint	2	$8.95	$17.90
29004M	Gauze Pads	10	$5.75	$57.50
32044M	J&J Coach 1.5 inch	30	$44.45	$1,333.50
21467	Foam Pre-Wrap	10	$39.45	$394.50
923574	Top of Form Clinic Paraffin Bath	1	$399.95	$399.95
	Pre-tax Total			**$2,203.35**
	Tax		8%	$176.27
	Shipping			$100.00
	Grand Total			**$2,479.62**

when evaluating bids to not assume every item requested was bid or that substitutions were not made. The athletic trainer should include a cover letter to the vendor that states explicitly the conditions of the bid, such as "no substitutions allowed," or "reserve the right to purchase all or part of the bid," or stating a bid deadline or other special instructions. Communicating openly with vendors allows the athletic trainer to negotiate certain points of the bid, such as shipping costs, delivery dates, giveaways, and discounts for bulk purchases.

Many vendors offer bid services directly through their website (i.e., shopping cart converted to a portable document [.pdf] or spreadsheet). This gives the athletic trainer an idea of how much purchasing supplies from that vendor will total. One disadvantage to shopping on websites is that it is time intensive and one vendor's bid sheet may not be able to be uploaded to a different vendor. If not using the vendor's website, the general steps of sending out bid sheets include using the vendor's catalog. When creating bid sheets, be sure to do the following:

1. Organize by the type of equipment and supplies. For example, all rehabilitation equipment is listed together, taping and bracing supplies are listed together, etc.
2. Describe the brand and type of equipment you desire, if any brand is acceptable, or substitutions are allowed be sure to specify that on the bid instructions.
3. Contact sales representatives and notify them of the forthcoming bid.
4. Delineate specific instructions on deadlines for receiving bids.
5. Once bids are received back from the vendors, review for any conditions from the vendor that may have been added before making a final decision.

Some vendors may ask for the opportunity to re-bid once they find out their bid was rejected. It is okay to let vendors re-bid. However, you should let all the vendors re-bid, and it is unethical to inform one vendor of a competitor's bid price.

Using local vendors may offer some unique advantages. When purchasing from local vendors the biggest advantage is usually reduced delivery costs. Often delivery is much sooner or even immediate, and delivery charges are often waived. Returning unused items is also much more efficient and less complicated. Some local vendors may even buy unused items back from you and restock them. Furthermore, purchasing from local vendors (even if a little more expensive) is a benefit to the local economy. Consider that more expensive items from local vendors may be offset by reduced shipping costs. Lastly, because access is much easier, having a good relationship with a local vendor may also cut down on your needed storage space.

Pooled Bidding

Pooled bidding is a model used by organizations with limited resources that allows for a larger size order to be made. **Pooled bidding** occurs when several smaller organizations join their resources to purchase a larger quantity of supplies. For example, a group of smaller regional hospitals, a group of local high schools, or an athletic conference may pool their money in order to buy larger quantities at a discounted price. When ordering in larger quantities, vendors are typically more willing to offer a "bargain" or reduced price per item. It is important when pooling resources to keep track of exactly how much each party ordered of each supply. Keeping accurate records may reduce any confusion when dividing up the supplies after they arrive.

Receiving and Stocking Inventory

Once the shipment of equipment and supplies arrives, be sure to thoroughly examine all the contents. Be sure everything paid for is there, that nothing is backordered, and that nothing is damaged. Cross-referencing the packing invoice with the actual contents of each box is an important step. Once all the ordered merchandise is accounted for it needs to be recorded (inventoried) and stocked.

Stocking merchandise requires thinking about access. Consider how accessible equipment and supplies need to be. If not needed immediately, it can be stored for later use at a remote location. Storing it where it will not be damaged or lost should be a high priority. For example, storing tape in a closet that gets very hot may ruin the tape. Once inventory is ready to be used, it becomes important to dispense it judiciously.

Dispensing and Recording Inventory

Athletic trainers should note when supplies are used and how much is left, then replace inventory by moving it out of a remote location or purchasing more. Every time an ankle is taped or a band-aid is used, inventory is reduced. Once inventory reaches a certain level, items will have to be replaced. Waiting until items are completely gone to reorder will mean everyone may have to go without until the new shipment arrives. Athletic trainers must monitor closely the inventory under their control. Generally speaking, inventory can be monitored by regulating use of certain items, restricting access to inventory, keeping all inventory is a secure central location, and tracking available inventory. Figure 9-2 is a schematic that outlines the inventory tracking and planning process.

Some athletic trainers may opt to order the same items every year or reuse their bid sheet template. While this may be a "time-saver," ordering the same amount of supplies every year regardless of use is not an efficient use of resources nor is it effective leadership.

Controlling Inventory

Controlling inventory can go a long way in helping to manage costs as well as ensure that what is needed is available. It is poor management to not have the equipment or supplies on hand when they are needed. The U.S. Small Business Administration[7] lists three methods used for controlling inventory that are appropriate for most athletic training settings. Visual control, tickler control, and click sheet control, are common methods used to control (or track) inventory.

Visual control is only used when inventory is small, dispensed from a single location, or seldom moved at all. This method enables managers to visually examine the inventory daily. Inventory is stored in one location where it can be easily seen and items are reordered when they appear to be at low levels.

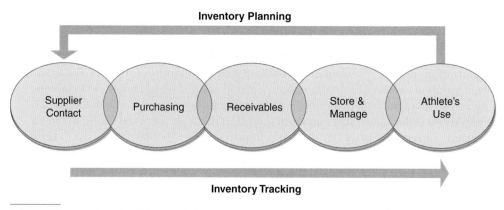

FIGURE 9-2 Inventory tracking and planning process

Tickler control requires the athletic trainer to physically count a small segment of the inventory each day. The advantage to this is each segment of the inventory is counted on a regular basis. The disadvantage is that it is very time consuming.

Click sheet control involves recording an item as it is used. Each time an item is removed from the central storage facility it is recorded. For example, once a predetermined number of cases of tape have been removed the head athletic trainer knows it is time to reorder. This method can be employed by hand or digitally using a barcode scanner. The most common way to implement this is to keep a list of supplies near the door to where inventory is stored and every time something is removed, note it on the sheet and have it initialed by whoever removed it. Obviously it is important to closely monitor who has access to the inventory.

Leadership Application

An athletic trainer at a small rural college has an open-door policy and is often in and out of the athletic training room all day. There are coaches and athletic training students who have access to all the athletic training facilities. Although his budget is tight and he sometimes goes without what other athletic trainers might consider essential supplies, he makes it work. This athletic trainer also has great rapport and works well with all the coaches, assistant coaches, and administrators. The problem is, since everything is so accessible things occasionally go "missing." These items are not stolen per se, but for example, on Friday afternoons several coolers are missing that show up again on Monday morning, or a fully stocked tape drawer is a few rolls short, or the bandages seem to run out earlier than normal, but he can not recall an increase of "scrapes and cuts" recently. It is obvious there is an inventory control problem, but the athletic trainer is afraid if he institutes too stringent an inventory control policy he will lose favor with administrators and coaches. His rationale is "After all, the athletic department ultimately is buying the stuff anyway, so why should access to coaches be limited if they truly need it?"

Critical Thinking Questions

1. Do you think this scenario is a problem, if so, how might you handle it? If not, why not?
2. What potential dangers or risks might occur if an inventory control policy was not implemented?
3. How can the trainer make coaches and administrators aware of these risks and how might he recruit administrators to help manage these risks?
4. How would you handle staff members or peers who were stealing inventory?

CHAPTER SUMMARY

Managing financial resources through understanding supply chain management, budgeting, and controlling inventory are important components of successful financial management and a critical managerial role for athletic trainers. Understanding the various application and uses for different types of budgets can help the athletic trainer make decisions based on what is best for their athletic training program given its unique circumstances. The three phases of implementing a budget, 1) initial preparation; 2) review and approval; and 3) implementation, can be employed regardless of budget type. Once the budget is implemented, purchasing, receiving, and managing inventory can have significant implications for future budgeting and departmental effectiveness. The athletic trainer who accurately tracks inventory, including tracking how inventory was used, is likely to minimize financial risks and increase the probability of making sound future financial decisions.

References

1. Borger C, Smith S, Truffer C, Keehan S, Sisko A, Poisai J, Clemens M. (2006). Health spending projections through 2015: Changes on the horizon. *Health Affairs* Jan-June, 61–73.

2. Dossett J. *Budgets and financial management in special libraries.* Accessed May 29, 2007 at http://www.libsci.sc.edu/BOB/class/clis724/SpecialLibrariesHandbook/ Budgets%20and%20Financial%20Management.htm

3. Levacic R. (1993). Assessing the impact of formula funding on schools. *Oxford Review of Education 19*(4), 435–458.

4. Liebler JG, McConnell CR. (2004). *Management principles for health professionals.* Boston, MA: Jones & Bartlett.

5. McConnell, CR. (2006). *Umiker's management skills for a new health care supervisor.* Boston, MA: Jones & Bartlett.

6. Minnesota Pollution Control Agency. *Inventory management.* Hazardous Waste Division Fact Sheet #2.62. Retrieved June 5, 2007 from http://www.pca.state.mn.us/waste/pubs/ 2_62.pdf

7. United States Small Business Administration. *Inventory management.* Management and Planning Series. Retrieved June 5, 2007 from http://www.sba.gov/library/pubs/ mp-22.pdf

8. Warner, A. S. (1992). *Owning your numbers: An introduction to budgeting for special libraries: An SLA self-study program.* Washington, DC: Special Libraries Association.

9. Westmoreland D. (2003). Managing costs and budgets. In: Yoder-Wise P, ed. *Leading and managing in nursing.* St. Louis, MO: Mosby 216–234.

Chapter 10

Reimbursement and Revenue

"I think the person who takes a job in order to live—that is to say, for the money—has turned himself into a slave."

JOSEPH CAMPBELL

CHAPTER RATIONALE

Role Delineation Study Components

Domain V: Organization and Administration

- Knowledge of reimbursement issues

Educational Competencies

- Describe the various types of insurance policies (HMO, PPO, fee-for-service), the common benefits and exclusions identified with these types of policies, and the procedures for filing health care insurance claims.

Key Terms

Accident: The direct result of a documented trauma that has an identifiable time and place.

Capitation: A reimbursement system in which the providers are paid a set amount for a certain number of patients in a given time frame regardless of number of visits or services to those patients.

Co-payment: The amount of money paid by the insured at the time any service is rendered; typically, a nominal fee for a doctor visit, emergency room visit, or prescription.

Deductible: The amount of money the insured (first party) is responsible to pay for any covered health-related expenses.

Exclusions: Health-related conditions that are not covered under the insurance policy.

Fee-for-service: The traditional reimbursement model in which the health care provider is paid by the patient when service is performed.

First party: The insured individual (or patient).

Health insurance: A policy held that will pay specified sums of money for medical expenses or treatments incurred as a result of covered injuries or illnesses.

Health maintenance organization (HMO): A group of health care providers intentionally organized to offer predefined services to members.

Health savings accounts: A form of self-coverage in which money can be saved for medical expenses in a tax-deferred status.

Health care common procedure coding system (HCPCS): Codes for items not covered in the CPT codes, such as, ambulance service, orthotics, and supplies.

Incident to billing: Billing under a licensed physician (or other health care provider).

Insurance: A system created to minimize financial losses to an individual or organization by transferring risk of loss from the insured to the insurer.

Medical insurance: Insurance that covers only medical expenses related to a diagnosed illness.

Preferred provider organization (PPO): A group of medical providers (similar to an HMO) who have contracted to provide care to a specific population.

Premium: A fee (usually monthly) paid by the first party to the insurance company for health care coverage.

Reimbursement: The amount of money a third-party payer is willing to pay for services rendered.

Revenue: The total amount of money generated by a business before any deductions are taken out.

Rider: An addendum to an insurance policy that expands coverage to include certain exclusions.

Second party: The health care provider.

Third party: The person who is contracted to pay.

Usual, customary, and reasonable (UCR): Signifies the reimbursement rate a third-party payer pays to a health care provider.

The span of practice for athletic trainers has grown dramatically since the profession's inception. In the traditional role, athletic trainers had little need of reimbursement. However, many athletic trainers now find themselves in venues where reimbursement and revenue are vital to their survival and longevity. Furthermore, innovative athletic trainers are finding ways to gain reimbursement in the traditional and in new athletic training settings. This growth has facilitated several innovations within the profession of athletic training.

The chance for reimbursement has created a huge opportunity for athletic trainers in terms of revenue generation. Today there are third-party payers and insurance companies who recognize the value athletic trainers provide their clients and are reimbursing athletic trainers for health care services. Therefore, it is important that the athletic trainer have a basic understanding of how insurance and reimbursement work within the health care industry. Furthermore, assimilating leadership behaviors such as communication, strategic thinking, and diagnosing, then integrating those leadership behaviors with important management skills can help make revenue generation and reimbursement a meaningful reality for athletic trainers.

In this chapter we will look into the issues of health insurance, third-party payers, reimbursement, and revenue. We will begin by examining the different types of insurance coverage, including primary and secondary insurance. Next, we will discuss the different types of third-party payers, such as health maintenance organizations (HMO) and Medicare. Finally, we will discuss reimbursement, coding, and billing for athletic trainers.

INSURANCE

The health care industry recognizes three parties. The **first party** is the insured or patient, the **second party** is the health care provider, and the **third party** is the payer. Most often the third party is an insurance company with which the patient (first party) has contracted. **Insurance** is a system created to minimize financial losses to an individual or organization by transferring risk of loss from the insured to the insurer. Insurance can be purchased to alleviate financial burden of replacing a home or automobile or to minimize risk of legal expenses (i.e., liability). Insurance can also be purchased to minimize loss due to medical or health related hardships.

Health insurance is a policy that will pay specified sums of money for medical expenses or treatments incurred as a result of covered injuries or illnesses. Health policies can offer many options and vary in their approaches to coverage. Health insurance is an agreed-upon contract between the holder of the policy and the insurance company. Most health insurance companies also offer additional benefits to the insured for efforts preventing sickness. Examples of efforts to prevent sickness may include routine well checkups or agreeing not to smoke. The primary way insurance companies offer these benefits is by covering a portion of the expenses related to preventive care or by providing non-smokers a lower premium than smokers. There are some insurers that may also provide a benefit (i.e., reimbursement of fitness club memberships) for living a healthy lifestyle. On the other hand **medical insurance**, which is slightly different from health insurance, typically only covers medical expenses related to a diagnosed illness. In other words, medical insurance typically will not give a benefit for maintaining good health or for preventive care.

The premise for either type of insurance is that the insured or client pays a premium. A **premium** is a monthly fee that the insured pays (whether sick or well) to the insurance company and in return, if the insured is ever sick or injured the insurance company pays a portion of the expenses of that sickness or injury. In other words, the insurance company assumes the risk for the bulk of any necessary health care expenses. How much the insurance company pays depends on an agreement between the insured and insurance provider. If the insured desires a higher level of payment by the insurance company then the premium is higher, because the risk is higher to the insurance company. If the insured agrees to assume a greater level of financial risk of any injury or illness then the premium can be negotiated down.

Most health insurance policies are written at an 80–20 percent ratio (but can vary). That is, the insurance company agrees to pay 80% of any medical expenses and the insured pays 20% of medical expenses and any deductible or co-pay. A **deductible** is the amount of the billed claim the individual must pay before the insurance company begins to pay. Another way for the insured to negotiate a lower premium is agree to pay a higher deductible. Deductibles usually have an annual maximum. Therefore, once the insured pays (out of his or her pocket) the entire deductible amount, the insurance company pays all other medical expenses accumulated that year. This way the insured is guaranteed that no matter what medical or health conditions arise in a year there is a maximum out-of-pocket amount that is not exceeded by the insured (patient). A **co-payment** (co-pay) is the amount of money paid by the insured at the time any service is rendered. Typically co-pays are a nominal fee for a doctor visit, emergency room visit, or prescription. The insurance company then pays the balance of any medical expenses accrued for that visit. Co-pays may or may not be considered part of the deductible.

In recent years there have many different attempts to regulate and reform this aspect of health care. Part of health care reform efforts has been to regulate insurance prices. In spite of the discussions on health care reform, few actual changes in policy have taken place. However, there has been a rise in the awareness of organizations and health care providers of the increased costs. This awareness has helped to foster innovation and creativity within the health care insurance system.

Primary Coverage

Most individuals will use primary insurance to pay for medical expenses. Primary insurance begins to pay as soon as any deductible is covered. Very large institutions that offer primary insurance to their employees or athletes typically do not have to pay an annual deductible, however premiums are usually higher. Most athletes and traditional patients are covered by their personal insurance policy. Very few athletic programs or institutions provide primary insurance for their athletes. Supplemental coverage, such a long-term or short-term disability, catastrophic, or accidental coverage, can be purchased to offset any expenses not covered by the primary policy. In respect to athletes, many universities defer to the athlete's (or their parent's) insurance policies for primary coverage. However, many athletic departments offer secondary coverage (for covered accidents only) to eliminate any out-of-pocket expense to the athlete (or their parents).

Exclusions and Riders

Many insurance policies have exclusions. **Exclusions** are health-related conditions that are not covered under the insurance policy. A typical exclusion might be for an injury with an insidious onset. Typically an **accident** is defined as something that is a direct result of a documented trauma associated with an identifiable time and place. Illnesses and overuse injuries typically have a difficult time satisfying this definition. Other exclusions may include pre-existing conditions. Pre-existing conditions include documented injuries that occurred before an insurance policy is enacted or, for an athlete, an injury that occurred outside of a sanctioned event. A **rider** is an addendum to a policy and is one way to expand a policy to cover exclusions. Riders are any additions to the insurance policy that covers conditions that normally might not be included in a health insurance policy. Riders are written and added to the insurance policy on a separate piece of paper, hence the term "rider." Adding riders increases the premium, but may be worth the extra expense in the case of known exclusions or pre-existing injuries. Another common rider is the multiple indemnity rider, which allows for a greater (double or triple) disbursement of funds to a beneficiary if certain conditions are met, such as accidental death.

Secondary Coverage

Secondary insurance is a type of insurance that pays only after all other insurances have paid their agreed-upon maximum. Many athletic programs offer secondary insurance. This means that the athletic department's insurance company only pays what is left of the bill after the athlete or athlete's parents submit the bill to their primary insurance. Let's say there is a $10,000 dollar insurance bill for an athlete's injury and the athlete's institution offers secondary insurance. That $10,000 bill would first be submitted to the athlete and his/her parent's primary insurance, which pays 80% of the bill, leaving a 20% balance. Secondary coverage would then be applied. When the athlete or parents receive the bill for the 20% balance, it is submitted to the athlete's university insurance policy (along with the Explanation of Benefits), which pays the remaining 20%. In this scenario, there is no out-of-pocket expense to the athlete or their parents. However, the athlete's personal insurance company is included in the payment process.

Self Coverage

Self insurance is an option when there is considerably less health risk to the individual. In essence, the individual assumes all of the risk. The "premium" that would normally be paid to the insurance company is retained by the individual and put into an escrow or personal savings account to be used for any medical expenses. Therefore, the individual saves the money that would normally be paid out to the insurance company. The benefit of this is that the individual earns interest on their own money instead of the insurance company and claims are easier to manage. Because there is no insurance company, the bill is just paid by the individual without any claims or insurance paperwork. One obvious disadvantage of self insurance is running out of money before all medical expenses are paid. The success of self coverage is also dependent on the individual's willingness and ability to actually set aside and save money for medical expenses every month.

Health savings accounts (HSA) are a form of self coverage in which money can be saved for medical expenses in a tax deferred status. In an HSA the patient pays a pre-set amount of medical bills directly. After that amount is satisfied, the HSA funds can be used to cover any tax deductible medical expense, this list of medical expenses is very broad. A benefit of HSAs is that the individual gets to keep money that is left over. HSA funds can be managed by the individual in one of two ways: 1) save money (tax-free) for future medical expenses and the interest that you accrue is also tax-free; or 2) withdraw money from the HSA at the end of the year, but would need to maintain a minimum balance. In HSA there is a severe penalty for using the money for non-medical expenses, such as paying full taxes and a 15% penalty.[2]

MANAGED CARE ORGANIZATIONS

Third-party payers are those groups (i.e., insurance companies) who pay for the medical expense. There are many types and styles of third-party payers also known as Managed Care Organizations (MCO). MCOs arrange any payments to health care providers in lieu of **fee-for-service.** Fee-for-service is the traditional reimbursement model in which the health care provider is paid by the patient when service is performed. Examples of third party payers include: Health Maintenance Organization (HMO), Preferred Provider Organization (PPO), Exclusive Provider Organization (EPO), and Point-of-Service (POS). Other third-party payers may include the government (i.e., Medicare or Medicaid), worker's compensation, or indemnity plans. Ultimately, the difference between each type of MCO is the availability and accessibility of health care providers.

HMO

A **health maintenance organization** (HMO) is a group of health care providers intentionally organized to offer predefined services to members. Participants in HMOs must select their primary care provider from an approved list of providers who participate in that specific HMO. Seeing a health care provider outside of that HMO requires pre-approval. In other words, care is restricted to certain providers, except in the case of an emergency. The HMO typically pays the medical provider on a sliding scale or on a per-patient basis (called capitation).

Capitation is a reimbursement system where the providers are paid a set amount for a certain number of patients in a given time frame regardless of number of visits or services to those patients.[1] Critics of capitation claim that the quality of medical care is threatened because the fewer procedures or services offered, or patients seen means less cost to the medical provider. Therefore, if services and visits are kept to a minimum, the medical provider potentially can make more money. Patients covered by HMOs (and other MCOs) also typically have to pay a co-payment for each office visit or other services, such as prescriptions or ER visits.

PPO

A **preferred provider organization** (PPO) is similar to an HMO, but consists of medical providers who have contracted to provide care to a specific population. PPOs offer a financial incentive (inexpensive co-pays and greater reimbursement) if the policyholder uses medical providers within the PPO. The policyholder has the option to use any provider they want, unlike an HMO, but they pay more (sometimes substantially more) for using providers outside of the PPO. In other words, PPO-approved providers agree to offer their services at a discount. Medical providers in a PPO are typically paid on a fee-for-service basis, instead of capitation. **Exclusive provider organizations** (EPOs) are very similar to PPOs. The only exception is that policyholders in an EPO cannot go outside of the EPO for medical care unless they are willing to pay 100% of the medical expense.

POS

Point-of-Service (POS) is a hybrid of the HMO and PPO models. POS plans allow policyholders to receive care from member medical providers, typically a family or general practitioner, however, policyholders have the option to receive medical care from other providers if certain conditions are met and a referral is made by their primary care physician. This type of system (like an HMO) is often referred to as a gatekeeper system. Gatekeepers help to coordinate patient care from a "central" location. The ideology behind a gatekeeper system is to prevent the patient from seeking unneeded or unwarranted medical care on their own.

Individual Practice Association

An **individual practice association** (IPA) is similar to an HMO. The primary difference is that care is given by a group of individual medical providers in their offices as opposed to a large medical facility. An HMO may contract with an IPA, which in turn contracts with local physicians to treat members at a pre-negotiated price. IPAs can consist of any specialty, but are primarily groups of general practitioners.

Other Third-Party Payers

Other third-party payers are administered by the government, worker's compensation, or indemnity plans. Governmental plans include Medicare and Medicaid. Medicare is a federally regulated program that pays for all or some (depending on qualification) for the elderly and disabled. Likewise, Medicaid is federally administered health care for low income patients. Worker's compensation is typically regulated by individual states and is paid if an employee has an accident at work. In worker's compensation, employers pay the premiums to special insurers who strive to get employees back to work sooner.[5] Theoretically, premiums paid by the employer cost less than time and productivity lost from employees not being on the job. **Indemnity plans** are the most traditional fee-for-service structure where the provider charges the patient (or insurance provider) on a set fee schedule. Therefore, allowing the patient to seek care whenever and wherever they choose.

EOB

Explanation of benefits (EOB) is a third-party payer's written response to a claim. Often the EOB can be confusing because procedural codes are used instead of descriptions of the services rendered. It is important that athlete's keep an EOB for reference and for future claims. Often a secondary insurance provider will ask for an EOB before they will provide payment for the remaining balance. Figure 10-1 is an example of an EOB with descriptions of how to interpret the information on the EOB.

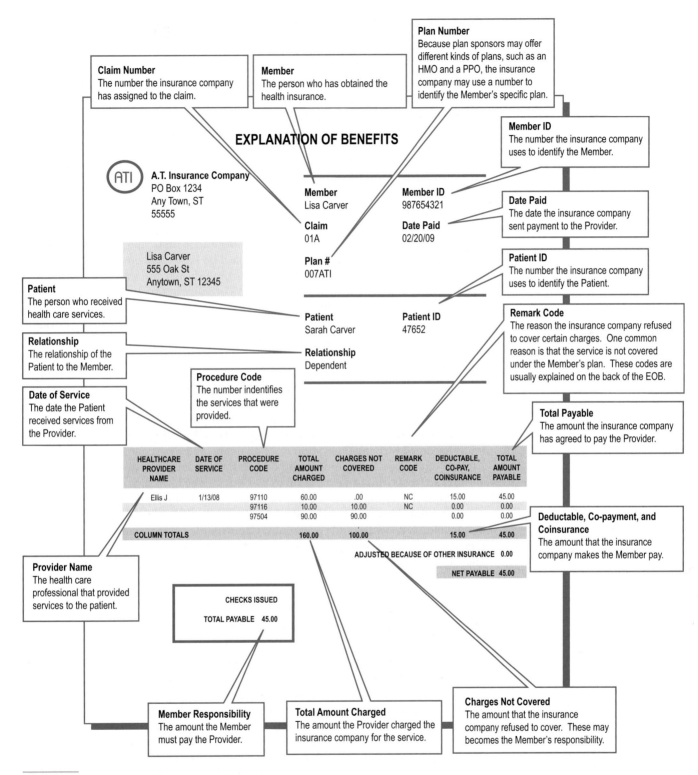

EXPLANATION OF BENEFITS

Claim Number
The number the insurance company has assigned to the claim.

Member
The person who has obtained the health insurance.

Plan Number
Because plan sponsors may offer different kinds of plans, such as an HMO and a PPO, the insurance company may use a number to identify the Member's specific plan.

Member ID
The number the insurance company uses to identify the Member.

ATI
A.T. Insurance Company
PO Box 1234
Any Town, ST
55555

Member
Lisa Carver

Member ID
987654321

Date Paid
The date the insurance company sent payment to the Provider.

Claim
01A

Date Paid
02/20/09

Lisa Carver
555 Oak St
Anytown, ST 12345

Plan #
007ATI

Patient ID
The number the insurance company uses to identify the Patient.

Patient
The person who received health care services.

Patient
Sarah Carver

Patient ID
47652

Remark Code
The reason the insurance company refused to cover certain charges. One common reason is that the service is not covered under the Member's plan. These codes are usually explained on the back of the EOB.

Relationship
The relationship of the Patient to the Member.

Relationship
Dependent

Procedure Code
The number indentifies the services that were provided.

Total Payable
The amount the insurance company has agreed to pay the Provider.

Date of Service
The date the Patient received services from the Provider.

HEALTHCARE PROVIDER NAME	DATE OF SERVICE	PROCEDURE CODE	TOTAL AMOUNT CHARGED	CHARGES NOT COVERED	REMARK CODE	DEDUCTABLE, CO-PAY, COINSURANCE	TOTAL AMOUNT PAYABLE
Ellis J	1/13/08	97110	60.00	.00	NC	15.00	45.00
		97116	10.00	10.00	NC	0.00	0.00
		97504	90.00	90.00		0.00	0.00
COLUMN TOTALS			160.00	100.00		15.00	45.00

ADJUSTED BECAUSE OF OTHER INSURANCE 0.00

NET PAYABLE 45.00

Deductable, Co-payment, and Coinsurance
The amount that the insurance company makes the Member pay.

Provider Name
The health care professional that provided services to the patient.

CHECKS ISSUED

TOTAL PAYABLE 45.00

Member Responsibility
The amount the Member must pay the Provider.

Total Amount Charged
The amount the Provider charged the insurance company for the service.

Charges Not Covered
The amount that the insurance company refused to cover. These may becomes the Member's responsibility.

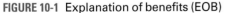

FIGURE 10-1 Explanation of benefits (EOB)

Other Types of Insurance Coverage

There are other types of insurance that are not typically covered under traditional health insurance policies, yet are often necessary for the individual to carry. For example, dental and optical insurance may have to be purchased as well as health insurance. Even though dentists and optometrists may be listed in the catalog of approved providers, a separate dental or optical policy is often needed. These additional insurance policies often function similar to health insurance, but require a separate policy of their own. For example, in the case of dental insurance basic and preventative dental cleanings, oral x-rays, etc. are provided to members. Any premium, deductible, or co-pay is the responsibility of the insured and service is provided by a group of dentists pre-approved by your dental carrier. In the case of optical, a premium is paid in exchange for routine office visits, eye exams, and prescription eye glasses.

Disability insurance is another type of insurance that may help recover lost income resulting from an accident or trauma. The basic concept of disability insurance is to replace a portion or all annual income should the insured be rendered unable to work. There is a huge diversity in coverage between disability insurance companies. Furthermore, definitions of disability vary between companies. The amount and type of disability often play a significant role in the benefit provided. For example, disability can be defined as not being able to perform any occupation at all or it can be limited to the insured's current occupation. In the latter definition, other employment may be allowed and the insured can still collect all or a portion of disability. Typically insurance companies will not pay for disability that is a result of a suicide attempt, drug abuse, war, or attempts to commit a crime. Pre-existing conditions also are not typically covered under disability policies.

Short-term disability is a policy that pays a benefit during the initial stages of an injury for time lost. Sometimes short-term disability can be part of the employee benefit package and allows for an uninterrupted break in income for extended time off, usually for two weeks, but can extend up to two years. Long-term disability coverage helps recover income for longer time-frames and may range from five years to retirement.

Catastrophic insurance, also called "major medical" insurance, typically has high deductibles, but low monthly premiums. Catastrophic plans usually cover major hospital and medical expenses above the deductible. The majority of catastrophic insurances cover expenses for hospital stays, surgery, and intensive care.

REVENUE AND REIMBURSEMENT

An important aspect of the insurance industry is reimbursement to the health care providers. Health insurance companies reimburse health care providers based on what is considered **usual, customary, and reasonable** (UCR). UCR helps to regulate health care provider charges by reimbursing only what another health care provider might charge. Many insurance companies use this system, but it was originally designed for the Medicare system. The UCR model was designed to protect the individual from excessive or inflated fees. This concept provides that the insurance company pay only what the *usual* fee is for similar services by other providers. Furthermore, it also provides for *customary* fees, that is the lowest of either the national average or 90th percentile. The 90th-percentile fee is the fee that 90% of all other medical providers charge in a given locale. Lastly, reimbursement is *reasonable*, which in this case means the lower of the two aforementioned aspects.

Revenue is the total amount of money generated before any deductions are taken out. **Reimbursement** is the amount of money a third-party payer is willing to pay for services rendered. Reimbursement can be complex to navigate initially. Until recently athletic trainers had little reason to concern themselves with revenue or reimbursement issues. However, as the profession of athletic training continues to grow and evolve and options for work settings continue open revenue generation has become something the athletic trainer needs to consider. Not all athletic trainers will need to generate revenue. However, athletic trainers in private clinics, rehabilitation or outpatient clinics, or occupational settings may benefit from revenue generation. Many athletic trainers' jobs can be justified by the revenue they produce. To stay competitive and increase job security, athletic trainers may need to be able to produce revenue for their employers.

Other models that the athletic trainer can employ to generate revenue include cash-based reimbursement, which bypasses third-party payers and bills patients directly. The difficulty with cash-based models is deciding a fare amount to bill patients. Two avenues to deciding appropriate pricing include UCR pricing and the second is based on the following equation, cost = time + materials + overhead + expenses + profit. There have been many athletic trainers who are able to generate enough revenue to sustain a viable sports medicine or rehabilitation business using cash-based reimbursement. However, the primary way many athletic trainers produce revenue is through third-party reimbursement. Taking advantage of third-party reimbursement requires knowledge of billing procedures.

NATA Committee on Revenue

The National Athletic Trainers' Association has established a standing committee with the sole purpose of dealing with reimbursement issues for the athletic trainer. The stated purpose of NATA's Committee on Revenue (NATACOR) is to pursue third-party reimbursement for athletic training services.[3] The NATACOR has six stated goals:

1. Continue to educate NATA members about reimbursement issues.
2. Encourage the establishment of reimbursement committees within each state athletic training association.
3. Approach national health care groups to seek NATA representation.
4. Approach payers on a national level to solicit support for reimbursement of ATCs.
5. Establish liaisons with appropriate groups to enhance the reimbursement efforts of ATCs.
6. Coordinate all reimbursement activities with the NATA Governmental Affairs Committee, the Clinical/Industrial/Corporate Committee, the Secondary School Committee and the College/University Committee.

Additional information on the role and function of the Committee on Revenue, as well as helpful information on gaining medical referrals can be retrieved from the NATA website.

Billing

Athletic trainers are entitled to bill third-party payers directly. Likewise, athletic trainers can bill "incident to" for non-therapy services. **Incident to billing** refers to billing under a licensed physician (or other health care provider). This means that the physician is billing the patient even though the service was performed by an athletic trainer. Most "incident to billing" requires that the actual service provider (in this case the athletic trainer) be licensed as well as the providing physician. In many cases this service is called physician extender (Box 10-1). Many third party-payers will

---

BOX 10-1   Common Physician Extender Tasks Performed by an Athletic Trainer

- Perform triage.
- Conduct initial patient medical history, brief injury evaluation, and prepare patient for physician evaluation.
- Assist physician in patient treatment.
- Answer patient questions after physician has left the exam or treatment room.
- Schedule special tests and procedures.
- Dictate examination and checkup notes.
- Perform gait training, crutch fitting, or orthotic fitting.
- Assist with therapeutic exercise and rehabilitation.
- Cast or the assist in casting of patients.
- Provide specific rehabilitation suggestions while the patient is evaluated by the physician.
- Prepare patient educational materials after the evaluation.
- Fit braces or medical supplies ordered by the physician.
- Provide rehabilitation and athletic training services in an outreach setting.

---

accept "incident to" claims. As the physician extender model of athletic training proliferates, this type of billing may increase for athletic trainers. It is critical that athletic trainers be familiar with their state's practice act as well as restrictions from individual payers if acting as a physician extender.

Direct billing is also a very good option for athletic trainers. To facilitate direct billing all athletic trainers are encouraged to register for a National Provider Identifier (NPI) number. Attaining an NPI number is an important step for the recognition of athletic trainers as legitimate health care providers. When billing athletic trainers need to be able to refer to specific diagnostic and procedural codes.

Coding

There are two types of codes athletic trainers need to be aware of and should take care to document correctly if planning to seek reimbursement from third-party payers. Diagnostic codes are those codes, which identifies an injury or illness. Procedural codes are those codes that identify a procedure, such as a modality, therapeutic procedure, or evaluation and assign it a numerical code. Both codes are necessary if reimbursement is desired.

Diagnostic Codes

The International Classification of Diseases (ICD) is published by the World Health Organization and is currently in its tenth edition, hence ICD-10. However, the ICD-9 (ninth edition) codes are currently being used in the United States. These codes are required by all third-party payers and uses standard language to identify the exact illnesses, injuries, or diseases that are being treated. The ICD-9 codes are organized as codes, sub-codes, and a condition. For example, sprains for the foot or ankle all require an 845 code and more specifically, a deltoid ligament sprain is coded 845.01. Table 10-1 is an example of a typical ICD-9 classification table. When communicating with third-party payers about billing, it is important to use the specific codes to ensure timely and correct reimbursement.

Procedural Codes

Used in conjunction with ICD-9 codes are Current Procedural Terminology (CPT) codes. CPT codes are a list of reference numbers published by the American

TABLE 10-1 ICD-9 Codes

Code	First Subcode	Second Subcode	Diagnosis/Condition
845			Sprains and strains of ankle and foot
	845.0		Ankle
		845.00	Unspecified site
		845.01	Deltoid (ligament), ankle
		845.02	Calcaneofibular (ligament)
		845.03	Tibiofibular (ligament), distal
		845.09	Other

Medical Association that correspond to specific medical procedures. These procedures are represented by an assigned number. Athletic trainers have their own CPT codes (i.e., 97001 – 97755 series). Athletic trainers can also use other physical medicine related codes. For example, when performing traction for an injury the athletic trainer would report to the third party payer CPT code 97012 instead of listing "traction." Table 10-2 is a list of CPT codes used by athletic trainers for reimbursement (note this is not a complete list). It is critical when submitting claims to third-party payers that the athletic trainer be diligent to use the correct diagnostic and procedural codes.

There are other codes that are used in health care examples e.g., DRG codes (Diagnosis Related Group). DRG codes are used to classify inpatient hospital services and are commonly used by many insurance companies and Medicare. There are also UB codes (i.e., universal billing), which are a list of reference numbers that refer to the types of services provided by hospitals.

Processing Claims

One of the most daunting tasks in the insurance process for an athletic trainer can be processing claims. Each third-party payer has specific idiosyncrasies to their claim

TABLE 10-2 Athletic Training CPT Codes

Category	CPT Code	Procedure
Evaluations	97005	Athletic training evaluation
	97006	Athletic training re-evaluation
Supervised Modalities		*Does not require direct (one-on-one) patient contact*
	97010	Hot or cold pack
	97012	Traction
	97014	Electrical stimulation
	97016	Vasopneumatic device (compression pump)
	97018	Paraffin bath
	97022	Whirlpool
Constant attendance		*Does require direct (one-on-one) patient contact for each 15 minutes*
	97032	Electrical stimulation
	97033	Iontophoresis
	97034	Contrast bath
	97035	Ultrasound

and filing processes. However, if the athletic trainer is thorough there is little reason to be intimidated about filing claims. Gaining experience with different third-party payers can facilitate the claim process. When filing claims it is important that the athletic trainer filing the claim be aware of their state's practice act. Obviously you do not want to commit fraud by submitting a bill for something that is not permitted for athletic trainers in your state. It will also be valuable to have the ICD-9, CPT, and **health care common procedure coding system** (HCPCS) manuals available for consultation. HCPCS codes are for items not covered in the CPT codes, such as, ambulance service, orthotics, and supplies. Codes from each of these manuals are likely to be required to accurately complete the claim form.

The specific forms used for filing claims vary according to third-party payer, but most third-party payers do accept the Center for Medicare and Medicaid Services (CMS) forms. The CMS 1500 is the standard claim form used by individuals or those not associated with a specific institution (Fig. 10-2). The UB 04 is the form that should be used by recognized institutions, such as a hospital (Fig. 10-3). The process for filing a claim needs to be done carefully to ensure correct and timely reimbursement.

After you get an NPI number, the first step in filing a claim should involve the knowledge of specific payer's claim time-lines. Payer's time-lines vary. Some payers may require filing a claim within 30, 60, or 90 days, after which all claims are denied or not eligible. When you submit a claim using either the CMS 1500, UB 04, or a payer's form, double check that the CPT and diagnostic codes are correct and that the treatment matches the diagnosis. It is also important to fill out the form in its entirety; be sure to include the patient's personal and insurance information. For this reason it is important to collect a copy of the patient's insurance card(s) and driver's license before any service or treatment is delivered. Once the form is completed, double check all the information that you are submitting for accuracy and correctness.

There are options available for submitting claims. The athletic trainer can always fill out the forms longhand or electronically and submit them, or a billing service can be hired. Some billing services require a fee up front and some will keep a percentage of what is collected. There is also software available that can be used via Internet and submitted directly to the payer.

The NATACOR has identified five common reasons payments may be ignored, denied, or reduced. Those five reasons are the following:

1. You have a contracted rate with a carrier and billed more than what was contracted.
2. You have billed the wrong codes.
3. The carrier only paid for partial services, because they deem some aspect inappropriate for the condition identified, or some of the services are not covered by the patient's policy.
4. The carrier is waiting for all the claims to come in for a specific claim.
5. You did not collect a co-payment charge and billed for the entire amount. The payer deducted the patient's portion of the bill.
    Other possible reasons for claim denial:
6. You are not an approved provider for the insurance company.
7. You did not have a physician's referral or order.
8. All the required paper work was not complete or submitted.

Ultimately, the EOB will give the exact reason for the denial or delay of any claim. If a claim is denied and the health care provider believes the denial was unjustified

1500

HEALTH INSURANCE CLAIM FORM

APPROVED BY NATIONAL UNIFORM CLAIM COMMITTEE 08/05

PICA

CARRIER

PICA

1. MEDICARE (Medicare #) MEDICAID (Medicaid #) TRICARE CHAMPUS (Sponsor's SSN) CHAMPVA (Member ID#) GROUP HEALTH PLAN (SSN or ID) FECA BLKLUNG (SSN) OTHER (ID) 1a. INSURED'S I.D. NUMBER (For Program in Item 1)

2. PATIENT'S NAME (Last Name, First Name, Middle Initial)

3. PATIENT'S BIRTH DATE MM DD YY SEX M F

4. INSURED'S NAME (Last Name, First Name, Middle Initial)

5. PATIENT'S ADDRESS (No., Street)

6. PATIENT RELATIONSHIP TO INSURED Self Spouse Child Other

7. INSURED'S ADDRESS (No., Street)

CITY STATE

8. PATIENT STATUS Single Married Other
Employed Full-Time Student Part-Time Student

CITY STATE

ZIP CODE TELEPHONE (Include Area Code) ( )

ZIP CODE TELEPHONE (Include Area Code) ( )

9. OTHER INSURED'S NAME (Last Name, First Name, Middle Initial)

10. IS PATIENT'S CONDITION RELATED TO:

11. INSURED'S POLICY GROUP OR FECA NUMBER

a. OTHER INSURED'S POLICY OR GROUP NUMBER

a. EMPLOYMENT? (Current or Previous) YES NO

a. INSURED'S DATE OF BIRTH MM DD YY SEX M F

b. OTHER INSURED'S DATE OF BIRTH MM DD YY SEX M F

b. AUTO ACCIDENT? YES NO PLACE (State)

b. EMPLOYER'S NAME OR SCHOOL NAME

c. EMPLOYER'S NAME OR SCHOOL NAME

c. OTHER ACCIDENT? YES NO

c. INSURANCE PLAN NAME OR PROGRAM NAME

d. INSURANCE PLAN NAME OR PROGRAM NAME

10d. RESERVED FOR LOCAL USE

d. IS THERE ANOTHER HEALTH BENEFIT PLAN? YES NO If yes, return to and complete item 9 a-d.

READ BACK OF FORM BEFORE COMPLETING & SIGNING THIS FORM.
12. PATIENT'S OR AUTHORIZED PERSON'S SIGNATURE I authorize the release of any medical or other information necessary to process this claim. I also request payment of government benefits either to myself or to the party who accepts assignment below.

SIGNED _____ DATE _____

13. INSURED'S OR AUTHORIZED PERSON'S SIGNATURE I authorize payment of medical benefits to the undersigned physician or supplier for services described below.

SIGNED _____

14. DATE OF CURRENT: MM DD YY ILLNESS (First symptom) OR INJURY (Accident) OR PREGNANCY(LMP)

15. IF PATIENT HAS HAD SAME OR SIMILAR ILLNESS. GIVE FIRST DATE MM DD YY

16. DATES PATIENT UNABLE TO WORK IN CURRENT OCCUPATION FROM MM DD YY TO MM DD YY

17. NAME OF REFERRING PROVIDER OR OTHER SOURCE

17a.
17b. NPI

18. HOSPITALIZATION DATES RELATED TO CURRENT SERVICES FROM MM DD YY TO MM DD YY

19. RESERVED FOR LOCAL USE

20. OUTSIDE LAB? YES NO $ CHARGES

21. DIAGNOSIS OR NATURE OF ILLNESS OR INJURY (Relate Items 1, 2, 3 or 4 to Item 24E by Line)
1. |___ , ___
2. |___ , ___
3. |___ , ___
4. |___ , ___

22. MEDICAID RESUBMISSION CODE ORIGINAL REF. NO.

23. PRIOR AUTHORIZATION NUMBER

24. A. DATE(S) OF SERVICE						B. PLACE OF SERVICE	C. EMG	D. PROCEDURES, SERVICES, OR SUPPLIES (Explain Unusual Circumstances) CPT/HCPCS MODIFIER	E. DIAGNOSIS POINTER	F. $ CHARGES	G. DAYS OR UNITS	H. EPSDT Family Plan	I. ID. QUAL	J. RENDERING PROVIDER ID. #
From MM	DD	YY	To MM	DD	YY									
1													NPI	
2													NPI	
3													NPI	
4													NPI	
5													NPI	
6													NPI	

25. FEDERAL TAX I.D. NUMBER SSN EIN

26. PATIENT'S ACCOUNT NO.

27. ACCEPT ASSIGNMENT? (For govt. claims, see back) YES NO

28. TOTAL CHARGE $

29. AMOUNT PAID $

30. BALANCE DUE $

31. SIGNATURE OF PHYSICIAN OR SUPPLIER INCLUDING DEGREES OR CREDENTIALS (I certify that the statements on the reverse apply to this bill and are made a part thereof.)

SIGNED _____ DATE _____

32. SERVICE FACILITY LOCATION INFORMATION
a. NPI b.

33. BILLING PROVIDER INFO & PH # ( )
a. NPI b.

NUCC Instruction Manual available at: www.nucc.org

PHYSICIAN OR SUPPLIER INFORMATION

PATIENT AND INSURED INFORMATION

APPROVED OMB-0938-0999 FORM CMS-1500 (08-05)

FIGURE 10-2 CMS 1500 claim form. Reprinted from U.S. Department of Health and Human Services, Centers for Medicare and Medicaid Services. Available at: http://www.cms.hhs.gov. Accessed November 7, 2008.

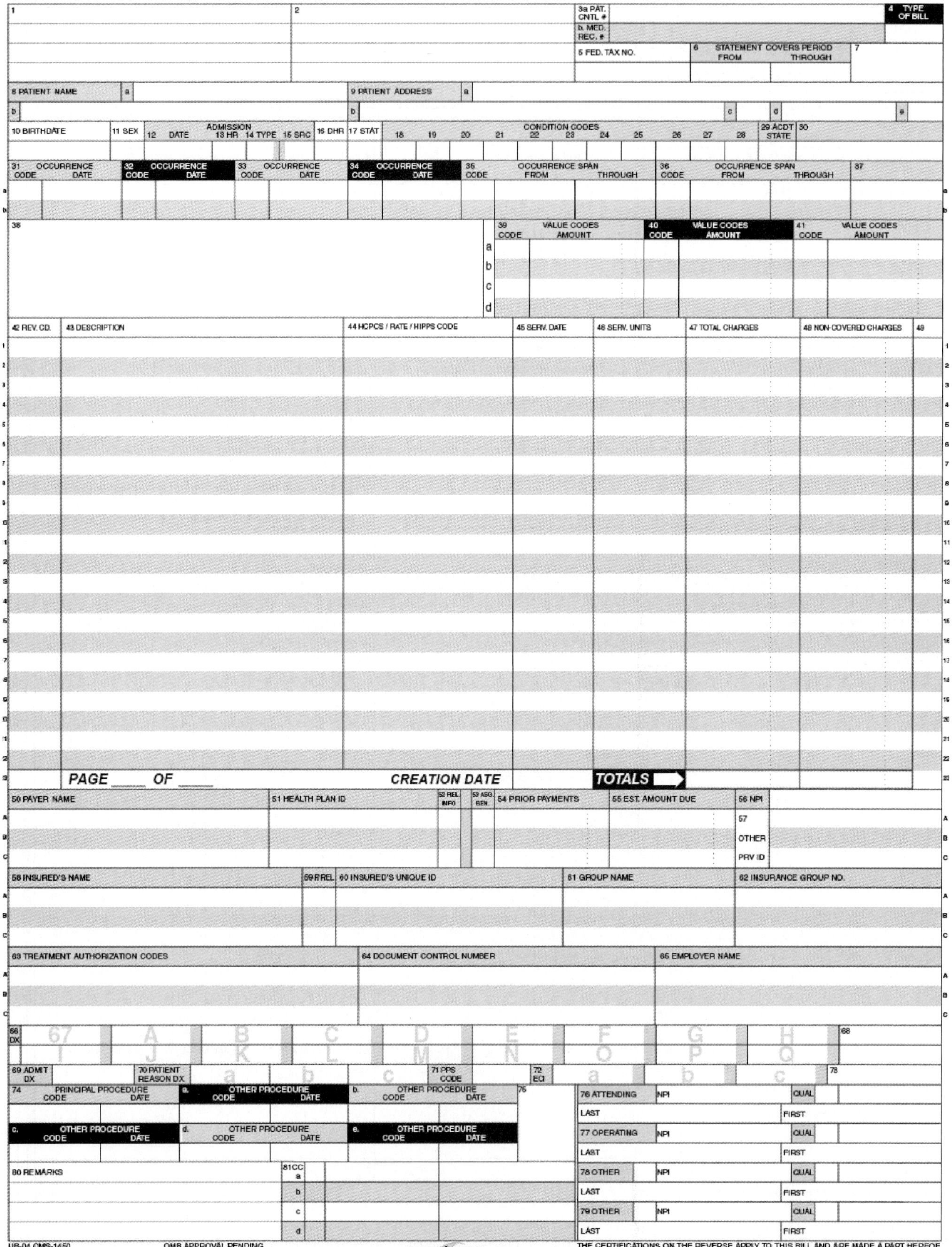

FIGURE 10-3 UB 04 claim form. Reprinted from Washington State Department of Labor and Industries. Available at: http://www.lni.wa.gov. Accessed November 7, 2008.

they can appeal the decision.[4] Appealing a denied claim will require writing a formal letter to the third-party payer that includes:

1. Policy's language in support of the treatment(s) rendered
2. Descriptions of the disorder and its medical nature
3. Facility information (location, accreditation, etc.)
4. Date of appeal and reminder of original date of the claim
5. Provider information (credentials and license number) and patient information
6. Date of service and total charges
7. Claim number
8. Reiteration of reason for denial
9. Explanation of why charges should be paid, include any evidence-based literature.

CHAPTER SUMMARY

Revenue and reimbursement can be intimidating to athletic trainers especially those not in a clinical context on a regular basis. However, understanding the nuances of third-party payment, managed health care organizations, and revenue and reimbursement are important aspects of athletic training. The importance of these issues will only increase as athletic training continues to define itself as a credible allied health care profession. Athletic trainers regardless of context or role benefit from understanding insurance and billing. Furthermore, managing third-party payers, generating a revenue stream, staying abreast of health care and coding regulations, navigating managed health care organizations, and accurately filing claims requires commitment and resolve. Athletic training needs its professionals to take leadership roles by promoting third-party reimbursement and innovating ways to generate revenue and gain reimbursement, doing so will add to the credibility of the profession.

 Leadership Application

Susan is an experienced ATC who works as a physician extender in a busy orthopedic surgeon's office. Susan's supervising physician allows her a lot of autonomy; she routinely conducts patient consultations, removes sutures, performs casting, conducts gait training, and supervises rehabilitation. She has always had very good success receiving reimbursement from third-party payers for these services. However, recently she has attempted to submit claims to an insurance company she has not previously billed before. This new third-party payer is denying her claims. Because she has little problem with other third-party payers, she is frustrated by this obstacle to her revenue generation.

Critical Thinking Questions

1. Is Susan's frustration warranted?
2. What are some steps Susan can take to try and discover the reason to these denials? What might she do to avoid denials in the future?
3. What steps might be necessary for Susan to get these denied claims reimbursed?

Leadership Spotlight

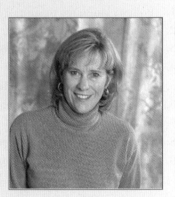

JULIE MAX

EDUCATION:

MEd, Physical Education Emphasis, Azusa Pacific University, Azusa, CA, 1985

Emergency Medical Technician, Santa Ana College, Santa Ana, CA, 1984

BS, Physical Education, California State University, Fullerton, CA, 1979

AA, Physical Education, Fullerton College, Fullerton, CA, 1973

CURRENT JOB:

Head Athletic Trainer, Department of Intercollegiate Athletics, California State University Fullerton, Fullerton, CA

I am responsible for the coordination and supervision of health care for 17 intercollegiate athletic teams, including prevention, treatment, assessment, and rehabilitation of all injuries and illnesses. Also, I am responsible for the overall supervision of three full-time and four graduate assistant certified athletic trainers, in addition to 20–25 athletic training students.

ATHLETIC TRAINING–RELATED AWARDS/HONORS:

- National Athletic Trainers Association, Julie Max Scholarship: presented to an undergraduate scholar at the NATA Annual Meeting and Clinical symposia, 2004–present
- California State University, Fullerton, Julie Max Scholarship: presented to an undergraduate scholar at the CSUF annual banquet, 2004–present
- Special Recognition Award, National Athletic Trainers' Association, for services rendered as the NATA President, June 2004
- District 8, Far West Athletic Trainers' Association, Most Distinguished Athletic Trainer, April 1999
- National Athletic trainers' Association Most Distinguished Athletic Trainer, June 1999
- California State University, Fullerton Student-Athlete Faculty of the Year Award, May 1997
- Special recognition Award, National Athletic Trainers' Association, for outstanding service to the association as a member of the Board of Directors, 1990–1996

ATHLETIC TRAINING–RELATED INVOLVEMENT:

- President, National Athletic Trainers' Association, 2000–2004. Elected first female president of a 26,000 member association. Served two terms and ran unopposed the second term.
- Director, District 8: National Athletic Trainers' Association. Director of the States of Nevada, California, and Hawaii. Re-elected to second three-year term, 1990–1996. The only female on a 10-member Board of Directors.
- Member: Education Committee, Continuing Education Subcommittee, National Athletic Trainers Association. 1997–2000
- Vice President: National Athletic Trainers' Association. First female elected. 1991–1992
- Chair: Budget and Finance Committee, National Athletic Trainers' Association. 1992–1996

Q & A

What first inspired you to enter the athletic training profession?

I have always been active in sports, and my love for this involvement was the first initial impetus behind my searching for an avenue within the sports community, where I could pursue a career. I was never interested in coaching, but I did have an interest in the "medical arena." Those two loves were probably the biggest influence in my deciding on athletic training. It allowed me to pursue the better of two very challenging and exciting interests of mine.

How would you define leadership in athletic training?

Leadership is defined in many ways by many people and for all professions. One definition that I think fits athletic training particularly well is, "Leadership is not POSITION, it is ACTION." An effective leader sees the big picture, is a visionary, and leads more by actions than by words. Our profession is one in which young people are visual learners, not only by observing the skills of our profession but also by observing how the leaders of the profession interact with many constituencies that cross our paths.

Who is the most influential athletic trainer in your professional life, and why?

This is a very difficult question for me because there have been so many leaders and true professionals that I have admired and that have influenced my life. Jerry Lloyd, who first hired me at California State University, Fullerton, would have to be at the top of this list. Jerry's influence on my life was tremendous because of the kind of person he was. He was a hands-on professional who taught me so many things by his dedication that he brought daily to the athletic training room. His ego never got in the way of him doing the best for every student athlete as well as every athletic training student. His desire to meet each of their medical and academic needs within the context of an intercollegiate athletic program always came first. He lived each day with a simplicity that has been difficult to duplicate in my life. His dedication and the excellence that he demanded from himself and from those around him left a lasting impression on my young mind. I hope that I have, to some extent, been able to continue in our program the legacy that he left.

What is the best advice you ever received from another athletic trainer?

I am not sure it is the "best advice," but it has served me well through the years that I have been a certified athletic trainer: "It is better to be **confident** than to always be right." The athletic world is a world of egos, and athletic training is no exception. To be confident, I have had to be willing to surround myself with professionals who complement my strengths and assist me in my weaknesses. Confidence comes with learning everyday from those young professionals as well as from those most experienced. Putting confidence ahead of ego has helped me stay grounded in this ever-changing profession.

What has been the most enjoyable aspect of athletic training?

Making a difference in young people's lives! Working with the student athletes and coaches in my early years was definitely a highlight of my career. While that is still very rewarding, educating the athletic training student has become another extremely valuable and enjoyable aspect of my day. Watching our students grow into mature, responsible, and skillful athletic trainers continues to be my daily mission.

What has been the least enjoyable aspect or your biggest challenge in athletic training?

The biggest challenge I face in my job is the lack of understanding and respect from the lay person regarding the profession of athletic training. It is a constant challenge to make "certified athletic trainer" a household term and to gain respect as an allied health care profession. Also, it is a challenge to consistently raise the level of awareness regarding the academic and clinical scope of practice for certified athletic trainers. We have made great progress, but we have yet to successfully reach the finish line.

What advice would you give a first-year athletic training student?

Explore all aspects of the profession of athletic training. Set the standard to be the best you can be. Learn from everyone you can. Make your mark and never forget your roots!

What advice would you give a brand new BOC-certified athletic trainer who is deciding between taking that first professional job or entering graduate school to pursue a master's degree in athletic training, and why?

Do your homework! Understand that over 70% of certified athletic trainers' have a minimum of a master's degree. That statistic alone affects the job market for every entry-level athletic trainer. Decide what is most important: short-term gratification or long-term career planning.

What other interests outside of athletic training have you pursued?

I have always loved animals and have investigated working with canines and equines medically, specifically in reference to orthopedic injuries. I am keenly interested in the advances that have been made in the area of "sports medicine" for animals. At one point early in my life, I had thought seriously about going into veterinary medicine. Perhaps down the road I will be able to devote more time to this other love of mine.

Where do you think (or hope) athletic training will be in the next 10 years?

Hopefully, athletic training will be the #1 allied health care profession in the next century! All 50 states will have some type of regulatory practice act, and the didactic and clinical standards will set the medical standard for health care. I am proud of how far we have come, but I am excited about where we have yet to go.

References

1. Albohm M. Campbell D, Konin J. (2001). *Reimbursement for athletic trainers.* Thorofare, NJ: Slack, Inc.
2. Blevins S. retrieved from http://www.forhealthfreedom.org/Publications/HealthIns/MSAs.html. Accessed October 12, 2006.
3. National Athletic Trainers' Association Committee on Revenue. http://www.nata.org. Accessed October 12, 2006.
4. Nicoletti B. (2006). Claims denials: Don't take No for an answer. *Medical Economics* 82(9):41.
5. Prentice W. (2008). *Arnheim's principles of athletic training.* Boston, MA: McGraw Hill.

Legal Issues and Risk Management

"Where there is no law, but every man does what is right in his own eyes, there is the least of liberty."

HENRY MARTYN ROBERT

Role Delineation Study Components

Domain V: Organization and Administration

- Knowledge of preparticipation screening policies and procedures
- Knowledge of legal standards and scope of practice
- Knowledge of guidelines for development of risk management policies and procedures
- Knowledge of statutory, regulatory, and other legal provisions pertaining to the delivery of health care services.

Domain VI: Professional Responsibility

- Knowledge of state statues, regulations, and adjudication that directly govern the practice of athletic training.
- Knowledge of federal and state statues, regulations, and adjudication that apply to the practice and/or organization and administration of athletic training.
- Knowledge of criteria for determining the legal standard of care in athletic training.

Educational Competencies

- Identify and describe the basic components of a comprehensive injury emergency care plan for the care of acutely injured or ill individuals, which include 1) emergency action plans for each setting or venue; 2) personnel training; 3) sideline emergency care supplies and equipment appropriate for each venue; 4) availability of emergency care facilities; 5) communication with onsite personnel and notification of EMS; 6) the availability, capabilities, and policies of community-based emergency care facilities and community-based managed care systems; 7) transportation; 8) location of exit and evacuation routes; 9) activity or event coverage; and 10) record keeping.
- Identify the components of a comprehensive risk management plan that addresses the issues of security, fire, electrical and equipment safety, emergency preparedness, and hazardous chemicals.
- Explain the basic legal concepts, such as, but not limited to, standard of care, scope of practice, liability, negligence, informed consent, and confidentiality, as they apply to a medical or allied health care practitioner's performance of his or her responsibilities.

Key Terms

Actual cause: Explicit proof that a breach of duty was the actual cause of damage to an individual.

Actual harm: Literal and real damage or loss (as opposed to potential damage or loss).

Adjudication: The decision of the court regarding a specific case or defendant.

Analytic jurisprudence: The philosophy of law that asks specific questions such as, "What is law?" or "What is the relationship between law and ethics or morality?" It seeks to analyze any differences between legal behaviors and other behaviors, such as ethical or moral behaviors.

Battery: A tort that involves deliberately bringing about a harmful or offensive contact without consent that is likely to cause injury or bodily harm.

Breach of duty: A finding that any duty or obligation owed to a harmed individual was violated.

Case law: The decisions made by judges in previous cases and that are recorded and used as precedent for other cases.

Causation: A finding that a breach of duty was the actual or proximate cause of any alleged harm, damage, or loss.

Civil law: The most common form of law in the world, based on abstract rules or notions, which requires a judge to interpret and apply to each case individually.

Commission: Performing an act that one is not legally permitted to perform.

Common law: Deals with the rights and responsibilities of individuals toward each other.

Comparative negligence: Assignment of negligence among multiple parties by considering all parties whose negligence contributed to a tort. The negligence is then allocated among the parties at fault and damages are assigned to the level each contributed toward the negligent action(s).

Duty of care: Proving that there is a responsibility to provide care based on the relationship between parties.

Family Educational Rights and Privacy Act (FERPA): A federal statute that delineates how to disseminate educational data.

Informed consent: The process of ensuring a patient is aware of all risks of having or not having a procedure or treatment, benefits, and any other possible outcomes associated with a given procedure.

Jurisprudence: The theory and philosophy of law.

Litigation: A dispute between parties that is argued in a court of law under the purview of a judge.

Natural law: The philosophy that there are unchangeable laws of nature that govern human behavior.

Negligence: The failure to act prudently or in a way that a reasonable person would act under the same or similar circumstances.

Normative jurisprudence: The field of law that considers obedience to the law and how law-breakers might be suitably punished within the proper uses and limits of regulations.

Omission: The failure to perform a duty.

Precedent: The prior decision of a judge that is used if another case has identical or similar legal questions.

Proximate cause: An action that leads to or ultimately ends in harm.

Regulatory law: The federal authorization necessary to establish rules and regulations to make a law effective.

Risk: The probability or potential for harm as a result of some action.

Scope of practice: Established practice boundaries of a profession that delineate to whom services can be provided and where those services are rendered.

Standard of care: The level at which a reasonable and prudent health care provider in a given community or context would practice.

Standing orders: A physician's (or other qualified, licensed health provider's) orders, pre-established and approved for use by an athletic trainer under specific conditions in the absence of a physician.

Statutory law: Rules and regulations imposed by regulatory bodies such as Congress, legislatures, or local governments.

Tort: A private wrong or injury suffered by an individual because of another individual's conduct.

thletic trainers are an integral part of an industry that involves risk.[10] With risk comes liability. Liability forces an awareness of legal standards and risk management. Therefore, the athletic trainer must be aware of existing practice standards and must understand the inherent risk for litigation and the implications that different types of law and legal precedent have on the daily practice of athletic trainers. The athletic trainer is not expected to be an expert lawyer, but each athletic trainer should be familiar with different legal considerations that pertain to the discipline and to the nature of our profession.

In this chapter we will cover the legal aspects of athletic training. We will begin with basic legal principles, followed by standards of care and scope of practice issues. Next we will discuss legal torts and include a discussion of liability, negligence, omission, and commission. After that, we will cover what athletic trainers can do to protect themselves from lawsuits, including specific risk-management behaviors such as responding to emergencies and conducting pre-participation physicals. We will conclude this chapter with a discussion of federal statutes of which athletic trainers need to be aware in their different professional roles.

LEGAL PRINCIPLES

Jurisprudence is the theory and philosophy of law, which has three primary areas. The first is **natural law**, popularized by Aristotle and Thomas Aquinas, and is the idea that there are unchangeable laws of nature which govern humans, and that institutions created by humans should try to match this natural law. Second is **analytic jurisprudence**, which deals with the philosophy of law and asks questions such as, "What is law?" or "What is the relationship between law and ethics or morality?" Analytic jurisprudence seeks to analyze differences between legal behaviors and other behaviors or motives, such as ethical or moral behaviors. The ideas associated with natural law are beyond the scope of this text and analytic jurisprudence fits better under discussions on ethics, which is covered elsewhere in this text. However, it should be noted that many legal systems are based on ethical suppositions and questions.

The third area of jurisprudence and the primary focus of this chapter is **normative jurisprudence.** Normative jurisprudence considers questions related to obedience to the law, such as "How might law-breakers be suitably punished?" It also considers the proper uses and limits of regulation. In other words, normative jurisprudence deals with how much freedom is removed from citizens as a result of having laws imposed on them and, in the case of a violation of the law, what is a suitable punishment.

Legal Paradigms That Influence Behavior

From a global perspective, there are three major legal systems that most people have to face, regardless of country of origin. Each legal system varies in importance from country to country or person to person. The three systems are civil law, common law, and religious law. Many countries develop their own variations or incorporate other aspects into their legal system, which results in many other forms and systems, but

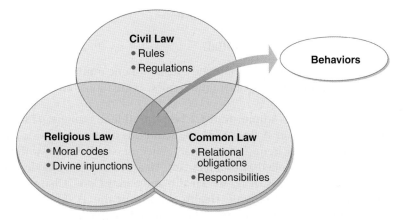

FIGURE 11-1 Illustration of how the three legal systems overlap to influence a person's behavior

most legal systems have their roots in some combination of these three legal paradigms.

Civil law is the most common form of law in the world. This form of law is based on abstract rules or notions, which require a judge to interpret and apply (or render judgments) to each case individually. **Common law** is concerned with the rights and responsibilities of individuals towards each other. Lastly, **religious law**, which from a global perspective is also widely accepted, is based on moral and ethical codes. While religious law may not have as obvious an impact on athletic training as civil or common law, it would be a mistake to think religious laws do not impact the practice of athletic training (see the From the Field in Chapter 15). Furthermore, it is important to realize that for some, religious law has significant punitive power. It is important to realize that civil, common, and religious laws all relate to influence an individual's behavior (Fig. 11-1).

LEGAL ISSUES FOR ATHLETIC TRAINERS

There are many legal concepts of which the athletic trainer needs to be aware. First are the three categories of law, which include statutory, regulatory, and case law. **Statutory law** is imposed by regulatory bodies.[6] These include regulatory agencies such as Congress, legislatures, or local governments. For example, the Occupational Health and Safety Act of 1970 was enacted to ensure a safe working environment and is regulated by the U.S. Department of Labor, Occupational Health and Safety Administration (OSHA). Athletic trainers must comply with many OSHA regulations. Other federal agencies which have regulations of which athletic trainers need to be aware include the following:[6]

1. The Department of Education
   a. Title IX – regulates equal opportunities for male and female athletes
   b. Family Educational Rights and Privacy Act (FERPA) – delineates how to disseminate educational data
2. Department of Health and Human Services - Health Insurance Portability and Accountability Act (HIPAA) – delineates how to disseminate medical information
3. Food and Drug Administration - Food and Drug Administration Act of 1938 – enacted to promote proper and safe use of drugs

4. Equal Employment Opportunity Commission
    a. Equal Pay Act of 1963
    b. Age Discrimination Act of 1967

Other rules include those of individual states. Each athletic trainer is responsible for becoming familiar with the athletic training rules, regulations, and definitions of their individual state.

For example, the Texas Administrative Code for athletic trainers, Title 22, Part 40, Chapter 871, Subchapter A Rule §871.13, Standards for Conduct, lists 26 provisions and several subpoints, item (f) states that "A licensee shall comply with the provisions of the Texas Controlled Substances Act, Health and Safety Code, Chapter 481, and the Texas Dangerous Drug Act, Health and Safety Code, Chapter 483, and any rules of the Department of State Health Services or the Texas State Board of Pharmacy implementing those statutes." This example explicitly outlines the fact that licensed athletic trainers (in Texas) have an obligation to understand certain regulations in addition to those outlined exclusively for athletic trainers. Other states may adopt similar statues. Therefore, an athletic trainer should investigate his or her state regulations for similar language.

The second legal concept is **regulatory law**, which is also based on federal legislation and authorizes different agencies to enact rules and regulations necessary to make a law effective.[6] Furthermore, states also may interpret and enact rules based on their codes.[6] Therefore, athletic trainers, regardless of state, need to know the different agencies that have jurisdiction over their professional practice.

The third legal concept is **case law.** Case law refers to the decisions made by judges in previous cases. If litigation has occurred, the decision of the judge is recorded and is used as precedent for other cases. **Litigation** is a dispute between parties that is argued in a court of law under the purview of a judge. **Adjudication** is the decision of the court regarding a specific case or defendant. **Precedent** is the prior decision of a judge that is used if another case has identical or similar legal questions. However, precedent is only binding in an equal or lower court in the same jurisdiction.[6] Therefore, a state is not bound by another state's case law. However, all federal and state courts in the United States are bound by decisions made in the U.S. Supreme Court. Statutory, regulatory, and case law may be used in athletic training litigation. Other considerations of litigation may include standard of care and scope of practice.

Standards of Care

A **standard of care** is an important legal consideration for athletic trainers. The standard of care for any health care provider is the level at which the reasonable, prudent provider in a given community or context would practice. For example, determining the standard of care of an athletic trainer would be determined based on the reasonable action of other athletic trainers within the same or a similar context or community. Basically, the standard of care refers to how other athletic trainers would have managed the patient's care under the same or similar conditions. From a legal perspective, the plaintiff must establish what the appropriate standard of care is or was and demonstrate that the standard of care was breached.

Scope of Practice

Scope of practice refers to established boundaries within a profession and details how that professional may perform his or her duties. Delineating scope of practice for athletic trainers answers the questions, "To whom can an athletic trainer provide services?" and "Where can those services be rendered?" It is imperative to understand that individual states delineate different scopes of practice for athletic trainers. Many states limit the practice of athletic training to those activities that fall under the direction of a licensed physician. However, there are states that identify other qualified licensed health professionals in addition to licensed physicians. Therefore, practicing outside of the direction of a licensed physician (or a qualified licensed health professional) is a violation of an athletic trainer's scope of practice. An athletic trainer's scope of practice is dependent upon the definitions employed by that state. Definitions such as "athlete," "injury," and "athletic trainer" vary by state. For example, under Texas Administrative Code, Title 22, Chapter 871, Subchapter A, Rule §871.2

> "an athletic trainer prevents, recognizes, assesses, manages, treats, disposes of, and reconditions athletic injuries and illnesses under the direction of a physician licensed in this state or another qualified, licensed health professional who is authorized to refer for health care services within the scope of the person's license. An athlete is a person who participates in an organized sport or sport-related exercise or activity, including interscholastic, intercollegiate, intramural, semiprofessional, and professional sports activities."

Licensed athletic trainers in the state of Texas are restricted to these definitions and the scope they delineate. Other states define and delineate these terms differently. For example, in New Mexico there is a broader scope of practice delineated for athletic trainers.

The New Mexico Athletic Trainer's Practice Act defines an "athlete" as a person trained to participate in exercise requiring physical agility and stamina; and an "athletic trainer" as a person who, with the advice and consent of a licensed physician practices the treatment, prevention, care and rehabilitation of injuries incurred by athletes. Compare New Mexico's scope of practice to Delaware's:

In the state of Delaware, scope of practice for athletic trainers is more restrictive. Delaware, Title 24, Chapter 26, Rule § 2602 states that,

> "Treatment of musculoskeletal injuries that are not defined as an 'athletic injury' will require direction from a physical therapist and direct supervision of every fifth treatment. An athletic trainer may not independently initiate, modify, or discontinue a physical therapy plan of care. Athletic training shall not include radiology, surgery, prescription drugs, or authorize the medical diagnosis of disease."

In that same rule an "athletic injury" is defined as "a musculoskeletal injury resulting from or limiting participation in or training for scholastic, recreational, professional or sanctioned amateur athletic activities." Suffice it to say, for states that regulate athletic training, each state's scope of practice for an athletic trainer is different. Athletic trainers just entering the profession or seasoned athletic trainers relocating to a different state after years of practicing in one state must obtain and assimilate the scope of practice and definitions of their state.

TORTS

A **tort** is a private wrong or injury suffered by an individual because of another individual's conduct.[7] Tort law is an aspect of statutory law and is considered a civil wrong. The law allows for any tort to be compensated through the recovery of damages.[7] However, damages as a result of failure to meet obligations established by a contract fall outside the scope of tort law. Concepts involved with tort law include liability, nuisance, and negligence. Nuisance is outside the scope of this chapter and deals with property and involves liability associated with hindering one's enjoyment of their personal property or land. However, liability and issues concerning negligence are far more likely to impact athletic trainers.

LEADERSHIP ACTIVITY

Find your respective state's rules and regulations pertaining to athletic training. The Board of Certification, Inc. website (http://www.bocatc.org) has a link to each state's regulations. If your state regulates the profession of athletic training find the definitions for the following terms "athletic trainer," "athletic training," and "athletic injury" (note: all states may not have definitions for each of these terms). If your state does not regulate athletic training, choose a state that does and find the definitions. After you have found these definitions, note any specific language that stands out about the definition, such as scope of practice, restrictions, inclusions, etc. Next, pick any other state that regulates athletic training and compare the definitions in your state to the other state you have chosen. Prepare a very brief essay (approximately 150 to 200 words) that attempts to explain in your own words any differences you noted.

Liability

Conceptually, liability is anything that detracts value or places someone at a disadvantage. Legally, liability denotes responsibility and accountability. In other words, when an athletic trainer is said to be "liable," it implies they have a responsibility and are accountable should something happen. For example, in athletic training having liability or being liable means there is an obligation or responsibility to an athlete or patient. The question may come up in a staff or departmental meeting of "Who is liable?" or "Where does the liability fall in that scenario?" Basically, the question is, "Who is at fault if something goes wrong?" Reducing liability implies practicing behaviors that inform or minimize risk.

Another aspect of liability includes **informed consent**. Informed consent is more than getting a patient to sign a waiver or consenting to a treatment. "Informed" is the operative word. The patient must be made aware, by the responsible party, of relevant information concerning the treatment or procedure. Relevant information includes risks of having or not having the procedure, benefits of the procedure, and any other possible outcomes for a given procedure. Furthermore, the patient must be legally competent to make sound judgment, and must be given an opportunity to ask any questions they might have concerning the treatment or procedure. The patient is then acknowledging that they have been made aware of these risks. Securing informed consent is a legal requirement with written statutes and case law in all 50 states; furthermore, the American Medical Association's holds informed consent as an ethical obligation for its members.

It is important to understand that having an informed consent does not remove liability from the athletic trainer. Failure to secure an informed consent prior to treatment can be considered **battery**.[2] Battery is a tort including deliberately bringing about a harmful or offensive contact without consent that is likely to cause an injury or bodily harm.

Negligence

Negligence is the failure to act prudently or in a way that a reasonable person would act under the same or similar circumstances. Negligence is an aspect of tort law that is based on the principle that those who have suffered loss or harm as a result of another individual's careless behavior or failure to act responsibly must be compensated for that loss or harm.[7] In order to be compensated, the person harmed must prove that negligence occurred. Stated another way, the burden of proof falls to the harmed individual. There are four elements that must be demonstrated in order to satisfy the legal requirements of negligence; duty of care, breach of duty, cause, and actual harm.

Duty of Care

The first element is duty of care. **Duty of care** is simply proving that there is a responsibility to provide care based on the relationship between the parties.[7] Typically, duty is easy to establish. By virtue of the athletic training profession and the profession's role in society, anyone an athletic trainer agrees to treat should be able to prove a duty of care exists.

Breach of Duty

The second element is breach of duty. **Breach of duty** is proving that the duty or obligation owed to the harmed individual was in fact breached. To establish breach of duty in athletic training, the athletic trainer is assessed against what is a normal and reasonable practice. This means the athletic trainer is expected to act in a way that other athletic trainers in similar situations and circumstances would act.[7] Because athletic trainers practice in a wide diversity of settings, the expected standard of care is based on expert testimony of other athletic trainers as well as published standards. Published standards used might include some of the following *The Standards of Professional Practice*, published by the Board of Certification, Inc., NATA's *Athletic Training Educational Competencies*, the BOC's *Role Delineation Study*, and individual state licensing requirements and standards of practice.

Cause

The third element is cause. **Causation** is more difficult to prove and must demonstrate that the breach of duty was the actual or proximate cause of the alleged harm, damage, or loss. **Actual cause** is explicit and evidence is presented that proves the breach of duty was the actual cause of the damage. **Proximate cause** is when the actions of the athletic trainer lead to or ultimately end in harm.[7] For example, clearing an athlete to return to competition with a known anterior cruciate ligament (ACL) tear or allowing a return to competition after failure to do an adequate assessment of the ACL for a suspected tear. These actions would be considered actual cause if additional damage occurred. On the other hand, failure to report suspicions of an ACL tear to the team physician can be a proximate cause. While the failure to report may not have been the actual cause of the damage, had it been reported to the team physician it could be reasonably argued that further damage would likely not have occurred.[7]

Actual Harm

The final element that must be demonstrated for negligence to be proven is **actual harm** (as apposed to actual cause). This is where the harmed individual must prove

---

▶ Leadership Application

Jim is the head athletic trainer in charge of football at a large Division 1 university. The football program at Jim's university has enjoyed a long tradition of success. One afternoon during two-a-day practices the starting quarterback and a likely Heisman Trophy® candidate, dislocates his shoulder. During the course of Jim's 15-year athletic training career he has watched his team physician reduce many dislocated shoulders and Jim assisted the team physician in reducing many of those shoulders. Furthermore, Jim enjoys a great relationship with his team physician and it is obvious to any serious observer that the team physician trusts Jim's professional judgment and his ability to handle any emergency. In fact on several informal occasions the team physician has given Jim verbal instructions that if he was ever not present, Jim could "reduce dislocations." In this particular case, the physician is not present and Jim knows he is unavailable to be reached. The quarterback is in obvious discomfort and the coach is now beginning to show signs of frustration over Jim's apparent lack of response.

Critical Thinking Questions

1. Should Jim reduce this shoulder dislocation on the spot? What if the physician can have been reached immediately?

2. What kind of pressure might Jim be feeling to be aggressive and reduce this shoulder, what kind of pressure might Jim be feeling to take a conservative approach?

3. How can you find out what restrictions are on Jim, concerning how he immediately manages this shoulder dislocation?

4. What are some possible repercussions of Jim's actions if he decides it is necessary to reduce this shoulder dislocation by himself? What if he reduces it and there are further complications? Are there repercussions of he reduces and there are no further complications?

5. If this same situation was in a small high school, only with a second string junior-varsity player, would any of the repercussions or sense of pressure be different, why or why not?

that there was actual or literal damage or loss, not just the potential for damage or loss. Once negligence is demonstrated, the injured party typically seeks to recover these damages or losses. Those areas include past, present, and future pain and suffering; medical expenses; and loss of earning capacity.[7]

Typically there are three kinds of damages that are awarded when negligence has been decided.[4] The first is punitive damages, which are intended to punish the negligent party. There are also economic damages, which are awarded to recover actual cost of the injury, such loss of wages or medical bills. The third, non-economic damages may also be awarded. Non-economic damages must be estimated and are intended to cover intangible losses, like pain and suffering, associated with the injury.[4]

Omission and Commission

Negligence can occur as an act of omission or commission. **Omission** is the failure to perform a duty. **Commission** is performing an act that one is not legally permitted to perform. For example, an act of omission may include failure to properly assess an injury and allow return to competition based on a poorly executed evaluation that results in additional damage. An act of commission might include reducing a dislocated elbow, suturing a minor laceration, or dispensing medications. Any act of omission or commission can be considered negligence and are grounds for legal action.

PROTECTING YOURSELF FROM LEGAL ACTION

Strategies to protect oneself from legal action should be an aspect of professional development athletic trainers should address. In the traditional athletic training setting, athletic trainers may be tempted to rely on the strong rapport they often enjoy with their patients as the only protection for litigation. While rapport and trust may be strong and often is a deterrent for an athlete in pursuing legal action, it is not enough protection from litigation. One practice to reduce risk of legal action is to clearly review and delineate any and all standing orders. **Standing orders** are a physician's (or other qualified licensed health provider's) orders, pre-established and approved for use by an athletic trainer under specific conditions in the absence of a physician. There are several additional behaviors that if practiced by athletic trainers will also limit the risk of a potential lawsuit.

1. Do not accept assignments or standing orders for which you are not trained.
2. Do not take shortcuts (especially when under duress).
3. Document all aspects of your care.
4. Never alter documents.
5. Do not make presumptions about patients or their injuries.
6. Try to consider the "big picture."[9]

These behaviors are suggestions that may help to reduce the risk of litigation by former patients. These suggestions reiterate the critical importance of knowing and staying within the defined scope of practice, being thorough in record keeping and documentation, and not being overly aggressive in patient care.

What to do if Sued

An athletic trainer who receives notice that a former athlete or patient is claiming that their care was negligent is disheartening. However, given the state of litigation today, receiving such an allegation is not uncommon. There are standard defenses that an athletic trainer can use when accused of negligence.

The first line of defense is often to try and prove that one of the four elements necessary to prove negligence was not present. For example, the athletic trainer may claim there was no duty, there was no breach of duty, there was no cause, or there was no actual harm. If these strategies are unsuccessful, another defense is assumption of risk.[7]

Assumption of risk is based on the premise that no harm can be done to someone who consents.[7] For example, an athlete with a known medical condition can assume their own risk, acknowledge awareness of their risk, and ultimately release liability of the athletic trainer. Athletic trainers who use assumption of risk as a defense must prove that,

1. The athlete knew of the risk (or a reasonable athlete should have known there was risk)
2. The athlete explicitly accepted their risk (in writing or orally) or implicitly accepted risk by participating.

However, many athletes, for a host of different reasons, including love of the game, prestige, peer pressure, or need for belonging[7], may waive the inherent risks of participation and play in spite of the risks. Simply because an athlete acknowledges risk and waives liability does not mean that the athletic trainer has no duty to the athlete. As an athletic trainer, there remains the obligation to provide the best possible athletic health care and the athletic trainer should do whatever is possible to limit risk for the athlete. This means that in the case of having to make treatment decisions, design rehabilitation programs, and make return to play decisions after an injury of an at-risk athlete, the athletic trainer is still responsible for using sound clinical judgment and evidence. Furthermore, just because an athlete waives liability and assumes risk it does not mean that negligence by the athletic trainer is automatically forgiven. Negligence can occur regardless of where the liability falls. There is the possibility of comparative negligence even after an athlete accepts liability and provides a waiver. **Comparative negligence** recognizes that damages should be paid by the negligent party, but are assessed against the level the athlete contributed to the damage.[7] This means that because an athlete contributed to the damage by participating, any award recovered for damages by the athlete (or patient) is at a lesser amount, proportionate to the degree of negligence.

Finally, immunity, such a Good Samaritan act, is a defense that is used based on the idea that a person performing a charitable act cannot be accountable for negligence.[2] This defense can be argued in schools that are established as a charitable institution with a religious affiliation.[2]

RISK MANAGEMENT

Risk is described as the probability or potential for harm as a result of some action (sometimes risk is also referred to as liability). Risk can be thought of as 1) the risk the athlete has in participating, for which the athletic trainer is present to minimize; and 2) the risk (liability) the athletic trainer assumes as a health care provider. Limiting both aspects of risk is an important professional behavior for athletic trainers.

Ultimately, the objective of all risk management practices is to reduce loss. Loss can be in any form (typically thought of as financial), but also emotional, physical, time, and any other area where loss can be felt. Managing risk involves any behavior that attempts to mitigate these risks. Therefore, risk management can be overt, such as employing an emergency action plan or practicing evidence-based medicine. Risk management can also be covert, such as implementing sound leadership behaviors and interpersonal skills.

For example, athletes can help to reduce their risk by knowing the rules of their sport, being in proper physical condition, practicing sound nutrition, developing rapport with coaches and teammates, and refining their sport-specific skills. An athletic trainer can engage in specific practices that reduces his or her liability as well as reduces the risks associated with participation for the athlete. Athletic trainers can help reduce an athlete's risk by ensuring the environment is safe for competition, e.g., by implementing NATA's position statements on lighting safety. Implementing a position statement can also help to reduce liability. Therefore, sound risk management practices benefit the athlete and the athletic trainer. One important risk management behavior is correctly responding to emergencies.

Responding to Emergencies

Properly responding to emergencies is a critical aspect of management and leadership for the athletic trainer. Failure to have and rehearse an emergency action plan (EAP) can be considered negligent.[3] Managing an emergency involves leadership skills such as confidence; organizational savvy; critical thinking; and clear, concise communication. Performing rehearsals of emergency situations is also prudent for the athletic trainer; this requires communication, foresight, and advance coordination. NATA has published a position statement on emergency planning in athletics that all athletic trainers should be aware of.

Serious injuries can occur without any advance warning. Further complicating emergency planning are the multiple venues in which many athletic trainers must oversee and manage. Each venue must have its own emergency action plan and emergency rehearsals. Figure 11-2 is sample emergency plan for different venues. Obviously, the proper care of the athlete is of primary concern, but emergency preparedness is also a legal concern for the athletic trainer and athletics department.[3] Preparation for emergencies involves:

1. Education and training of athletes and staff
2. Availability and maintenance of emergency equipment
3. Appropriate use of personnel
4. The formation and implementation of an emergency action plan[3]

Each of these issues falls within the domain of the athletic trainer and involves aspects of good leadership and management.

NATA's position statement on emergency action plans identifies 12 items of an emergency plan. Box 11-1 is a list of those 12 items. In addition to these 12 items, NATA recommends eight components be included in emergency planning.[3]

1. Implementation of an emergency plan. This component involves three phases, writing it, educating staff on it, and rehearsing it.
2. Notify all personnel involved. First responders vary greatly in an emergency. Each person with potential involvement should be educated on the plan and rehearse the plan.
3. Accessible equipment. All necessary emergency equipment needs to be available and accessible to any of the personnel who may be involved. Therefore, emergency equipment should not be kept under lock and key, with only limited access during practices and competitions.
4. Clear communication. Proper and prompt communication is essential in an emergency. Communication devices (cell phones or two-way radios, etc.) and back-up plans must be made available to personnel.

Sample Venue-Specific Emergency Protocol

_____University Sports Medicine Football Emergency Protocol

1. Call 911 or other emergency number consistent with organizational policies
2. Instruct emergency medical services (EMS) personnel to "report to _____ and meet _____ at _____ as we have an injured student-athlete in need of emergency medical treatment."
   University Football Practice Complex: _____ Street entrance (gate across street from _____) _cross street:_ _____ Street
   University Stadium: Gate _____ entrance off _____ Road
3. Provide necessary information to EMS personnel:
   - name, address, telephone number of caller
   - number of victims; condition of victims
   - first-aid treatment initiated
   - specific directions as needed to locate scene
   - other information as requested by dispatcher
4. Provide appropriate emergency care until arrival of EMS personnel: on arrival of EMS personnel, provide pertinent information (method of injury, vital signs, treatment rendered, medical history) and assist with emergency care as needed

Note:

- sports medicine staff member should accompany student-athlete to hospital
- notify other sports medicine staff immediately
- parents should be contacted by sports medicine staff
- inform coach(es) and administration
- obtain medical history and insurance information
- appropriate injury reports should be completed

Emergency Telephone Numbers
_____ Hospital   _____ - _____
_____ Emergency Department   _____ - _____
University Health Center   _____ - _____
Campus Police   _____ - _____

Emergency Signals

Physician: arm extended overhead with clenched first
Paramedics: point to location in end zone by home locker room and wave onto field
Spine board: arms held horizontally
Stretcher: supinated hands in front of body or waist level
Splints: hand to lower leg or thigh

FIGURE 11-2 Sample EAP for a sports venue source. Reprinted with permission from National Athletic Trainers' Association Position Statement: Emergency Planning in Athletics. (2002). _Journal of Athletic Training 37_(1):99–104.

5. Establish transportation. Emergency transportation should be available at all high risk events and emergency vehicle response time should be factored into emergency plans.

6. Rehearse at each venue. Many athletic departments host practices and events at different venues. The athletic trainer should have a specific plan for each venue.

7. Notify Emergency Care Facilities. It is sound practice to notify any local health care facility (i.e., hospital, urgent care center, or ER) that they are part of your emergency plan for a specific venue. It is also wise to advise that facility in advance when events are occurring at a venue in close proximity.

8. Correct documentation. Written emergency plans should be reviewed by institutional administrators, other members of the sports medicine team, and legal counsel.

In addition to responding to emergencies, having an appropriate pre-screening process is an important risk management behavior.

BOX 11-1   NATA Position Statement on Emergency Planning

1. Each institution or organization that sponsors athletic activities must have a written emergency plan. The emergency plan should be comprehensive and practical, yet flexible enough to adapt to any emergency situation.

2. Emergency plans must be written documents and should be distributed to certified athletic trainers, team and attending physicians, athletic training students, institutional and organizational safety personnel, institutional and organizational administrators, and coaches. The emergency plan should be developed in consultation with local emergency medical services personnel.

3. An emergency plan for athletics identifies the personnel involved in carrying out the emergency plan and outlines the qualifications of those executing the plan. Sports medicine professionals, officials, and coaches should be trained in automatic external defibrillation, cardiopulmonary resuscitation, first aid, and prevention of disease transmission.

4. The emergency plan should specify the equipment needed to carry out the tasks required in the event of an emergency. In addition, the emergency plan should outline the location of the emergency equipment. Further, the equipment available should be appropriate to the level of training of the personnel involved.

5. Establishment of a clear mechanism for communication to appropriate emergency care service providers and identification of the mode of transportation for the injured participant are critical elements of an emergency plan.

6. The emergency plan should be specific to the activity venue. That is, each activity site should have a defined emergency plan that is derived from the overall institutional or organizational policies on emergency planning.

7. Emergency plans should incorporate the emergency care facilities to which the injured individual will be taken. Emergency receiving facilities should be notified in advance of scheduled events and contests. Personnel from the emergency receiving facilities should be included in the development of the emergency plan for the institution or organization.

8. The emergency plan specifies the necessary documentation supporting the implementation and evaluation of the emergency plan. This documentation should identify responsibility for documenting actions taken during the emergency, evaluation of the emergency response, and institutional personnel training.

9. The emergency plan should be reviewed and rehearsed annually, although more frequent review and rehearsal may be necessary. The results of these reviews and rehearsals should be documented and should indicate whether the emergency plan was modified, with further documentation reflecting how the plan was changed.

10. All personnel involved with the organization and sponsorship of athletic activities share a professional responsibility to provide for the emergency care of an injured person, including the development and implementation of an emergency plan.

11. All personnel involved with the organization and sponsorship of athletic activities share a legal duty to develop, implement, and evaluate an emergency plan for all sponsored athletic activities.

12. The emergency plan should be reviewed by the administration and legal counsel of the sponsoring organization or institution.

Reprinted with permission from National Athletic Trainers' Association Position Statement: Emergency Planning in Athletics. (2002). *Journal of Athletic Training* 37(1):99–104.

Preparticipation Physical Exams

Ensuring a properly administered pre-participation physical exam (PPE) for each athlete is another critical risk strategy. This practice will help to limit the liability of the athletic trainer as well as possibly prevent the athlete from participating in an activity that is too risky. Unfortunately, many PPEs are not sufficient as a medical screening process.[5] In other words, many PPEs are not thorough enough to identify areas where athletes might be at risk if allowed to compete unrestricted. The minimal objectives of a standard PPE should include the following:

1. Determination of the overall state of health and treatment of remedial conditions
2. Determination of and recommendations for the level of physical fitness (i.e., flexibility, strength, power, and cardiovascular fitness)
3. Assessment of size and maturation to aid in determining the safety of participating with peers
4. Evaluation of preexisting injuries and recommendations for rehabilitation where appropriate
5. Restriction of activity or disqualification from specific sports when contraindicated by physical limitations or disease that would preclude safe participation
6. Recommendations for appropriate activity when participation has been restricted[2,8]

In reference to restriction or disqualification from athletic activity the American Academy of Orthopaedic Surgeons has identified six classifications for sport participation that is to be determined during the PPE:[1]

1. Passed = unrestricted activity.
2. Passed with conditions = requires a follow-up (likely with a specialist) before full clearance.
3. Passed with reservations = there are restrictions to participation (usually collision or contact sports).
4. Failed with reservations = not cleared for requested sport, may seek participation for an alternate activity.
5. Failed with conditions = medical conditions must be addressed and then a full reevaluation is required.
6. Failed = no participation is allowed.

Common conditions that may result in failure or participation restrictions might include, loss of vision, repeated head traumas, one kidney, one testicle, or Marfan's syndrome.[1]

Types of Physicals

Physicals can be performed in any number of contexts. Two popular ways physicals are conducted are the station-based, which can be performed in any large facility capable of facilitating several different stations, and the office-based physical. As the name implies, office-based physicals are conducted by a physician in his or her office.

In station-based physicals athletes systematically filter through any number of different stations, one at a time. These types require many volunteers as well as properly trained and educated personnel to work each station. Stations may include any number of areas, including:

1. Health history (usually a written questionnaire)
2. Vital signs (height, weight, blood pressure, heart rate, and can include Snellen eye chart)
3. Internal conditions (i.e., physician exams)
4. Fitness (sub-max stress, e.g., the 3-minute step test)

LEADERSHIP ACTIVITY

Read NATA's Position statement entitled "Emergency Planning in Athletics" (this can be accessed on NATA's website at http://www.nata.org). Next, in conjunction with a classmate review an existing EAP for one of the sports you have covered recently, you are not to critique the EAP, you are only re-familiarizing yourself with the outlined procedures. Next, outside of class consult with your current (or a recent ACI) and arrange and implement a full-scale rehearsal of an emergency situation following the guidelines and suggestions of NATA's position statement.

5. Muscular endurance and strength (1-minute sit up or push-up tests)

6. Orthopedic conditions (musculoskeletal, range of motion, and joint integrity exams)

7. Socio-demographic characteristics (typically a private screening room to discuss sex, drugs, birth control, depression, or other related issues)

8. Exit interview (to answer specific questions restricted to disqualifying conditions).

Other stations may include assessments by optometrists, to perform a more extensive eye exam and dentists, perhaps to fit customized mouth guards. There is no limit to the number of stations that can be used in this delivery model. An advantage to this style is the limitless possibilities of what can be examined. However, a drawback is that this type of physical requires a lot of human resources, planning, and time.

Office-based physicals are typically not as extensive. For example, many office-based physicals do not include orthopedic evaluations or fitness exams, elements which are critical to a sport's physical. Furthermore, physicians usually do not have the staff or time to be as extensive as they would like and the patients may not have the resources (or insurance) to get all the screenings their physician would prefer. It is also a possibility that the primary care physician may not have the necessary background in sports medicine needed for thorough sports-related PPEs. However, office-based physicals allows for more privacy and candidness between patient and physician.

FEDERAL STATUTES

There are many federal statutes that have implications on athletic trainers and the practice of athletic training. Some of those statues are listed elsewhere in this text and earlier in this chapter. However, FERPA and HIPAA deserve a more detailed explanation.

Family Educational Rights and Privacy Act (FERPA) is a federal statute that delineates how to disseminate educational data. The greatest impact of FERPA to athletic training is in relation to athletic training education. Basically it makes provision for all students to be notified and give permission in writing for academic records to be viewed. This includes students giving permission for accrediting agencies, such as CAATE personnel, to view their educational files. Furthermore, FERPA also impacts how athletic training instructors disperse student grades. Grades are not to be posted outside offices or class doors nor should students be allowed to pick up grades from a collective spot.

The Department of Health and Human Services regulates the Health Insurance Portability and Accountability Act (HIPAA) also known as the Buckley Amendment, which delineates how to disseminate medical information. Athletic trainers must comply with HIPAA regulations. HIPAA regulations apply to most athletic trainers and have particular interest to those in occupational settings. HIPAA strives to maintain confidentiality of a patient's medical records, including disclosure to parents and guarantee that records can be transferred to other healthcare providers. The patient must sign a HIPAA release for all medical records and designate each party they wish their information to be disclosed to Figure 11-3 is a sample HIPAA release form that can be used in athletic training. Furthermore, athletic training students should be well versed in HIPAA requirements before they are assigned to any clinical education responsibilities.

I, _____, hereby authorize _____
(Please print name)   Name of My Institution
and its physicians, athletic trainers and health care personnel to disclose my protected health information and any related information regarding any injury or illness during my training for and participation in intercollegiate athletics to my parents/guardians.

_____
(Please print name, address & telephone number of parent(s)/guardian(s) to whom the information may be released)

I understand that my injury/illness information is protected by federal regulation under with the Health Information Portability and Accountability Act (HIPAA) of Family Education Rights and Privacy Act of 1974 (the Buckley Amendment) and may not be disclosed without either my authorization under HIPAA or my consent under the Buckley Amendment. I understand that my signing of this authorization/consent is voluntary and that my institution will not condition any benefits on whether I provide the consent or authorization requested for this disclosure. I also understand that I am not required to sign this authorization/consent in order to be eligible for participation in NCAA or conference athletics.

This authorization/consent expires 380 days from the date of my signature below, but I have the right to revoke it in writing at any time by sending written notification to the head athletic trainer at my institution. I understand that a revocation is not effective to the extent action has already been taken in reliance on this authorization/consent.

_____
Printed name of student   Signature   Date

FIGURE 11-3 Sample HIPAA release form

CHAPTER SUMMARY

There are several general legal principles that athletic trainers need to be aware of to practice the profession effectively, including civil and common law. Within the profession of athletic training, all athletic trainers should be acutely aware of Standards of Practice and any Scope of Practice outlined by the state in which one practices. Additionally, athletic trainers need to be aware of certain aspects of tort law including liability, negligence, including omission and commission, as well as the specific aspects one must demonstrate in order to prove negligence, such as duty of care, breach of duty, cause, and actual harm. Athletic trainers are also responsible to demonstrate knowledge of legal defense in the case of litigation. Furthermore, athletic trainers should practice behaviors that minimize risk and reduce personal liability, such as delineating, implementing, and rehearsing an emergency action plan and ensuring complete and thorough pre-participation physical exams for all participants. Finally, each athletic trainer is responsible to adhere to and abide by any state and federal statues, including HIPAA and FERPA regulations.

> ## Leadership
> ## Application

Below is an excerpt from the opinion for the legal case Pinson v. State, 1995, Tennessee Court of Appeals, Dec. 12, 1995. Additional details and the specific rulings of the case can be found by searching Tennessee's court opinions at http://www.tsc.state.tn.us/.

In August 1984, Pinson enrolled at UTM and reported to football camp for practice. He passed his physical examination and began participating in practice. On August 25, 1984, Pinson suffered a blow to the head during a football practice. He walked to the sidelines, said that he had been "kicked in the head," and collapsed, unconscious.

During the time that Pinson was unconscious, the UTM athletic trainer, James Richard Lyon (Lyon), examined Pinson. Lyon's personal notes from the day of Pinson's injury show that Lyon found palsy on the left side of Pinson's face, no control of the left side of his body, unequal pupils and no response to pain, sound or movement. These notes also show that Pinson remained unconscious for a period of 10 minutes.

After his examination of Pinson, Lyon summoned an ambulance which transported Pinson to the Volunteer General Hospital in Martin, Tennessee. Lyon did not personally accompany Pinson to the hospital but had a student trainer [sic] accompany Pinson. Lyon did not give the trainer [sic] any instructions about the information that the trainer [sic] should give the emergency room doctor. Hospital records show that the trainer [sic] informed an emergency room nurse that Pinson lost consciousness for about two minutes. Although Lyon visited the emergency room shortly after Pinson arrived, Lyon did not speak to a doctor about the neurological signs he had observed on the practice field.

At Volunteer General, Pinson's head was X-rayed and found to be normal. No CT scan was ever done. Pinson was assigned to Dr. O. K. Smith for follow-up care and was admitted to the hospital for observation. Although all neurological checks were normal, hospital records show that Pinson complained of headaches to the hospital staff. Pinson complained that one of these headaches was so severe that it made him sick to his stomach.

On August 26, 1984, Dr. Smith telephoned Lyon and told him that Pinson should not participate in football practice for a week and that, if any further trouble arose, Pinson should return to Dr. Smith or another physician. On that same day, Dr. Smith released Pinson to Lyon, and Lyon transported Pinson from the hospital to UTM.

When Lyon picked up Pinson, he complained to Lyon of a headache. Lyon did not record this headache in the UTM records. On August 27, 1984, Pinson complained of a headache and was given Empirin by Lyon. On August 28, 1984, Pinson told Lyon that he had a headache, but that it was milder than the one he had on the previous day. Lyon's notes of August 30, 1984, which refer to Pinson, contain the statement "Headache!"

On September 3, 1984, Lyon contacted Dr. Ira Porter, the UTM team physician. Lyon told Dr. Porter that Pinson was asymptomatic for a concussion on September 3. Lyon did not tell Dr. Porter about Pinson's headaches on the 26th, 27th, 28th, or 30th. Relying on Lyon's report of Pinson's condition, Dr. Porter concurred with Dr. Smith's prior advice that Pinson could return to practice if there were no further problems.

On September 3, 1984, Pinson returned to practice. He participated in practice, traveled as a member of the team and played in at least two games. Testimony from Pinson's mother, roommate and girlfriend, indicated that Pinson suffered headaches and complained of dizziness, nausea and blurred vision throughout this three week period from September 3 to September 24. Lyon did not report any of these symptoms to Dr. Porter. On September 24, Pinson walked to the sideline during a practice, stated that he had been "kicked in the head" and collapsed, unconscious.

Pinson was eventually taken to Jackson-Madison County General Hospital where he underwent brain surgery. Surgeons there found that Pinson had sustained a chronic subdural hematoma of three to four weeks' duration of several hundred cubic centimeters and an acute subdural hematoma of approximately 25–30 cubic centimeters and a shift of mid-line structures of almost 1.5 centimeters. Pinson remained in a coma for several weeks and was transferred to the Lamar Unit of Baptist Hospital in Memphis for intensive rehabilitative treatment. As a result of his injuries, Pinson suffered severe and permanent neurological damage.

Critical Thinking Questions

1. Did the athletic trainer student have any significant role in the case? (If so, what; if not, why not?)
2. What was the athletic trainer's duty to the athlete in this case? Was his duty performed, or was there some duty that was neglected?
3. Do you think there was any contributory negligence on the part of the athlete in this case? (If yes, why?; If no, why not?).
4. What, if anything, should the athletic trainer have done differently?
5. What defense could the athletic trainer use in court?
6. What published standard of care should be used as a baseline to establish how the athletic trainer should have responded in this case?
7. What was the role of the physician's in this case and was there any negligence on their part?

References

1. American Academy of Orthopaedic Surgeons. (1991). *Athletic training and sports medicine.* Rosemont, IL: AAOS.
2. American Academy of Orthopaedic Surgeons. (1999). *Athletic training and sports medicine.* Rosemont, IL: AAOS.
3. Andersen JC, Courson R, Kleiner D, McLoda T. (2002). National Athletic Trainers' Association Position Statement: Emergency Planning in Athletics. *JAT 37*(1):99–104.
4. Berntsen K. (2005). Looking beyond tort reform toward safer healthcare systems. *Journal of Nursing Care Quality 20*(1):9–12.
5. Carek P, Mainous A. (2002). The preparticipation physical examination for athletics: A systematic review of current recommendations. *BJM 2*:661–664.
6. Mickle A. (2007). The legal parameters defining the role of the certified athletic trainer. *ATT 12*(1):10–13.
7. Osborne B. (2001). Principles of liability for athletic trainers: Managing sport-related concussion. *JAT 36*(3):316–321.
8. Puffer JC. (1982). Sports medicine – Objectives of the preparticipation evaluation. *The Western Journal of Medicine 137*(1):58–59.
9. Roman L. (2007). Nurse attorneys tell you: How to stay out of legal hot water. *Registered Nurse 70*(1):27–31.
10. Streator S, Buckley W. (2001). Risk management in athletic training. *ATT 6*(2):55–59.

Program and Facility Management

Chapter 12

Forming and Planning a Program

"Apathy can be overcome by enthusiasm, and enthusiasm can only be aroused by two things: first, an ideal, which takes the imagination by storm, and second, a definite intelligible plan for carrying that ideal into practice."

ARNOLD TOYNBEE

Role Delineation Study Components

Domain V: Organization and Administration

- Knowledge of strategic planning and goal setting

Educational Competencies

- Describe vision and mission statements to focus service or program aspirations and strategic planning (e.g., "weaknesses, opportunities, threats and strengths underlying planning" [WOTS UP], "strengths, weaknesses, opportunities and threats" [SWOT]) to critically bring our organizational improvement.

Key Terms

Hoshin Kanri (or planning): A Japanese phrase that is translated "direction setting" and is the systematic process by which an organization sets and achieves specific long-term goals with respect to quality.

Intuition: A compressed expertise; or instinctive knowledge that comes from instantly accessing and assimilating years of experience or a lot of experiences in a moment.

Mission statement: The athletic training program's statement of its reason for existence in respect to present-day clientele, distinct services offered, philosophy, and geography.

Planning: The act of delineating behaviors intended to bring about a predetermined or expected course of actions.

Strategic planning: The process of diagnosing the organization's external and internal environments, articulating values, vision, and mission, developing overall goals, implementing action steps, and allocating resources to achieve goals and promote values.

SWOT analysis: The thorough assessment of a program's specific strengths, weaknesses, opportunities, and threats.

Vision statement: An ideal image of the future one seeks to create.

T*he opportunity for an athletic trainer to integrate leadership and management is perhaps at its all-time high during the formation, planning, and implementation of an athletic training program. Leaders are often expected to think strategically, while managers are often required to implement strategy. Forming and planning an athletic training program requires both the strategic intent and thinking of a leader as well as the implementation and assessment of a manager.*

Planning an athletic training program from beginning to end is no small task. Athletic trainers must take intentional actions when creating and establishing athletic training programs. These actions should meet patient's needs, meet financial obligations, achieve needed clinical outcomes, promote the integrity of the profession and the allied health care industry, as well as provide a satisfying environment for any staff.

The overall strategic process is multi-faceted and includes delineating organizational, stakeholder, and individual values, creating vision statements and mission statements, setting goals and objectives, program analysis, and an established decision-making process. Therefore, in this chapter we will examine important leadership roles necessary in establishing and strengthening an athletic training program. We will begin by discussing the first aspect required to establish a strong athletic training program: determining stakeholders and delineating values. Next, we will discuss drafting vision and mission statements, followed by setting goals and objectives. After we discuss these elements, we will look to strategic planning and how to implement an S.W.O.T. (Strengths, Weaknesses, Opportunities, and Threats) analysis. Finally, we will discuss the role of innovation in program planning as well as decision-making strategies.

STRATEGIC CONCEPTS

Strategic thinking requires conceptualizing the past, present, and future. This requires understanding any relevant history, including the factors that helped or hindered the process up until the present day. Relevant present-day activities that are occurring locally, professionally, or globally (i.e., perceptions, new research, changing regulations or reforms) must also be accounted for. Only after historical information and the present-day environment has been evaluated can the process of planning for the future and implementing decisions proceed. Furthermore, planning for the future must include innovation and a willingness to navigate change.

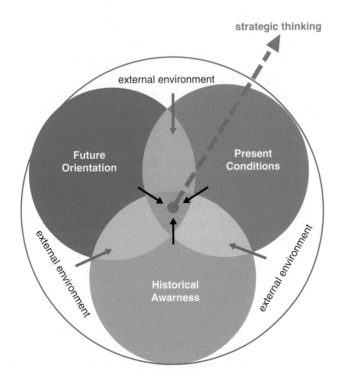

Therefore, athletic trainers who are planning programs should be aware of the historical evolution of the profession, a department, or a program, the current contextual variables that inform the present-day attitudes, as well as future expectations. Only after these three conceptual elements have been assimilated is the strategic backdrop properly prepared.

PROGRAM FORMATION

No one can convincingly argue that planning is not a fundamental aspect of long-term success, or that lack of planning is a considerable contributor toward failure. Therefore, it is paramount that planning be taken seriously by athletic trainers wishing to establish a new, revamp, or sustain an existing athletic training program. The principles of planning work in any athletic training context. **Planning** is the act of delineating behaviors intended to bring about a predetermined or expected course of action. For athletic training programs, key planning behaviors should include the following:

1. Determining stakeholders
2. Delineating values
3. Creating a vision
4. Drafting a mission
5. Establishing goals and objectives

Determining Stakeholders

All enterprises in every industry across the globe have stakeholders. Stakeholders are anyone that is affected by the actions or plans of an organization, department, or even an individual. A fundamental component to proper planning is to realize that all decisions and actions affect something or someone. Therefore, decision makers must take responsibility for their actions. Not all actions equally impact all stakeholders, but they have an affect nonetheless. In athletic training, stakeholders can include athletes, patients, parents, students, staff associates, coaches, physicians, the community, friends and loved ones, other members of the sports medicine team, and other medical or health professionals.

When planning, athletic trainers must take the time to determine which stakeholders will be impacted by any decisions or ensuing actions. In other words, athletic trainers must ask and answer the question, "If we do this particular action who (from the greatest to the least) will be impacted, and to what degree?" Different programs will have different stakeholders and not all stakeholders are as important as others, but all should be considered. Determining stakeholders early on in a program's forming and planning process can facilitate an easier implementation of any plans. Furthermore, determining stakeholders will help inform the values of the program and ultimately help ensure longevity and satisfaction. After stakeholders are identified, the next step is determining the values of those stakeholders.

Delineating Values

Delineating values can be a long and hopefully fun process. Values are those practices or attitudes which are predetermined to be celebrated.[2] Values are a list of ideals on which the organization focuses its time, attention, and resources. Later on, it will be values that guide the creation of the vision and mission statements. In essence, values are the framework to the entire strategic planning process (Fig. 12-1).

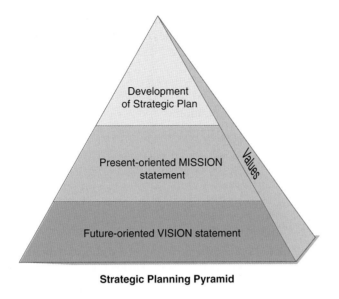

Strategic Planning Pyramid

FIGURE 12-1 Strategic planning pyramid

Values are delineated based on input from stakeholders and critical self-reflection. First try and delineate the values of stakeholders. This can be a formal or informal process. A formal process includes interviewing and questioning stakeholders about what they deem to be important and how the athletic training program you are creating or reorganizing can facilitate those values. An informal process includes casually observing stakeholder's behaviors and forming an educated guess as to how they might react to the program's actions. Next, it is important to decide your values (or your team's values) as they relate to the athletic training program. Being able to critically and accurately self-reflect is a necessary skill to determine values.

Actions should be informed by 1) the values of key stakeholders; and 2) the personal values of the creating team. For example, it would be illadvised to violate the values of referring physicians, especially if the program is dependent on referrals for revenue. Likewise, to ignore personal values could potentially create ethical or moral dilemmas and even conflict. On the other hand, having a clearly defined list of values can help inform actions and guide decisions. For example, if an opportunity violates or simply does not promote a core value deliberation over a course of action is easier; or if there is a new opportunity that promotes one or all of the values then that too helps to inform any decision. However, if no values have been defined, it becomes much more difficult to make decisions or decide which opportunities to pursue.

Identifying Values

How many values does an athletic training program need? There is no set number of values required, however, the longer the list of values the greater the risk of some of those values conflicting. Conflicting values (either internally or among stakeholders) can be extremely problematic and can paralyze decision making. Values can be identified by asking stakeholders or team members to critically reflect and analyze behaviors or attitudes they deem critically important to success. Because success means different thing to different people, expect the list to long and varied. Part of the process of identifying values involves honing down the list to a manageable size. It is a good idea to have approximately three to five values, any more than this and it becomes difficult to clearly articulate a concise vision statement.

Values can be anything from behaviors to attitudes. Experience, personal conviction, and ethics are the only necessary guides to establishing values. A list of values in athletic training might include:

- Cost-effective treatment
- Empathy toward patients
- Safe and timely return to competition
- Quality health care
- Service orientation
- Profit
- Teamwork
- Empowerment
- Promoting diversity

Without clearly articulated values, the meaning of a vision statement is lost.

Creating a Vision

Leadership expert Peter Senge[1] reminds us that, "without a vision people perish." Meaning a clear and articulate vision is essential for the successful operation of any enterprise. A **vision** is an ideal image of the future one seeks to create.[1,2] It is the goal or direction an organization, individual, or team strives toward. This concept of vision suggests an orientation toward the future, and a key leadership practice is to visualize an ideal future. Athletic trainers and students can facilitate the advancement of their program and their profession by maintaining a vision of a desirable future for athletic training.

Vision statements are important because people need to know where they need to be in order to act in a reasonable manner to get there.[3] Articulating a clear picture of the future with a vision statement is important for every athletic training program. However, creating a clear and concise vision statement is not as easy as one might initially believe. Nearly 75% of vision statements do not provide an adequate picture of the future.[4] Many vision statements are filled with contemporary jargon and catch-phrases, which is difficult to translate into tangible action.[4] Therefore, it is important to use stated values as the framework for vision.

The vision statement should be created through consensus, not as an edict from senior leadership. Buy-in of the vision statement by all involved parties is extremely important because accomplishing the vision requires a combined effort. Although the senior leadership may ultimately decide on the exact wording of the vision statement, the ideas and values presented in the statement should come from key stakeholders.

Drafting Vision Statements

Once the leadership is satisfied with delineated values, the process of drafting the vision statement begins. The vision statement itself is a concise, one or two sentences, describing the values the athletic training program wishes to propagate for the future of the program. Ultimately it is the vision statement, based on the program's values, that determines the effectiveness of the program. On a regular basis the athletic training program should be evaluated based on its stated vision.

Vision statements have at least five characteristics:[4]

1. They are brief – typically one or two sentences.
2. They are verifiable – at least 10 people should be able to recognize if the vision is being accomplished.
3. They are focused – they remind others of one or two issues critical for success to your target population.

4. They are understandable to everyone – clearly articulated and free from industry or organizational specific jargon.

5. They are inspiring.

Sample Vision Statements

The following are examples of vision statements from various sports medicine and athletic training settings. In the university setting, a sample vision statement might read,

> "The department of athletic training services at XYZ University is dedicated to the comprehensive health care needs and the highest quality injury management for our athletes."

An industrial athletic training program's vision statement might read,

> "IQ Industries sets a standard within our industry for least number of work hours lost due to on-site injuries and is committed to the overall wellbeing of all employees."

An example of an occupational or outpatient rehabilitation's vision statement might read,

> "XYZ Hospital's Athletic Training Services will be the leading provider of athletic training coverage and injury rehabilitation services to the high schools of Metro city."

Finally, using three of the values identified earlier (i.e., service orientation, empathy toward patients, and safe and speedy return to competition) a vision statement might read,

> "to provide affordable, accessible, and uncompromising health care to the active population in our community."

Drafting a Mission

After the vision statement has been developed the next step is to develop a mission statement. Mission statements expand on the vision statement by adding "how" the vision will be accomplished. There is a fundamental difference between vision and mission statements: The vision statement is future oriented, and the mission statement is oriented toward current services and conditions; visions challenge, missions anchor.[7] The mission statement keeps the athletic training program focused on who it is serving and how it is serving them. A clearly defined mission can help drive leadership decisions and actions.[6] The following elements are often found in many health care related mission statements:

- Customer definition (stakeholders)
- Product/service definition
- Organizational philosophy
- Description of public image
- Geographical area
- Distinctive competencies.[5]

Based on these elements we will define **mission statement** as the reason for existence in respect to present-day clientele, distinct services offered, philosophy, and geography. An example of an effective mission statement might be:

> "Mercy Hospital's Athletic Training Department exists to provide high quality sports medicine services to the physically active and student–athletes in our local community by providing: injury prevention, clinical evaluation and diagnosis, immediate injury care, treatment, rehabilitation, reconditioning, and community education that is competent, efficient, and professional and to ensure a safe and timely return to activity at or beyond their normal level of involvement and competition. We intend to accomplish this by providing easy access to sports medicine clinics, and a tangible presence at community-based sporting events, and by providing certified athletic trainers to each High School within the local community."

Drafting a mission statement is similar to drafting a vision statement. Begin with the vision and simply explain how that vision will come to past for the current stakeholders or target population. In the sample mission statement above it is easy to identify what the vision statement was…. "to provide high quality sports medicine services to the physically active and student-athletes in our local community." In other words, the mission was drafted by including the "where" and "how" of their existing vision statement. After vision and mission are articulated, next is the establishment of goals and objectives related to those statements.

Establishing Goals and Objectives

As the process of determining stakeholders, listing values, drafting vision and mission statements nears the end, it is important to compile a list of goals and objectives. For effective planning and strategizing, it is important to state goals and objectives clearly. While some debate exists as to the difference between goals and objectives, generally speaking objectives are the ultimate end one hopes to achieve. Therefore, objectives are usually generalizations of what is expected or hoped for.

On the other hand, goals are more specific and include time-specific and measurable language. Goals should answer the questions of "who," "what," "when," "where," and "how" of the objectives. In other words, goals are specific action steps. You should strive to create S.M.A.R.T. (specific, measurable, achievable, realistic, and time-oriented) goals. The reader of the goals should easily be able to identify each of the S.M.A.R.T. elements within the statement.

Typically each goal is based on a larger objective. For example, the more general objective of "to be a premier sports medicine provider" may be further explained by the following goal, "to be one of the top three most profitable sports medicine providers in the county by the end of the fiscal year." Note that the objective is general and lacks measurable language. On the other hand the goal is measurable and includes time-oriented language.

Another example of an objective may be to "reduce the amount of injuries on the job." The goal to meet that objective might be twofold: 1) to hire an athletic trainer to introduce a validated injury prevention education program to be attended by 90% of employees by December 31; 2) hire an athletic trainer to conduct and publish a work-safety analysis of each division on a quarterly basis. These goals help to accomplish the objective and are specific, measurable, achievable, realistic, and time oriented.

STRATEGIC PLANNING

Strategic planning is the process of diagnosing the organization's external and internal environments, deciding on a vision and mission, developing overall goals, creating and selecting general strategies to be pursued, and allocating resources to achieve the organization's goals.[8] Athletic trainers of all levels and ranks participate in strategic planning, both formal and informal. In its purest form, strategic planning is undertaken to gain a competitive advantage over competition. Stated another way, strategic planning involves developing innovative strategies to perform similar tasks differently than competition. This has particular relevance to entrepreneurial initiatives of athletic trainers in the marketplace (i.e., clinic owners). However, athletic trainers in not-for-profit arenas such as high schools or public universities also need to plan strategically to ensure buy-in and participation of others.

The process of strategy includes answering the questions, where do you want to go, and how do you want to get there? In athletic training programs, strategy may

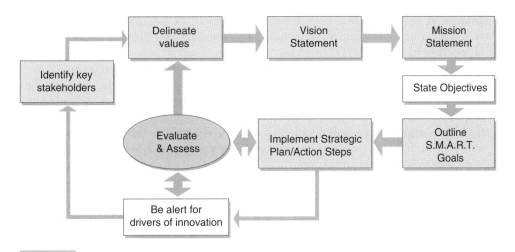

FIGURE 12-2 Strategic planning cycle

involve evaluating current delivery models and comparing those to competitor's delivery models, then coming up with a viable plan to implement that model. For example, in a large metropolitan area there are likely to be several companies offering athletic training services to local high-schools. A sound strategic planning process can help set one athletic training company above its competitor(s).

A majority of the strategic planning process includes what has been previously discussed, i.e., stakeholders, values, vision, mission, objectives and goals. However, the crucible of strategic planning comes when it is time to implement those stated goals. Once implementation begins, strategic planning is not over. Strategy must be continually monitored and evaluated. An important part of monitoring the strategic plan includes conducting a SWOT analysis. Figure 12.2 shows the strategic planning cycle.

SWOT Analysis

The strategic plan includes evaluating and assessing internal strengths and weaknesses, and external opportunities and threats. Many strategists call this a **SWOT**

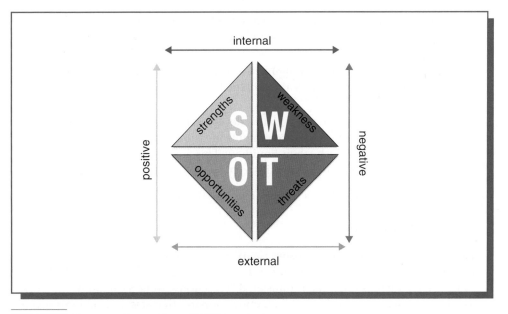

FIGURE 12-3 Common layout for a SWOT analysis

analysis. A SWOT analysis is an internal assessment of Strengths and Weaknesses (i.e., SW), and an external assessment of Opportunities and Threats (i.e., OT); combined, they become a SWOT analysis.

It is important to articulate values, vision, mission, and goals before a SWOT analysis is performed, as it is important to have a baseline measurement. Even though there are similarities between many athletic training programs, values and objectives are individualized and as such threats and opportunities may differ significantly. Furthermore, opportunities need to be examined in the light of values and goals otherwise time and resources may be wasted on things that may not help in accomplishing objectives or worse wasted on opportunities that do not promote the values of the organization or team.

The SWOT analysis has two distinct phases. First, the internal SWOT in which assessment is focused on the organization's strength and weaknesses. The second part is the external SWOT in which the environment is assessed for opportunities and threats. Figure 12-2 shows a common layout for performing a SWOT analysis. In addition to conducting a SWOT analysis, other tools or models used in strategic planning include strategy mapping and Hoshin planning.

Strategy Mapping

A strategy map can show how different aspects of a strategic plan work together.[10] It is specifically useful for assigning a value to intangible skills. In other words, a strategy map can help create a visual representation of how seemingly unrelated values are related. A properly developed strategy map can prevent others from developing a myopic or biased view of an individual's worth or contribution. For example, an athletic trainer in an outreach setting who is only valued or assessed by generated referrals could use a strategy map to illustrate how his or her "other" skills add significant value to the organization. Another example in an outreach setting might include the athletic trainer who has responsibility for several high schools and therefore can only triage injuries once or twice a week at each high school. A strategy map could depict how pulling away from a multiple venue system and focusing on how having a major presence in one high school adds more value than having a minor presence in many schools.

Strategy mapping involves the following three parts.[10]

1. Describing the intangible asset – An example of an intangible asset in athletic training might be several leadership competencies, such as excellent communication ability and people skills.

2. Aligning and integrating intangible assets – This means identifying which aspect of the organization's strategy the athletic trainer's leadership competencies can best enhance.

3. Defining how intangible assets can be developed or promoted – You measure intangible assets the same way accountants measure other assets, by how fast they can be converted to cash (their liquidity). This means providing opportunity for the athletic trainer to use these skills to promote the organization's goals.

Figure 12-4 is a sample of how a strategy map can be used in athletic training, and

Hoshin Planning

Hoshin planning (also called **Hoshin Kanri**) is a Japanese form of strategic planning that is sometimes used in the health care industry, especially in hospitals. Hoshin Kanri is a Japanese phrase that is translated "direction setting" and has been defined as "the systematic process by which an entire organization sets and achieves specific long term goals with respect to quality."[11]

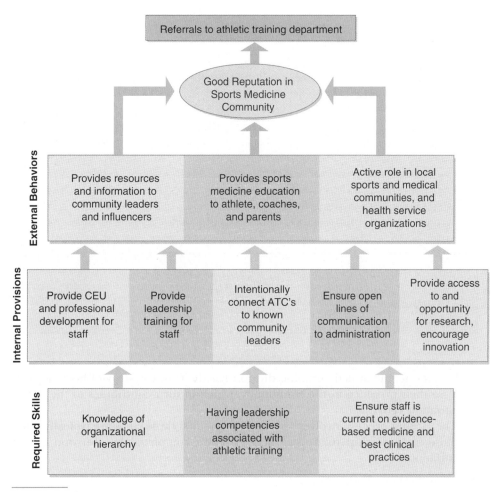

FIGURE 12-4 Strategy map

Hoshin planning is a top-down approach to strategic planning, where decisions and directions are primarily set by organizational leaders.[12] However, Hoshin planning does allow for a team-based process. For example, decisions are based on feedback, input, and implementation from many organizational members and stakeholders. Hoshin planning relies heavily on each member of the organization sharing a common vision. This common vision is often implemented through group interaction and consistent feedback referred to as "catchball" (i.e., throwing around ideas and goals until everyone buys in).

Hoshin planning is essentially a two-pronged process. The first prong involves long-range planning for the entire organization. This is typically completed by those with formal leadership or management roles. Once long-range plans are articulated, the next prong involves tracking how departments or divisions are implementing those plans.[9] For example, within a large hospital there can be several areas of specialty, such as "sports medicine," and within sports medicine there might be physicians with differing specialties such as therapists, physiologists, and athletic trainers. Once the plans are set for the entire hospital, it is up to individual departments or specialties (i.e., athletic training) to determine how they can best contribute to and accomplish those plans. For instance, if the hospital has a plan for increasing their presence in the local community, then the athletic training division is left to decide how they can best do that. Obviously what athletic trainers might do to accomplish that plan is different from what another branch of medicine might do. When all is

> ### ✏️ *From the Field*
>
> *For financial reasons, a local hospital I had worked for decided to eliminate its sports medicine department, leaving me and four other athletic trainers who had long histories in the community without jobs. Because the values that drove our athletic training department were community and service oriented, all the athletic trainers provided more than merely athletic training coverage. We were vested into the high schools (in fact most of us were alumni of the schools we served, which was intentional), therefore, we went above the call of duty, not only event and practice coverage, rehab, and injury diagnosis but routinely volunteering to teach courses, supervising the strength programs, creating and supervising student aides, and covering camps, etc. Ultimately, the hospital's financial decision to drop athletic training had additional long-term negative impact. This was demonstrated by the fact that within 24 hours of our being notified our services were no longer needed, we were all employed by competitors and each of us retained our schools. The hospital's reputation in the sports medicine community was tarnished badly. Rehabilitation referrals, once taken for granted, were now referred elsewhere, and even the physicians and orthopedic surgeons associated suffered financially. This is an example of how failure to recognize other intangible assets that athletic trainers contributed to the overall mission of the hospital ended in financial loss and an tarnished reputation in the sports medicine community.*

said and done, the athletic training division has their own strategy of how they can increase their presence in the community, which in turn contributes to the entire organization's goal.

The Hoshin process involves seven steps. The first three steps are typically done by those in leadership roles, and steps 4–7 are completed by everyone in the organization:

1. Identification of critical issues
2. Establishment of objectives to address these issues
3. Definition of the company's over-all goals
4. Development of strategies that support the over-all goals
5. Definition of sub-goals (objectives) that support each strategy
6. Establishment of indicators for measuring process performance
7. Establishment of fundamental measures[12]

Strategy Pitfalls to Avoid

Careful strategic planning is not a guarantee of success. If care is not taken to prevent some of the common mistakes, time, effort, and momentum can be wasted or lost. Among the most common offenders are:[9]

1. Setting unrealistic or arbitrary goals
2. Failing to focus on real values
3. Allowing goals to become "wishes"
4. Lacking common values among team players
5. Planning sessions being treated as events
6. Having inadequate or outdated data
7. Relying too much on expert and experienced planners
8. Leaders failing to take responsibility for outcomes
9. Relying too heavily on financial outcomes as a basis for decision making.

DRIVERS OF INNOVATION IN FORMATION AND PLANNING

Innovation is the creation or introduction of something brand new. Conceptually, innovation is typically framed around future action or intention. On the other hand, change (which is usually mentioned in conjunction with innovation) is typically conceptually associated with a historical fact or behavior. This is perhaps why many people generally resist change, but often embrace innovation. Furthermore, organizations that intentionally practice and are committed to innovation are often the most successful.[13] Innovation is a prerequisite for longevity.

In athletic training, innovation can help create new ways to offer "athletic training services" to the non-traditional athlete or in non-traditional settings. This can be a tremendous asset to the formation and planning of athletic training programs. Peter Drucker[13] has identified seven drivers of innovation:

1. Unexpected occurrences
2. Incongruities
3. Process needs
4. Industry or market changes
5. Demographic changes
6. Changes in perception
7. New knowledge

While all of these drivers of innovation deserve attention, four have an obvious relationship to athletic training: new knowledge, changes in perception, industry or market changes, and demographic changes.

New Knowledge

Athletic trainers who perform research and disseminate their findings and the athletic trainers who implement those findings are innovators who are ensuring the profession's future. New knowledge and discoveries can be great sources of innovation that can help athletic training make a permanent mark in the health and medical industries. As athletic training knowledge expands, it fosters another driver of innovation: changes in perception. As other professions change their perception (positively or negatively) of athletic training (based on this new knowledge and the quality of it), further innovation is likely to follow. Therefore, since athletic trainers have decided to create a culture of discovering knowledge, innovation will be a natural by-product.

Changes in Perception and Industry

Another driver of innovation in athletic training is changes in perception. Changes in perception can be positive and negative, and anything at any time can contribute to a change in perspective. Therefore, these specific drivers are often unanticipated. If a perception changes that is threatening to the profession, an innovation can occur in retaliation. If a perception shifts that benefits the profession, such as a new state's licensure, there is likely to be innovation as well. Either way, athletic trainers must respond to changes in how we are perceived with new ideas on how to forge ahead in light of those perceptions.

Industry changes can also drive innovation. For example, athletic trainers who identify a new work setting or practice niche as a response to new or revised regulations, accreditation outcomes, educational reform, or law suites, ultimately benefit the profession and the organizations that employ them.

Demographic and Market Changes

Another opportunity to innovate occurs when demographics change. For example, the aging populations, many of whom still want to remain active, or the growing number of ethnically diverse patients and clients, all need athletic training services. As the demographic characteristics (i.e., age, gender, education, ethnicity) of a population change, athletic trainers will be forced to create new practice settings, delivery models, or create new recruitment models that attract more ethnically diverse students to the profession; this will accommodate the changing demographic or expand into a new arena made up of a new demographic. Innovating as a result of changing demographics and target markets will help ensure athletic trainers remain on the cutting edge.

Performing a thorough SWOT analysis and paying close attention to the external opportunities and threats is one way to stimulate innovative ideas. Leaders in the athletic training profession take advantage of these opportunities to innovate, but it is the strategic process that often alerts someone to these drivers of innovation.

ANALYTICAL AND INTUITIVE DECISION MAKING

Forming and planning an athletic training program requires decision making. Furthermore, the practice of innovation requires decisions. Leaders cannot afford to be squeamish about making decisions. Making the right decisions fosters trust and increases credibility. Failure to make the right decisions or even hesitating to make decisions undermines the decision maker's credibility and can jeopardize morale.

Leaders need to have a process for making decisions. Risk and emotion are inescapable parts of every decision.[14] The presence of human emotion in the decision making process can be what makes them so risky. Ironically, reducing risk is often the goal of many decisions. Therefore, a keen sense and understanding of one's emotional state of mind is critical before making a decision. It has been said that decision' implies the end of deliberation and the beginning of action.[14] This deliberation is a multi-stage multi-layered phenomenon that involves analytical, rationale, and intuitive processes.

Analytical Decision Making

Mack, Crawford, and Reed[15] have delineated an analytical and rationale seven-step model for making healthcare-related leadership decisions (note: this is distinct from clinical decision making). The seven steps are:

1. Understand the organization.
2. Define the objective of the decision.
3. Identify and prioritize the factors that will influence the decision.
4. Collect information needed to make the decision, and generate decision options.
5. Evaluate options and make the best choice.
6. Develop an action plan, and implement the decision.
7. Monitor decision's effects, and revise as appropriate.

Understanding the Organization

Understanding the organization implies knowing the organizational culture (i.e., its politics, symbols, policies and procedures, and influencers) as well as how decisions have historically been made. Often an organization takes on a personality of its own with different symbols, beliefs, and unwritten values weaved into its culture. The conscientious decision maker will take time to learn and assess the organization's culture.

Defining the Objective of the Decision

Defining the objective of the decision involves determining what outcomes are expected from the decision, i.e., what should be different after the decision is made. For instance, expectations for decisions made in a crisis or medical emergency might be different from day-to-day operational decisions or long-range strategic decisions.

Identifying and Prioritizing the Factors That Will Influence the Decision

Identifying and prioritizing the factors that will influence the decision simply implies recognizing any obstacles that may impede the decisions implementation. This step involves brainstorming with key stakeholders. Prioritizing involves ranking (i.e., assigning a point value) to the factors that will influence the decision then tallying those points to determine the most significant factors.

Generating Decision Options

Collecting information needed to make the decision, and generating decision options means to collect as broad a range as possible of all available options or possible outcomes. This step also should involve multiple stakeholders' interests, which may require input from several sources. It is a good idea to get input from trustworthy stakeholders with opposing points of view.

Evaluating Options and Making the Best Choice

Evaluating options and making the best choice involves evaluating the pros and cons of each potential decision (or option). This step involves listing all options then assigning pros and cons to each option. Each pro is assigned a point value and each con is assigned a negative point value the option with the highest point total is theoretically the "best" decision. These points are not assigned arbitrarily. Point values are assigned to each option based on the objectives set in step 2. For example, an athletic training department needs to find a way that motivates staff to make better clinical decisions and reduces medical errors. Therefore, two options arise and a decision needs to be made between paying overtime or reducing the work load. Each decision will have individual outcomes. Both may produce "happier" staff (+1), but option one (paying overtime) means less personal time (−1) and therefore more fatigued staff (−1); and option two (reducing work load) means more personal time (+1) and allows more time to read evidence-based literature at work (+1), points are assigned to each option's objectives and totaled. The best decision is the option with the highest points; option one (overtime) totaled −1; option two (reduced load) totaled +3, therefore, it appears option 2 is the best decision. This process works for an infinite number of options.

Developing an Action Plan and Implementing the Decision

Developing an action plan and implementing the decision involves obtaining buy-in from stakeholders as well as deciding how to deal with the obstacles identified earlier. Part of this involves establishing priorities, setting target dates, delegating authority and assigning responsibilities, and determining how the decision will be evaluated. Follow-through is critical at this juncture. Planning is only as effective as the degree of implementation. Some experts indicate that success is 20% planning and 80% implementation.[15] Decisions are worthless and time is wasted without proper implementation. For example, in the earlier example of deciding that it is best to reduce staff work load is worthless unless there is a strategy in place to actually implement reduced workloads.

Monitoring the Decision and Revising

No decision is without its flaws or blind spots. Hopefully the flaws can be minimized and discovered during the previous six steps, but it is unrealistic to believe no other obstacles will arise. A decision is only as good as its ability to be flexible and adaptable. Therefore, once a decision is implemented it is important to assess its effectiveness.

One drawback to the above seven-step process is the time required to implement them. If a quick decision is needed obviously these seven steps can not occur in a few minutes or even in a day. In the above case the decision-making process is deliberate and occurs in stages that involve input from multiple stakeholders and may take significant time. This is as it should be. However, the luxury to take time and involve multiple stakeholders is not always an option. Another drawback to analytical decision making is that it can present too much information, which can create blind spots or lead to faulty conclusions. Therefore, an acceptable alternative to a purely analytical approach is to include intuition in the decision-making process.

Intuitive Decision Making

Another aspect of the decision making process is intuition. Intuitive decision making is well documented in scholarly literature.[16,17,18,19,20] Intuition is the skill of focusing on potentially important but often faint signals that fuel imagination, innovation, and creativity.[17] **Intuition** has also been explained as "compressed expertise" or instinctive knowledge that comes from instantly accessing and assimilating years of experience or a lot of experiences in a moment.[16]

Intuition plays an important part in every decision regardless of how much time is available to make it. Intuition is a pronounced aspect of decision making in experts.[21] Therefore, the greater the expertise of the leader or the clinician the more one can expect to rely on intuitive sensing (or the proverbial "gut" reaction). However, regardless of experience there is a certain level of intuitive insight expected of those in leadership roles.

While there is evidence to support intuitive decision making as a viable process, there are shortcomings to relying purely on intuition and most researchers suggest utilizing a combination of intuition and analytical processes. The most obvious shortcomings of intuitive decision making are the lack of reproducible methods. However, intuitive decision making has a place, has been documented to be very effective, and has been demonstrated to be more effective at times than purely analytical or "rational" decision making.[16]

Traps of Decision Making

Decision making can be as much an art as it is science. Within the art and science of decision making, athletic training leaders can fall into several traps. Some of the more common things that hinder effective decision making are described below.

Anchoring

A common trap in decision making includes anchoring, which is when the mind places too high a value on the first information it receives.[22] The most common anchor is the past, specifically past successes or failures. Often these successes or failures bias us from seeing other viable decision options. Anchoring tends to bias the decision maker toward repeating similar decisions or avoiding logical ones.

Status-Quo Trap

The status-quo trap is also very prevalent in sabotaging decisions and its probability of occurring increases as the number of choices increases.[22] The status quo trap is very powerful and displayed in actions intended to "not rock the boat." Examples of the status-quo trap include tabling decisions until later, waiting for a situation to "stabilize" which further entrenches current behaviors, decisions based on trends, or historically justified decisions. Status-quo traps are particularly attractive because omission (doing nothing) appears to have less consequence than commission (doing something).[22]

Sunk-Cost Trap

The sunk-cost trap is another way decisions are sabotaged. The sunk-cost trap is making a decision in order to justify a previous decision.[22] For example, hiring an unqualified employee, and later needing to give extra training, mentoring, and development money in order to get that person qualified. Another example might be pouring money into the maintenance of equipment that is never used, but was lobbied hard for in the past. The best way to avoid this trap is to admit to the failure of a past decision and cut losses.

Confirming-Evidence Trap

The confirming-evidence trap is when we place too much value on information and evidence that supports our original premise and too little value to equally as reputable, yet conflicting or contradictory evidence. There are usually valid sides to every option or opinion. The "side" of the evidence you "embrace" is likely biased by your experience(s). This in turn entrenches your decisions further. Confirming-evidence trap is also seen when asking peers for opinions and justification of decisions. For example, let's say you want to build a 5000 square foot athletic training room (ATR), but are not sure if your institution actually needs or ever will need that much space. As part of the decision making process you phone a good friend and peer who has just built a 5000 square foot ATR and she tells you how great it is to have that much space and the all the new options available with that space, etc. A wise decision maker should not allow that conversation to be the sole source of input as it is likely subject to confirming-evidence bias.

CHAPTER SUMMARY

Strategic planning is a critically important process in the creation, development, and implementation of an athletic training program regardless of context. The elements of strategy include identifying key stakeholders, delineating stakeholder and personal values, and drafting vision and mission statements. Following the drafting of the mission statement is identifying general objectives and S.M.A.R.T. goals that are measurable and time-oriented. Once objectives are clarified it is important to act on them and implement the plan, being sure to measure and evaluate the plan's effectiveness.

Leadership
Application

You are a new member of the athletic training staff at a large community sports medicine clinic. You were hired because of your 18 years of experience with athletes, in a large collegiate setting. It is your second week of work in the clinic and you are unexpectedly invited by the owner to attend an annual strategic planning meeting with the clinic's senior staff. The senior staff is surprised to see you at the meeting, but seem glad of your presence. The senior staff consists of one athletic trainer, two physical therapists, one occupational therapist, one massage therapist, and the owner, an orthopedic surgeon. The agenda includes an open brainstorming session, where any and all new ideas are encouraged. The brainstorming session is specifically intended to generate ideas for new revenue streams. As an athletic trainer at a large university for several years prior you are new to this idea of generating revenue.

Critical Thinking Questions

1. What experiences might you be able to draw upon to help you generate ideas for revenue production?

2. How might the senior staff respond to your ideas?

3. Identify external stakeholders you can now target because of your addition to the staff.

4. What is the benefit of having you present at the meeting, what are some risks?

Innovation and decision making are also important aspects of the strategic process. Without innovation it is difficult to sustain longevity. Finally we discussed the decision making process and emphasized both an analytical and intuitive process. Being mindful of common traps such as anchoring, status-quo, confirming-evidence, and sunk-cost traps can help the decision making process be more effective.

References

1. Senge P. (1996). Leadership in living organizations. In: Hesselbein, F., Goldsmith, M., & Somerville, I. *Leading beyond the walls.* San Francisco, CA: Jossey-Bass.

2. Kouzes J, Posner B. (1995). *The leadership challenge.* San Francisco, CA: Jossey-Bass.

3. Tichy N. (1997). *The leadership engine.* New York: Harper Business.

4. Brown MG. (1998). Improving your organization's vision. *The Journal for Quality and Participation 21*(5):18–21.

5. Bart C, Hupfer M. (2004). Mission statements in Canadian hospitals. *Journal of Health Organization and Management 18*(2/3):92–110.

6. Umbdenstock R, Hageman W, Amundson B. (1990). The five critical areas for effective governance of not-for-profit hospitals. *Hospital & Health Services Administration 35*(4):481–492.

7. Pointer D, Orlikoff J. (2002). *The high performance board: Principles of nonprofit organization governance.* San Francisco, CA: Jossey-Bass.

8. Hellriegel D, Jackson SE, Slocum JW. (2002). *Management, a competency-based approach.* Mason, OH: South Western Thomson Learning.

9. Tennant C, Roberts P. (2000). Hoshin Kanri: A technique for strategic quality management. *Quality Assurance 8*:77–90.

10. Kaplan R, Norton D. (2004). The strategy map: Guide to aligning intangible assets. *Strategy and Leadership 32*(5):10–17.

11. Melum M, Collett C. (eds.) (1995). *Breakthrough leadership: Achieving organizational alignment through Hoshin planning.* Chicago: American Hospital Publishing.

12. Kenyon D. (1995). Strategic planning with Hoshin process. *Quality Digest 26*(5): Retrieved from http://www.qualitydigest.com/may97/html/hoshin.html

13. Drucker P. (1998). The discipline of innovation. *Harvard Business Review* November-December:149–157.

14. Buchanan L, O'Connell A. (2006). A brief history of decision making. *Harvard Business Review* January:32–41.

15. Mack K, Crawford MA, Reed M. (2004). *Decision making for improved performance*. Chicago: Health Administration Press.

16. Sauter V. (1999). Intuitive decision-making. *Communications of the ACM 42*(6):109–115.

17. Sadler-Smith E, Shefy E. (2004). The intuitive executive: Understanding and applying 'gut feel' in decision making. *Academy of Management Executive 18*(4):78–91.

18. Claxton G. (2001). The anatomy of intuition. In Atkinson T, Clayton G. (Eds). *The intuitive practitioner*. Buckingham, England: Open University Press: 32–52.

19. Hogarth RM. (2001). *Educating intuition*. Chicago: The University of Chicago Press.

20. Shaprio S, Spence M. (1997). Managerial intuition: A conceptual and operational framework. *Business Horizons* January/February: 63–68.

21. Benner P. (2000). *From novice to expert: Excellence and power in clinical nursing practice*. Upper Saddle River, NJ: Prentice Hall.

22. Hammond J, Keeney R, Raiffa H. (2006). The hidden traps of decision making. *Harvard Business Review* (January): 118–126.

Chapter 13

Facility Design and Management

"A great architect is not made by way of a brain nearly so much as he is made by way of a cultivated, enriched heart."

FRANK LLOYD WRIGHT

Key Terms

Business plan: A document that spells out the expected course of action of an existing or new enterprise for a certain period of time.

Construction management: An approach in which a general contractor is involved early on in the design process.

Contrast: The degree of difference between the lightest and darkest elements in a room; poor contrast makes it difficult to distinguish details of an object or room as a result of paint colors that are too similar in the background or foreground or poor lighting.

Design-bid-build: A construction process in which the design and building of a project is completed by several different groups (or sub-contractors).

Design-build: A construction process in which a single entity is used for all of the construction processes.

Ergonomics: The science of increasing work productivity by designing work stations that are comfortable for any person.

Foot-candle: The amount of light that a candle generates one foot away.

Glare: Inability to distinguish details or focus eyes on an object as a result of too much light or too many reflective surfaces.

Material safety data sheet (MSDS): A form from manufacturers that contains all the necessary data (including handling and storage, hazards, chemical ingredients, and exposure care) regarding the properties of a particular substance.

Regional investigations: Evaluations that include data about the surrounding environment and local community and that outline possible interactions.

Site investigations: Evaluations of different geographical sites or locations for the facility.

Specifications: Facility drawings with all of the details included, such as outlet locations, drainage, plumbing, ventilation, etc.; everything that is supposed to be in the final product should be included in the specifications.

Traffic flow: The relationship between the different services or designated spaces within the facility.

Deciding to build or remodel an athletic training facility can be an exciting time. It usually means that growth and change are imminent. While growth and expansion can be fun, creating and managing an athletic training facility requires patience and planning. Integrating leadership and management skills can help ensure that the planning, design, and building phases are successful.

One goal for building and planning a facility is to meet the existing needs of the users. It is also important to provide for future growth and expansion. Like many other aspects of leadership, having a conceptual grasp of the present and the future is important in this process. Conceptually the athletic trainer needs to know how an existing space is being used and how the planned space will meet current needs and future projections. To properly conceptualize the present and future facility requires an awareness of what did and did not work in the past facility. Therefore, that athletic trainer needs to strategically think of the facility in terms of the past, present, and future, which requires a leadership mindset. Furthermore, management techniques, such as controlling costs, organizing resources, effectively communicating with the design and building teams, as well as other relevant stakeholders requires planning, budgeting, and coordination. When these leadership behaviors and management skills are integrated, opening a new facility can be an exciting and rewarding experience.

In this chapter we will discuss important aspects of designing and maintaining an athletic training facility. We will begin with discussing the five steps of the preliminary planning process, followed by development and design considerations, giving special attention to space allocation, safety, lighting, traffic flow, hiring an architect, and other important aspects of design. Then we will discuss important considerations during the construction phase. Finally we will look into management and maintenance of the facility.

THE PLANNING AND BUILDING PROCESS

Building a new facility requires knowledge of the overall construction process. There are three primary methods used in a construction bidding process. The methods are design-bid-build (or lump sum), design-build, and construction management. **Design-bid-build** is the most traditional method. This method involves retaining an architect (or engineer) to design and produce drawings of the proposed facility. Early on the architect consults various engineers including mechanical, civil, and electrical. After consulting with engineers and other professionals such as landscapers and plumbers, a drawing is rendered. Then various contractors bid on the right to build the facility as rendered by the architect. Once a contractor is selected, building begins. Often the contractor will hire specialized workers (sub-contractors) for different aspects of the building project. The primary benefit of this method is that the least expensive workers can be hired, and usually it is less expensive then design-build; however, a "cheaper is better" mindset may propagate poor quality or a propensity to cut corners. Therefore, it is important for the athletic trainer to communicate closely with the architect and contractor during the entire process.

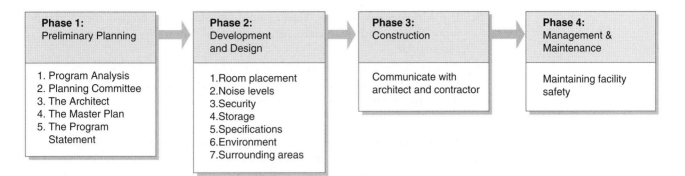

Figure 13-1 Phases of the facility design process

An alternative method is the design-build method. **Design-build** (also known as "Master Builder") process varies slightly from the traditional method. This method involves all aspects of construction being contracted and completed by a single entity. In other words, the designer is the builder and the builder employs a range of professionals who can complete any specialized work. Advantages to the design-build model include greater accountability by the builder to the athletic trainer and single-source delivery (instead of having to visit and communicate with various contractors and sub-contractors, there is one contact who is knowledgeable about the whole project). However, design-build contracts typically do not allow for many changes or alternations once building commences.

One other construction model is the construction management model. This model is a hybrid of the design-build and design-bid-build models. In **construction management,** the general contractor is hired early and is involved in the design process early on. A contractor is still hired by the architect or engineer to build, however the contractor is able to have some input into the design process. Regardless of method, the building of a new facility typically will involve at least four phases. Each of the phases has accompanying steps to help implementation. Walker[6] identified those four phases as 1) preliminary planning; 2) development and design; 3) construction; and 4) management and maintenance. These first two phases are of the utmost importance and can significantly reduce the risk of delays and setbacks during the final two phases. Figure 13-1 shows a flow chart delineating the phases of facility design.

PRELIMINARY PLANNING

Before an athletic trainer can make informed decisions about design and construction, he or she must have a realistic sense of available resources. Advance budgeting will facilitate a smoother design and building process. A major risk of building or remodeling a traditional athletic training room or clinic is spending too much money on unplanned items. As design features are added or upgraded, several minor costs can result in large financial consequences. Some tips to reducing or avoiding unexpected costs while building include:

1. Avoid time delays from the master plan. Stay on schedule with the building. Delays on one phase or portion will inevitably delay other aspects, which can cost time and money.

2. Keep upgrades and plan changes to a minimum. The more upgrades or features added outside of original plan means there is less money available for planned features.

3. Use simple space layouts. Having uniquely shaped or angled rooms requires more labor and materials; when possible keep floor layout square or rectangular.

4. Be aware of hidden costs. Be ready to pay for inspector, certificate, and application fees. While not a way to keep cost down, being aware ahead of time that there are often several fees associated with different aspects of building will reduce cost surprises.

Raising money for construction is also an important aspect of facility planning. It is important to begin saving and raising money as far in advance as possible. In the more traditional athletic training settings (i.e., high schools or colleges) resources for building or remodeling may come from the county, city, or state development funds, tax or levy dollars, a grant, an endowment, or major donations from capital campaigns. For smaller or private clinics, fund raising for facilities may require grants, personal savings, or business-based loans. Banks, local chambers of commerce, and some private lenders (or philanthropists) usually offer loans with special incentives for new or private businesses.

In order to secure funding from an external source (i.e., loan), it is very likely a business plan or prospectus will be required. A **business plan** is a document that spells out the expected course of action for a specified period of time (at least one to five years). Business plans usually include outlining risks, strategic plans, proposed products or services, the target market, the industry needs, management policies, and production or financial needs. With a good business plan many lenders are more willing to take a financial risk on the proposed facility.

Preliminary planning can be very involved and entails several steps. Walker[6] advocates a five-step process for the initial planning phase. These steps include 1) analyzing the program; 2) establishing a planning committee; 3) choosing an architect; 4) creating a master plan; and 5) creating a program statement. These steps are intended to occur in sequence. However, sequential order is not an absolute necessity and some steps may overlap slightly.

Step One: Program Analysis

A program analysis begins with identifying the needs of the facility as well as an assessment of the current programs and services offered in the facility. This is not a small task. The typical athletic training room (or clinic space) provides space for several services. Some of those services include:

1. Practice or game preparation
2. Injury treatment and management
3. Triage and emergency treatment
4. Physician or physical exams
5. Administration
6. Rehabilitation
7. Storage
8. Education
9. Research
10. Counseling

Figure 13-2 is a sample bubble diagram of typical functions within an athletic training room. After needed areas are identified, an assessment of how the current facility is being used is necessary. It is at this time when strengths and weaknesses in the current design should be noted. During this analysis step, it is also appropriate to

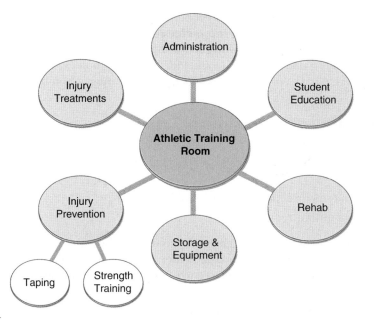

Figure 13-2 Bubble diagram of the functions of an athletic training room

revisit the program's strategic plan (values, vision, goals, or S.W.O.T. analysis) so that the facilities features promote the overall values of the department or organization and capitalize on strengths while addressing any weaknesses.

Once all of the uses of the facility have been identified and evaluated, it is important to consider each stakeholder's interest in the new facility. This also takes time. There are several people who have a vested interest in the facility, each having a specific goal or purpose for being involved. Taking into account each stakeholder's interest will help guide the construction, design, and layout of the facility. Stakeholders include the facility's users and non-users. Facility users include staff, physicians, and patients. Non-users include equipment and supply vendors, emergency medical personnel, administrators, maintenance crews, technology personnel, and accrediting agencies (e.g., Commission on Accreditation of Rehabilitation Facilities).

Other aspects of the initial program analysis are regional investigations, site investigations, and a functional analysis. **Regional investigations** include data about the surrounding environment and local community and outlines possible interactions. **Site investigations** include evaluating different geographical sites or locations for the facility. Deciding on a site for the facility is an important task. Questions to be addressed during a site investigation include access to roads, proximity to community services such as hospitals or parks, as well as ease of attaining utilities, such as water, Internet, and electricity (if in a remote location). Facility planners should visit other locations of different sites that serve similar populations and have similar goals. Obviously one cannot visit every site, but sound initial planning includes allocating resources to visit sites that have features you may wish to include in your facility. Be sure to plan time to speak with the workers and managers of these other sites so that there is ample time to discuss pros and cons of their design and layout. Finally, a functional analysis entails how specific spaces within the facility are related. An important part of the facility analysis includes determining access to specific spaces from various locations throughout the facility.

Step Two: Planning Committee

Forming a planning committee is the next step in preliminary planning. Most of the time, the planning committee is established after the initial program analysis.

However, sometimes the planning committee will be appointed before a program analysis is initiated. The planning committee consists of several stakeholders who will be using or impacted by the new facility. If there are several services being offered within the facility it may be difficult to include every stakeholder. Stakeholder groups that may need to have representation on a facility planning committee include:

1. Administrators
2. Athletic training staff/employees
3. Coaches
4. Athletes or patients
5. Educators
6. Emergency medical professionals
7. Local community representative

Obviously, once an architect or engineer is hired he or she will also become a member of the planning committee. Each stakeholder group may not require a spot on the committee per se, but should be allowed to offer feedback during the analysis phase.

Step Three: Hire an Architect

After the planning committee is formed and a needs analysis is completed or under-way, the planning committee's next task is to hire an architect. Once hired, the architect takes on the primary role as the leader in the planning, schematic design, bidding, and construction processes.[7] Therefore, hiring the right architect for the job is a major consideration. It is recommended that the planning committee evalu-ate several different architects. Evaluating architects may include visiting and touring facilities the architect has designed, asking architects to submit preliminary or con-ceptual drawings of the proposed facility, interviewing, and checking references. As important as the architect is to this process, Walker[6] suggests that hiring an architect too soon, before the planning committee has thoroughly digested and delineated recommendations from the program analysis, can be problematic. An architect may not be familiar with the committee's specific obligations or goals and may inadver-tently steer the design in a different direction.

During the interview process it is important to ask the potential architect the right questions. The following are a few examples of some questions to ask potential architects.[1]

1. How long have you been in business?
2. Do you have a valid architect's license? If so, what is your license number?
3. What percentage of your practice involves the type of structure I intend to build?
4. Do you carry insurance? If so, what type(s)?
5. How long have you carried each type and what are the policy limits?
6. Have you recently designed the type of structure I intend to build?
7. When and what was your most recent project?
8. May I see examples of your previous projects that are similar to my project (sketches, photos, plans)?
9. May I have the names, addresses, and telephone numbers of the clients for these previous similar projects?
10. What was the actual construction cost versus budgeted cost for these projects?

Furthermore, when checking the references of architects, be sure to ask the follow-ing questions:[1]

1. Did the architect adhere to required schedules and budgets?
2. Were you pleased with the architect's services and your working relationship with the architect?
3. Did the architect listen to your concerns and attempt to resolve them?
4. Would you hire the architect again?
5. What problems surfaced during the project?

Making the right choice in architects can be a tremendous asset to your program as you prepare for the future.

Step Four: Create a Master Plan

The next step is creating a master plan. This step may or may not require the input of an architect and can therefore take place earlier in the phase. The master plan is the assimilation of all of the information garnered from the program analysis. The master plan should be constructed from the vantage point of the facility and how it can meet the needs of the programs and not how programs can be manipulated to accommodate the facility.[6] When developing the master plan there are a number of important points to consider:

1. Do not overextend the budget—build the best with the available resources.
2. Consider multiple points of view—do not limit yourself to a few ideas. Discuss design and layout with several colleagues and peers and visit other athletic training facilities.
3. Do not compromise with the architect—keep the aspects you feel are critical to the facility.
4. Make sure the facility meets federal compliance regulations (i.e., Americans with Disabilities Act).
5. Minimize errors of omission by multiple feasibility studies (i.e., legal, user, financial, administrative, design-flow, etc.).
6. Map out how designated spaces interface with each other to get an overall conceptual framework for flow and traffic.
7. Reflect on how the physical facility needs to be managed. Consider flow, access, visual lines, and placement and location of storage and maintenance spaces.
8. Plan and anticipate change. Plan so that the space can be updated and changed in the future to accommodate growth or changes in goals and values.
9. Understand the environmental impact of the facility.[6]

Step Five: Create a Program Statement

The last step in the preliminary planning phase is creating the program statement. The program statement is the creation of a written report for the architect. The architect uses this report, in conjunction with interviews and dialogue, as a framework for design. This report may also be useful as a marketing tool or for justification to stakeholders. Basic components of a program statement should include:

1. The objectives of the facility
2. Basic assumptions about the facility and its use
3. Current building trends that influence planning and design
4. Space allocations
5. Special needs and relationships
6. Expected usage

7. Equipment and furniture lists
8. Environmental considerations.

This report can then be used to create marketing documents, which might include shortcomings of the existing facility; benefits (direct and indirect) of the new facility; a summary of special features, projected costs, or budgets; and a projected timetable.

DEVELOPMENT AND DESIGN

The second phase includes development and design. Once all the preliminary planning is completed, the architect has been hired and the master report has been submitted, the fun begins. It is important to maintain close dialogue with the architect during this second phase. It is during this second phase where initial schematics and drawings are altered or modified. Evaluating and changing drawings can be an exciting time, but it is important not to lose sight of the initial vision and plan. The planning committee must closely evaluate the drawings relative to the special needs and requirements set out in the program analysis and master report. While it is almost guaranteed that minor changes will occur during the development process, it is important not to violate the integrity of the facility's intended uses. This responsibility typically falls to the planning committee.

Furthermore, development includes creating and strictly adhering to realistic timetables. In conjunction with the architect, the planning committee delineates timetables for construction and relays and enforces those timetables to contractors. It is also important to set a realistic cost estimate as well as realistic projections for space allocations and square footage. For example, if the athletic training room is a stand-alone structure then space must be allocated for storage, maintenance, administration, and other essential spaces. However, if the athletic training room is being constructed as a smaller part (or room) within a larger facility, storage and physical plant space may be located elsewhere in the facility and may not need to take up functional athletic training room space.

Determining the Appropriate Size

When determining square footage for an athletic training room it is especially important to be mindful of current needs as well as potential needs. Size should be appropriate for the number of users. It is important to keep in mind that athletic training programs change. Some of these changes include responding to the addition or reduction of sports teams, accreditation standards, federal or state regulations, educational reform, addition or subtraction of personnel, etc. Even new facilities can quickly become obsolete or inadequate. For example, an existing athletic program may currently complete at the NCAA Division III level, it is feasible that in the future that institution may want to compete at the Division II level. This transition from DIII to DII or from NAIA to NCAA may require an addition of some athletic teams. Compliance to Title IX regulations may also require the addition of teams. Either of these scenarios means altering existing space to accommodate these changes. Locker rooms may need to be added or altered and the athletic training room may need to be expanded or modified to accommodate additional athletes and teams. Therefore, it is important to consider how the space might be designed so that if more space is needed in the future it can be easily accommodated. Likewise, within a clinic setting new services such as work hardening or occupational therapy may be added, which would also require additional space.

The amount of space required for a functioning athletic training room or rehabilitation facility should be based on the number of users. In determining space needs the following formula has been suggested, number of patients at peak divided by 20 per table per day, multiplied by 100, equals total square footage (TSQF)[5] or (number of patients/20) $\times$ 100 = TSQF.

For example, 200 athletes require a minimum of 1,000 square feet [200/20 = 10, 10 $\times$ 100 = 1000].

Allocating that 1000 square feet for specific functions requires additional planning. Depending on the context, more space may be required for certain functions. For example, in a small suburban high school the athletic trainer may not require a large space for rehabilitation or need space for large therapy pool. However, an athletic trainer in a self-owned rehabilitation clinic requires a much larger and more functional rehabilitation area and direct access to and from a therapy pool to dressing rooms.

Many athletic training rooms have specific allocated spaces, this is not to say these are the "only" spaces necessary, but these are at least standard to most athletic training rooms. Those spaces include:

1. An area for treatment of injuries—first aid stations, post-event treatments and modalities.
2. A hydrotherapy or wet area—a place to keep hydrocolators, whirlpools, pools, ice machines, and water outlets for filling and washing coolers.
3. A rehabilitation area—for therapeutic exercises and conditioning.
4. An administration area—office space for general administration tasks, correspondence, and storing of medical records.
5. A storage area(s)—for ease of access and to keep inventory of supplies and equipment.
6. A preparation area—for pre-event taping and bracing.
7. A private exam room—for physician evaluation and physicals.

From the Field

Athletic training rooms can vary in size based on the perception of importance administrators place on them. I have worked in several athletic training rooms; some were portable trailers or converted closets and others spacious state of the art facilities. As an undergraduate athletic training student our athletic training facility was a "temporary" trailer (it was "temporary" for at least two decades). Later, I was part of a university athletic training staff that operated two athletic training rooms. I was responsible for two teams, each one based out of a different athletic training room, but they were in relatively close proximity to each other. I also worked at a high school with two athletic training rooms. Unfortunately, these athletic training rooms were about five miles apart. One was at an off campus location (i.e., the football stadium) and other was adjacent to the gymnasium. Managing a remote location with zero staff proved to be challenging. After I moved on from that job my next athletic training room was literally a storage cabinet housed in the athletic director's (AD) office. That entire first year I used whatever space I could find. Typically, I worked off of the gymnasium's bleachers or out of the hallway using folding chairs outside the AD's office. The next year at that same high school I was given the old football helmet storage room (a 5 $\times$ 6 closet) as my athletic training room. The third year I was given the adjoining closet. I knocked out the dividing wall and had a 5 $\times$ 12 space. The point is athletic training room sizes, locations, and functions vary considerably and one must always be prepared to be able to work effectively in any size athletic training room.

A clinic may also require a common area for staff to congregate or eat as well as a waiting or lobby area for patients. How much space is needed for each area depends on daily usage. Estimates should take into account the size of equipment, number of pieces of equipment, and ease of movement between and around equipment. If equipment is large and bulky, space estimates may have to be increased to accommodate the size of certain pieces of equipment. It is a good rule of thumb to add 1–3 feet between tables or equipment. This allows for greater freedom of movement and multiple users. For example, if the taping area has five stations, then there could maximally be 10 people at once occupying the space (five athletic trainers taping and five athletes getting taped), using the TSQF equation this might require at least 50 square feet (or a 10 × 5 space). However, the taping tables alone (2 feet wide × 4 feet long) takes up nearly all that space leaving 1 square foot per taper to stand and move and no extra space for those being taped. Therefore, adding a foot on either side of the tables or arranging the taping area in an open space might be beneficial.

Space Allocation and Design Considerations

The size and location of the athletic training room have an obvious impact on how it is managed.[3] Athletic training rooms vary considerably in size. Large facilities or having to administrate multiple facilities require management considerations that smaller facilities might not. For example, line of sight, traffic flow, access, privacy, signage, electrical outlets, acoustics, and lighting are special considerations for many facilities.

Line of Sight

Line of sight is an important aspect of larger facilities with multiple uses. An athletic trainer should have an unobstructed visual line to all areas of the athletic training room from his or her office or anywhere else in the athletic training room. Those designated spaces with elevated risks, such as rehabilitation and hydrotherapy are specifically important to design with visual inspection in mind. One way to facilitate line of sight is to include large windows in offices or in rooms and use half-walls when delineating spaces is necessary. If walls are not necessary, consider open spaces and delineate them by equipment or furniture arrangement or different carpet or tile colors.

Traffic Flow

One important aspect of allocating space is planning for traffic. **Traffic flow** is the relationship between the different services or designated spaces within the facility. It is important that spaces have a rational relationship to one another. One way to help determine this is to ask how important is accessibility to this location from the other areas within the facility or how important is supervision of this location? Spaces that have a strong relationship should be placed closer together. Spaces that are less related need not be close. For example treatment and rehabilitation spaces have a high relationship and should be placed closer together. This allows for easier movement to and from with less obstacles. On the other hand, the rehabilitation and storage areas have little relationship and need not be placed as close together. For example, a common design consideration in many athletic training rooms is where to place the preparation or taping space. Placing the taping area close to a main doorway immediately off the hallway may be desirable for keeping the athletic training from becoming a "waiting room" for athletes needing only to be taped. However, this same design feature may cause a "clogging" effect at the facilities main access or exit point. An athletic trainer must carefully consider the pros and cons of where to place certain service areas in relation to traffic flow and peak hours.

Another consideration for deciding traffic flow is the need for supervision. If the athletic trainer knows they will be spending a lot of time in a certain area during busier times then it would be important to place any supervision intensive areas (i.e., hydrotherapy or rehabilitation) closer to those spaces. For example, an athletic trainer who is aware that a significant amount of time during the day will be spent in his or her office, placing the treatment area nearby and with an open line of sight from the office is important.

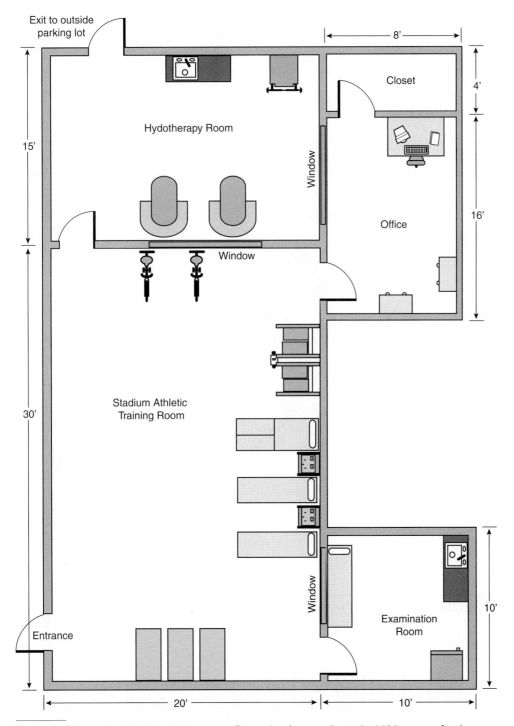

Figure 13-3 Sample athletic training room floor plan (approximately 1400 square feet)

Access

Where to place access points (entrances and exits) requires strategic foresight and should include consulting the emergency actions plan (EAP). If the EAP is already created for an existing facility that is being renovated consulting the plan is important for determining necessary changes. If the facility is brand new and the EAP has not been created, design the space so that emergency transportation can be easily facilitated (i.e., there must be quick access available for emergency medical personnel). Therefore, it is recommended that whenever physically possible the athletic training room have immediate access to an outside parking area via a double doorway (to accommodate a gurney or stretcher). Access also includes facilitating admission to other spaces outside of the athletic training room, such as locker room, storage, practices areas, or outside water spigots with minimal interference or distance (Figs. 13-3 and 13-4).

Exam Rooms

Private exam rooms can be an important element to include when designing an athletic training room. There are many times when offering privacy is the best practice during examinations or treatments. When designing a clinic space or a traditional

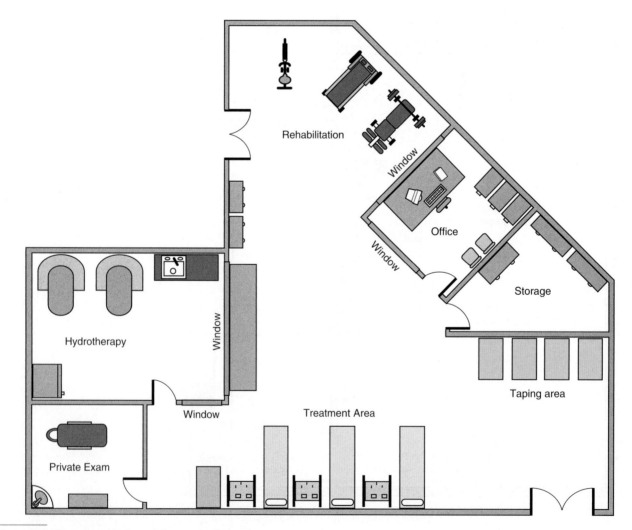

Figure 13-4 Sample athletic training room floor plan

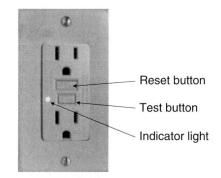

Figure 13-5 Ground fault interrupter

athletic training room it may be necessary to include at least one private exam room for the team physician to perform confidential evaluations. If designing a rehabilitation facility, it may be necessary to have several private exam rooms to accommodate multiple evaluations and treatments.

Signage

Signage is an essential design consideration in all facilities. Signs within the athletic training room that delineate spaces are not as essential as signs directing people to the athletic training room. However, there are several signs that could be beneficial in an athletic training room. Signs that need to be included in the athletic training room include location of Automated External Defibrillator (AED), warning and danger signs, high voltage signs, exits, athletic training room rules, and any specific facility guidelines that are remanded by Occupational Safety and Health Administration (OSHA) or accrediting agencies. Signs should be large enough to see from a distance, brightly colored, and when possible, should incorporate graphics.

Outlets

While most of the time standard electrical outlets are sufficient wet areas or areas where there is a risk of water coming in contact with an outlet requires a Ground Fault Interrupter (GFI). Electrical code requires GFIs in spaces near or above sinks, whirlpools, swimming pools, hydroculators, ice machines, or other wet areas. A GFI is a special outlet that cuts power off immediately if there is a surge. Without GFI outlets the risk of electrocution is increased. A typical circuit breaker interrupts the circuit at 20 amperes, but it takes only about 100 milliamperes to electrocute a person. The GFI is designed to detect currents of a few milliamperes and trip a breaker at the receptacle or at the breaker panel to remove the risk of electrocution. A typical GFI has a test button to reset if it is tripped. Figure 13-5 is a photo of a GFI outlet. Other outlet considerations include knowing the types of plugs that will come with equipment. Often commercial equipment has plugs with different arrangement of prongs to prevent them from being used just anywhere. If equipment comes with special plugs, be sure to arrange outlets in the appropriate places.

Acoustics

Acoustics may be a necessary design consideration. In many buildings, noise is cited as an impediment to productivity or added stressor.[2] Athletic training rooms that are located next to or near gymnasiums or busy weight rooms may have to consider acoustics. Therefore, designing spaces that minimize echo and reverberation are important. OSHA standards state that if a facility's noise exceeds 90 decibels it requires a remedy. Excess noise can be a result of poorly designed rooms, poor choice of

LEADERSHIP ACTIVITY

Design an athletic training room for a fictional high school with a limited budget (your instructor may assign a budget limit). Begin by estimating the total square footage needed to accommodate a potential maximum of 139 athletes in the athletic training room at once. Once that is determined, plan spaces for the following areas: taping and preparation, storage, treatment, administration, private exams, wet or hydro area, and rehabilitation. Be sure to consider the size of the equipment and supplies in the space, given your space limitations and the relationship of how each area interacts, as well as access and visual lines. Draw this design on graph paper to scale, draw in all equipment, and include entrances, exits, any walls, and windows. After your drawing is complete, exchange it with a peer and let him or her critique it for space allocation, traffic flow, and overall aesthetic appearance.

building materials, or misplacement of equipment such as HVAC (heating ventilation air conditioning) or ice machines. Strategies for reducing unnecessary noise include placing noisy equipment at an appropriate distance from workers, use sound absorbing materials for walls, enclosing noisy equipment, and using open floor plans.

Lighting

It should go without stating, but lighting in any health care facility needs to be adequate. Adequate lighting tends to increase productivity and safety. Light is measured in **foot candles**. One foot-candle (a.k.a. lumen per square foot) is the amount of light that a candle generates one foot away. Standard lighting requires approximately 30 foot candles at four (4) feet above floor level. However, athletic training facilities may require additional light sources called "supplemental" light. Supplemental light provides greater light for smaller work stations, such as task lighting in offices or a lamp for diagnostic uses. An example where lighting may need to be greater is during a physical examination where observing minor changes in skin color or pupil size might be necessary, or when reading x-rays. Natural lighting is also very desirable. Patients may feel more at ease and comfortable when they are exposed to natural light. Designing with natural light involves including several windows or glass doors to the outside.

There are two common lighting problems that need to be addressed during design and construction, glare and contrast. **Glare** is a result of too much light or too many reflective surfaces. When glare is a problem, focusing on smaller objects in less light is difficult. Reduce glare by using less intense light, cover light fixtures or bulbs, increase brightness of nearby areas, position fixtures to reduce reflected light, use low-gloss paper for office work, and paint walls with semi-gloss or flat paint. Improper **contrast** is also a lighting issue that may need attention during the design portion of building and constructing a facility. Improper contrast is often due to light intensity changes or having background or foreground colors too similar. Poor contrast may contribute to poor depth perception, which can be especially problematic during rehabilitation or functional testing. Making sure lighting, glare, and contrast are part of the design considerations from the beginning can help maintain a safer and more productive work environment.

Safety and Ergonomics

Each facility must plan for proper safety features, which includes a detailed emergency action plan (EAP). Details of an EAP are outlined in Chapter 11. However, other safety features necessary when planning and designing any health care facility include allocating visible and accessible spots for AEDs, fire extinguishers, and other emergency equipment (such as spine boards and splints). Ergonomics is another consideration in the design of athletic training facilities.

Ergonomics is the science of increasing work productivity by designing work stations that are comfortable for the worker. Designing comfortable and ergonomically correct work spaces increases productivity and reduces the risk of accumulative stresses on the body. One example of ergonomics in the athletic training room includes the use of taping tables. Taping multiple ankles on standard treatment tables can cause significant back discomfort, however, just increasing the height of the table can ease or eliminate that pain entirely. Other ways ergonomics can be incorporated into a workspace is by adjusting office space or work stations to fit each individual person who uses that space. For example:

1. Adjusting the position of a computer keyboard to prevent carpal tunnel syndrome.
2. Using adjustable height computer monitors to reduce tension on upper back and neck muscles.

3. Being sure that the height of a desk chair allows feet to rest flat on floor.
4. Making sure office chairs include support for the lumbar region of the back.
5. Learning the right way to lift heavy objects to prevent back injuries.

CONSTRUCTION PHASE

The third phase in the facility design and building process is the actual construction. This phase accounts for a majority of the time spent on building a facility. During the construction phase, it is important to rely on the expertise and experience of the

From the Field

Several years ago I served on a planning committee of a very large recreation and fitness facility. This was joint project between the hospital I worked for and the recreation/fitness facility. I worked for the hospital's athletic training and performance enhancement team. My responsibility as a planning committee member was the sports performance areas. Once construction began, I was on-site a few times a week, usually in the mornings before practices began at my high school. As planned, early one morning all the sports medicine staff met to unload our new state-of-the-art sports training equipment. The shipment and delivery dates had been planned for weeks. The shipment of equipment was arriving from out of state via semi-truck. Each piece was custom made, therefore, it was bulky, awkwardly shaped, and heavy. Our intent was to unload the equipment onto the parking lot and have a crane and crane operator (which we rented by the hour) lift each piece of equipment to the second floor through a very large opening set to be a bay window (it was not our choice to put this equipment on the second floor). Much to our chagrin, we arrived that morning to find the panes of glass installed and the liquid track floor that was not scheduled to be poured for days had been poured the previous evening around the entire perimeter of the second floor and needed 72 hours to set. Furthermore, the glass was not to be installed until we notified the contractor that our equipment was in place. Needless to say, tempers flared and several discussions with contractors and administrators ensued. What had happened was that the some of the subcontractors, who had no idea of the time tables, were not able to finish one of their other jobs because of weather. So, instead of losing a day of work due to inclement weather they decided to install the large bay window. After they installed the window and according to the planned sequence called the guys to pour the liquid track floor (because the window was in). They had no idea we had six pieces of equipment coming the next morning, the lightest of which was 2000 lbs. After much discussion and deliberation, the decision was made to move the equipment in as planned, which required breaking out the window and ruining part of the poured track. The window was reinstalled later and a portion of the track had to be re-poured.

A few days later there was another issue. The electrician, wanting to reduce costs installed standard electrical outlets that were left-over from one of his previous worksites. He either forgot or was not aware that commercial grade treadmills with special prongs were ordered. When the treadmills arrived, two weeks later, the treadmill's plugs would not fit into the standard outlets. Two weeks had passed since the installation and the electrician was on another job and unavailable to return to install the specified outlets. Each of these minor fiascos was very frustrating for everyone involved and ended up costing the contractor time and money. Several lessons can be learned here, the most important being to remain flexible and gracious during the construction process. Also, it is important to ensure that specifications are clearly delineated in writing as well as explicitly articulated in writing that an installation schedule has some allowance for delays.

architect for advice and counsel. However, do not discount your own experience or let the the architect modify or alter plans without the expressed consent of the planning committee.

The construction process is facilitated by two important documents, the working drawings or schematics (i.e., blueprints) and specifications (i.e., specs).[4] **Specifications** include an enormous amount of detail, but these details are essential to ensure that the building is constructed as envisioned.[4] Everything that you want to see in the final product should be included in the specifications.[4] The Construction Specification Institute mandates 50 specific divisions, each area needing to be represented in the final specifications. For a detailed list of those specifications, visit http://www.csinet.org/masterformat.

Once construction is underway the architect and members of the planning committee should visit the construction site regularly. The purpose of these site visits is to ensure appropriate progress is being made and to stay abreast of the latest facility developments. Often a contractor will hire out subcontractors to do the labor based on their specialties. For example, masons, electricians, plumbers, etc. maybe subcontracted to do labor that the contactor is not able to do. These subcontractors are often not aware of the entire plan (or the big picture) and may not appreciate timetables or sequencing (for an example see the case in point below). Therefore, frequent visits to the construction site are important.

MANAGEMENT AND MAINTENANCE

The first three phases involve planning, design, and construction. The fourth and final phase takes place independent of the first three and is management and training. Once construction is completed or near completion, it is important to consider how the facility is going to be managed. Obviously there are operation and administration issues such as staffing, staff training and orientation, and operational policies and procedures that need to be carefully considered and articulated. In an athletic training room or rehabilitation facility, managing and planning for basic health and safety of those using and working in the facility is important.

Safety concerns, such as what to do in an emergency, are an important aspect of facility management. One important safety and maintenance action is to calibrate all equipment on a regular basis. Modalities should be calibrated at least annually. It is also prudent to be sure that all rehabilitation or exercise equipment is well maintained. For example, cables for exercise equipment should be monitored and replaced if frayed, pulleys should be lubricated, treadmill belts aligned, and seat cushions, mats, and tables all should be maintained on a regular basis.

Most athletic training rooms tend to be have a naturally welcoming environment. While this is admirable, the athletic training staff must resist the temptation to allow the athletic training room to become a lounge.[2] Keeping the athletic training room or a rehabilitation facility clean and sanitary at all times is important. While this is important for professional appearance, sanitary conditions can limit risk associated with airborne or bloodborne pathogens, viruses, and bacteria. Athletic training rooms must adhere to the OSHA regulations for the operation of health care facilities. These guidelines can be found at http://www.osha.gov. Prentice[3] recommends the following rules be implemented to help in managing the hygiene and sanitation in an athletic training room:

1. Cleated shoes should not be allowed into the facility.
2. Game or practice equipment should be kept outside.
3. Shoes should be kept off of the treatment tables.

4. Athletes should shower before receiving any treatment.
5. Food, smoking, or smokeless tobacco should be strictly prohibited.
6. Facility should be cleaned daily (certain pieces of equipment should be cleaned after each use).

Another management consideration is scheduling the use of facilities for practice times, events, and outside events. In athletic training rooms scheduling is typically not an issue with which athletic trainers need to deal. However, it is important to communicate with coaches and athletic training personnel to avoid overlapping treatment and pre-practice preparation times when large numbers of athletes are expected.

Manufacturers' Operational Guidelines

Manufacturers' operational guidelines are recommendations for use, care, and maintenance of any equipment that might be used in an athletic training room or rehabilitation clinic. Manufacturers of athletic training equipment typically supply information for equipment they manufacture or have manufactured if discontinued. Athletic trainers should keep operational guidelines with each piece of respective equipment or at least keep a file that contains all the operational guidelines for easy retrieval. Keeping operational guidelines on hand can help to reduce risk and increase the impact and the longevity of equipment. Lost operational guidelines can often be downloaded or replacement copies requested from a manufacturer's web site.

In addition to following operational guidelines it is important to keep information on any hazardous materials in the facility. Facility managers should keep a **Material Safety Data Sheet** (MSDS) book available for all employees. MSDS is a form that contains the necessary data regarding the properties of a particular substance. MSDS

▷ Leadership Application

State High School is planning to build a new sports facility including two gymnasiums, locker rooms, team room, coach's offices, and an athletic training room. Construction is slated to begin in six weeks. Julie is the head athletic trainer and to date has not been consulted by any party on the design and layout of the new athletic training room. Julie has been waiting patiently and even has a few pencil drawings she has doodled of her ideal athletic training space in the new facility. She has calculated needing at least 1200 square feet to meet the current demands of the teams. Later that day she is finally called to come to a meeting on the construction. She arrives and is surprised to find out that several preliminary meetings have already taken place and this meeting is to approve the third draft of schematics from the architect. Realizing she was not included in any previous meetings, she anxiously looks for the athletic training room on the floor plan, but none is labeled. Trying to hide her disappointment, Julie despondently asks the architect if there is an athletic training room in the plan and he enthusiastically replies, "Yes, of course" and points to a 700 square foot trapezoid-shaped room in an obscure place of the proposed facility with no outdoor access or water supply.

Critical Thinking Questions

1. Should Julie mention to the architect this late in the planning that this "space" is not adequate for an athletic training room?
   a. Or should she keep quiet and go directly to her administrators for an explanation?
   b. How might Julie mention this to her administrators and the architect?
2. If the space is unable to be altered or resigned, how might Julie make the best of this situation, and what other options might she have to increase her space and make it more functional?
3. How could Julie have avoided this situation from the beginning?

contains information on how to handle and store materials, as well as active and inactive chemical ingredients, and how to administer care if exposure to the materials occurs. MSDS are available from manufacturers and many are also available on the Internet. Keeping an accurate and up-to-date MSDS book helps reduce risk and is a necessary facility management practice.

CHAPTER SUMMARY

Building, planning, designing, or redesigning a facility can be fun and exiting. In the midst of the excitement of a new facility, it is important not to lose sight of the importance of planning and foresight. Conducting a thorough program analysis, establishing a competent building committee, and hiring the right architect for the job are crucial. After the designs and specs are created, continuing to monitor the construction process throughout the entire project is essential. Ultimately a well-designed facility will promote health and safety and reduce risk to employees and users. Making sure that all staff are well versed in the facility operations policy and procedures, including safety procedures, will make the new or redesigned facility a more enjoyable place.

Leadership Spotlight

JACK RANSONE

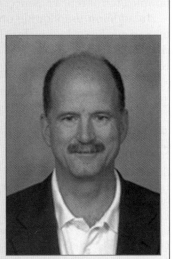

EDUCATION:

PhD, Exercise Science, University of New Mexico, Albuquerque, NM, 1991

CURRENT JOB:

Professor and Director of Athletic Training, Department of Health, Physical Education, and Recreation, Texas State University

FIRST ATHLETIC TRAINING JOB:

Graduate Assistant, University of Oklahoma

PROFESSIONAL INTERESTS/RESEARCH FOCUS:

Sports physiology, overtraining, and ergogenic aids

ATHLETIC TRAINING–RELATED AWARDS/HONORS:

National Athletic Trainer Association "Most Distinguished Athletic Trainer" Award

ATHLETIC TRAINING–RELATED INVOLVEMENT:

- Athletic Trainer for U.S. National Track and Field Team – XXIII and XXIV Olympic Games
- Former member of the NATA graduate council, CAATE site reviewer

Q & A

What first inspired you to enter the athletic training profession?

Personal injuries that occurred during my athletic career

How would you define leadership in athletic training?

In my opinion, leadership in athletic training is being an effective role model in both professional and personal behaviors to students, young professionals, and peers.

Who is the most influential athletic trainer in your professional life, and why?

I'm still searching for that. I have made many good friends, though.

What is the best advice you ever received from another athletic trainer?

Always make time for your family.

What has been the most enjoyable aspect of athletic training?

Interaction with coaches and athletes.

What has been the least enjoyable aspect or your biggest challenge in athletic training?

Long hours and balancing professional with personal life.

What advice would you give a first-year athletic training student?

Meet as many athletic trainers as possible.

What advice would you give a brand new BOC-certified athletic trainer who is deciding between taking that first professional job or entering graduate school to pursue a master's degree in athletic training, and why?

Take the job experience; hands-on experience always exceeds what is learned in the classroom.

What other interests outside of athletic training have you pursued?

My family has always been a top priority.

Where do you think (or hope) athletic training will be in the next 10 years?

A respected health profession.

References

1. California Architect's Board. (2006). *Consumer's guide for hiring an architect.* Sacramento, CA: CAB.

2. Carisa, T. (2002). Designing workspaces for higher productivity. *Occupational Health and Safety 71*(9), 192–194.

3. Prentice W. (2006). *Arnheim's principles of athletic training: A competency-based approach.* Boston: McGraw Hill.

4. Sawyer, TH. (1999). Construction Documents and Bidding. In Sawyer, T.H. (ed.). *Facilities planning for physical activity and sport: Guidelines for development.* Dubuque, IA: Kendall-Hunt.

5. Secor M. (1984). Designing athletic training facilities or "where do you want the outlets?" *Athletic Training 19*(1),19–21.

6. Walker M. (1997). The Planning, Design, Construction, and Management Process. In Walker, M. and Stotlar, D. (eds.). *Sport facility management.* Boston: Jones and Bartlett.

7. White H, Karabetsos J. (1999). Sports Medicine and Rehabilitation. In Sawyer, T.H. (ed.). *Facilities planning for physical activity and sport: Guidelines for development.* Dubuque, IA: Kendall-Hunt.

Ethical and Global Issues

Chapter 14

Professional Ethics

"Relativity applies to physics, not ethics."

ALBERT EINSTEIN

CHAPTER RATIONALE

Role Delineation Study Components

Domain VI: Professional Responsibility

- Knowledge of NATA Code of Ethics
- Obtaining, interpreting, and applying NATA Code of Ethics

Educational Competencies

- Differentiate the essential documents of the national governing and accrediting bodies, including, but not limited to Standards of Practice of the Profession, Code of Ethics

Foundational Behaviors of Professional Practice

- Understand and comply with NATA's Code of Ethics
- Understand the consequences of violating the NATA's Code of Ethics
- Understand and comply with other codes of ethics, as applicable

Key Terms

Applied ethics: The study of the use of ethical values and actual behaviors.

Code of ethics: The rules, standards, or principles that dictate proper behavior among members of a profession.

Conflict of interest: A situation in which a person has a private or personal interest that appears to influence or influences the objective exercise of his or her official duties as an allied health care professional.

Deontology: A branch of moral philosophy that underscores the duty or obligations of an individual to act; what a person ought to do regardless of outcome.

Ethics: A systematic inquiry and judgment about the moral dimensions of human conduct.

Meta-ethics: The study of the philosophy or concept of ethics, dealing with relativism and the meaning of "good," "bad," "right," and "wrong."

Morals: The values or principles rooted in an individual's philosophy, culture, or religion used to determine right or wrong conduct.

Normative ethics: The study of how to determine ethical values; concerned with what "ought to be."

Teleology: A branch of moral philosophy that underscores the importance of the outcome. Appropriate actions are based on the outcome; i.e., the end justifies the means.

Utilitarianism: An approach in which the good of the many outweighs the good of the one; i.e., the larger group benefits more than any single person or smaller group.

Whistleblower: A person who reports inappropriate behavior of members to an entity or organization that presumably has the power and authority to take corrective action.

E thics is an essential element of all professions everywhere. This is especially true of athletic training. Many athletic trainers frequently face situations that require ethical consideration. How athletic trainers respond to ethical situations speaks volumes about him or her and the profession. Therefore, athletic trainers must practice their profession according to a code of ethical behavior and principles.

A code of ethics is important because athletic trainers are entrusted with the public's interests. A **code of ethics** is a set of guidelines, rules, standards, or principles established by a professional body that conveys moral tenor and is designed to govern the conduct of members.[6]

To live and practice by a code of ethics implies the athletic trainer is aware of an external accountability beyond personal standards. It is necessary to have an external code because an individual's personal ethics may be less stringent. The external code also serves to delineate principles of ethical behavior, because no ethical code could possibly cover all of the possible scenarios of ethical situations. Therefore, the principles espoused in a code of ethics can be used in situations that are not clear cut. The foundation for all ethical behavior is rooted in the fact that decisions and behaviors will impact others. Determining who those "others" are and how they are impacted is a central concern of ethical decision making.

Consistent and deliberate ethical behavior is one way athletic trainers can earn and keep the trust of their many stakeholders. It is fundamental to athletic training that all athletic trainers demonstrate ethical behavior at all times, regardless of the role or setting. These ethical behaviors should even transcend the work context and be applied even when not acting in an official athletic training capacity. One incident of unethical behavior may cast a long-lasting or perhaps permanent shadow on the athletic trainer, the profession, or employer.

We will begin this chapter by discussing the nature of ethics and the different aspects of ethics. We will follow that with a brief discussion of moral development and philosophy, followed by discussing ethical standards within athletic training. The discussion of ethics within athletic training will include the National Athletic Trainers' Association (NATA) Code of Ethics, Commission on Accreditation of Athletic Training Education (CAATE) Code of Ethics, Board of Certification (BOC) Standards of Professional Behavior, and NATA's Foundational Behaviors for Professional Practice. We will conclude the chapter with a brief discussion on ethical decision making.

WHAT IS ETHICS?

Ethics is closely associated with professional behavior and is a branch of philosophy that studies the values and customs of a person or group. By definition, **ethics** is a systematic inquiry and judgment about the moral dimensions of human conduct or morality.[6] **Morals** are the values, principles, and judgments applied to guide right or wrong conduct. Morality is based on cultural, religious, or philosophical concepts.[6] Together, ethics and morality cover the analysis and implementation of concepts such as right and wrong, good and evil, and responsibility.

Ethics is divided into three primary areas. **Meta-ethics** is a broad concept that examines the concept of ethics itself. Meta-ethics tends to deal with relativism and asks, what does "good" or "bad," "right," or "wrong" mean? Another branch of ethics is **normative ethics**, which is the study of how to determine ethical values and asks about what "ought to be." The third aspect is **applied ethics**, which is the study of the use or application of ethical values. Applied ethics deals with behaviors. Athletic trainers will primarily deal with applied ethics as they pertain to professional behaviors and practice. Applied ethics is an approach to ethics that focuses on the rightness or wrongness of actual behaviors, as opposed to the rightness or wrongness of the consequences of those behaviors. Applied ethics can be described as having a perceived duty or obligation to behave in a certain way. Applied ethics is often closely associated with legal action (i.e., duty and breach of duty).

Applied ethics in athletic training is about delineating intentional actions to ensure certain ethical principles are practiced. For example, the ethic of human rights can be applied to athletic training by ensuring or making arrangements for patients' confidentiality and ensuring patients are aware of all associated risks with a particular treatment.

Athletic trainers need to be familiar with ethical principles (i.e., outlined by NATA) so that actions can be informed. Ignorance is rarely accepted as a viable defense of unethical behavior. Unfortunately, too often ethics is left to abstract concepts and theories that have little practical value in terms of demonstrated behavior, leaving much of ethical behavior subject to interpretation, which increases the risk of violation.

Applied ethics is much more than defining legal and illegal actions. The study and application of applied ethics require the very difficult responsibility of classifying behaviors, even if legal. Unfortunately, the luxury of having purely black and white behaviors is rare. It is difficult to say that a certain behavior is always and without exception unethical. For example, intimate relationships with athletes or patients. How is an "inappropriate" relationship defined? Are all relationships that extend outside of a professional context (including close friendships) unethical, or only those of a sexual nature? Furthermore, how does disclosure of any relationship affect the ethical tenor of the circumstance? Why do many athletic training programs have policies forbidding or discouraging athletic training students from dating athletes?

In addition to intimate relationships, athletic trainers are faced daily with other ethical situations. Think through and discuss the following list of ethical situations:

1. In treating an injury, could it be construed as unethical to discuss the injury or treatment to an unrelated third-party?
2. In treating an injury, could it be construed as unethical to not disclose all of the available treatment options or side effects to an athlete or patient?
3. What is the ethical responsibility of the athletic trainer to find out all of the possible side effects or alternatives to a certain treatment or intervention?
4. What is the ethical responsibility of the athletic trainer to ensure all treatments and interventions are based on available evidence?
5. Is it ethical to change the initial injury date for an athlete so that school insurance will cover the injury?
    a. What loss might there be to the insurance company?
    b. What benefit is there for the athlete?

6. In treating an injury, could it be construed as unethical to extend treatment beyond what is absolutely necessary simply because insurance allows more treatments?

7. In treating an injury, could it be construed as unethical to discharge or discontinue a patient who clearly requires additional rehabilitation, but is beyond the number of visits that the insurance provider covers?

Moral Philosophy

Morals have a greater association with demonstrated behaviors as compared to ethics. Morals are based on tacit knowledge derived from an individual's culture, religion, or philosophy. There are two primary branches of moral philosophy that deal with behavior. The first is deontology. **Deontology** is a line of reasoning that supposes duty or obligations determine the worth or value of an individual's decision. In other words, it is what a person ought to do regardless of outcome; hence the phrase, "do the right thing." Directly opposed to deontology is a second branch of moral philosophy, teleology. **Teleology** underscores the importance of the outcome, instead of obligation or duty. Therefore, to a teleologist, appropriate actions are solely based on the outcome; in other words, the end justifies the means. This type of reasoning leads to a "do whatever you want as long as nobody gets hurt" mentality that is dangerous and often leads to justifying the use of lies, conflict of interests, and other normally unethical practices.

Conflict of Interest

Many athletic trainers are faced with conflict-of-interest scenarios. A **conflict of interest** is a situation in which a person has a private or personal interest that appears to influence or actually influences the objective exercise of his or her official duties.[3] In other words, it may be a conflict of interest to receive financial or other type of gain by recommending a product or service to a patient. For example, recommending to a patient additional services deemed necessary (i.e., massage, orthotics, personal training, etc.) is perfectly fine, however receiving money from a provider for referring patients only to that provider could be considered a conflict of interest, especially if those services can be considered unnecessary. It is typically not considered a conflict of interest if your company has a referral agreement with a provider, however, if you personally broker an exclusive agreement or are approached to form an exclusive agreement with another provider outside of your employer's knowledge, then that may be considered a conflict of interest. Another example of the potential for conflict of interest comes during the athletic training program accreditation process. For example, the CAATE has specific measures in place to make sure that among other things, alumni do not serve on the site-review team of their alma mater. Finally, for obvious reasons, dating or perhaps even being close friends with patients or athletes for which you are providing care can be a conflict of interest. Conflicts of interest in athletic training occur more often than one might originally think.

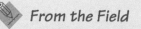

From the Field

Early on in my professional career, I would earn extra income in the summer months by coaching sports camps and taking on personal training clients. It was at this time that I was approached by a fledgling supplement company and invited to help this company grow by recommending supplements to my clients. I would be paid for clients I referred when they purchased the supplement. Their sales pitch included the ease of having a ready-made clientele; all I would need to do was talk up the supplements during our sessions, ask a few well-placed questions to convince them they needed the supplement, and the money would make itself for me. I immediately recognized this for what it was and rejected the offer, specifically citing it as a conflict of interest. I knew that if I accepted this offer that my motivation toward my clients and my purpose for meeting with them in the first place would be compromised, and I would be tempted to forfeit their best interest.

ATHLETIC TRAINING ETHICAL STANDARDS

The profession of athletic training adheres to codes of ethics, which are based on certain ethical principles. Of the professional organizations and agencies that govern athletic training, two have specific codes of ethics and the other has a delineated standard of practice. NATA has a Code of Ethics that should govern member's behaviors. Also, the CAATE has a code of ethics that governs associated athletic training education programs and the ethics of the agents acting on behalf of CAATE (i.e., CAATE members). The BOC has delineated Standards of Professional Practice that also have implications in the athletic trainer's ethical behaviors. Furthermore, many state practice acts and athletic training by-laws have ethics codes or behavioral standards included in their regulations.

NATA Code of Ethics

The preamble to NATA's Code of Ethics delineates specific overarching principles of ethical behavior that should be followed by all athletic trainers. The purview of NATA's Code of Ethics is restricted to NATA members, but in principle, these Codes are for all athletic trainers whether NATA members or not. The NATA Code of Ethics is intended to establish and maintain high standards and professionalism in athletic training. It is important to mention that, "when a conflict exists between the Code of Ethics and the law, the law prevails."[6] It is important to realize that there are situations in athletic training when ethics and law are in conflict. Therefore, it is possible to behave unethically without violating the law. To prevent unethical (albeit legal) behavior, the athletic trainer should strive to adhere to some basic ethical principles.

The NATA Code of Ethics strongly advocates four overarching principles. These principles may not cover every possible situation, but represent the spirit in which ethical decisions should be made. These ethical principles include:

1. Respecting the rights, welfare and dignity of all.
2. Complying with the laws and regulations governing the practice of athletic training.
3. Maintaining and promoting high standards in their provision of services.
4. Avoiding conduct that could be construed as a conflict of interest or that reflects negatively on the profession.

These principles are intended to be practiced at all times. These principles are not exhaustive and should be considered in conjunction with the BOC's Standards of Professional Practice, and NATA's Foundational Behaviors of Professional Practice, which do have purview over all certified athletic trainers, whether members of NATA or not.

The four principles of the NATA Code of Ethics are delineated in more detail in the actual code (Box 14-1). The Code also identifies some specific behaviors that embody the principle. The implicit nature of a "principle" is that it is interpreted and implemented in every situation. For example, "Principle 1" is fundamentally about respecting others and includes the following behaviors, but is not limited to only the following behaviors:

1. Not discriminating against any legally protected class (i.e., the principle supersedes legally protected classes and in theory is enacted regardless if legally protected or not; the principle is not to discriminate against anyone at all, most of all legally protected classes).
2. Being committed to providing competent care.
3. Preserving confidentiality.

It is important to realize that practicing these three specific behaviors does not guarantee that the spirit of the principle is being honored. It is up to the individual to

BOX 14-1 NATA Code of Ethics

PRINCIPLE 1:

Members shall respect the rights, welfare and dignity of all.
1.1 Members shall not discriminate against any legally protected class.
1.2 Members shall be committed to providing competent care.
1.3 Members shall preserve the confidentiality of privileged information and shall not release such information to a third party not involved in the patient's care without a release unless required by law.

PRINCIPLE 2:

Members shall comply with the laws and regulations governing the practice of athletic training.
2.1 Members shall comply with applicable local, state, and federal laws and institutional guidelines.
2.2 Members shall be familiar with and abide by all National Athletic Trainers' Association standards, rules and regulations.
2.3 Members shall report illegal or unethical practices related to athletic training to the appropriate person or authority.
2.4 Members shall avoid substance abuse and, when necessary, seek rehabilitation for chemical dependency.

PRINCIPLE 3:

Members shall maintain and promote high standards in their provision of services.
3.1 Members shall not misrepresent, either directly or indirectly, their skills, training, professional credentials, identity or services.
3.2 Members shall provide only those services for which they are qualified through education or experience and which are allowed by their practice acts and other pertinent regulation.
3.3 Members shall provide services, make referrals, and seek compensation only for those services that are necessary.
3.4 Members shall recognize the need for continuing education and participate in educational activities that enhance their skills and knowledge.
3.5 Members shall educate those whom they supervise in the practice of athletic training about the Code of Ethics and stress the importance of adherence.
3.6 Members who are researchers or educators should maintain and promote ethical conduct in research and educational activities.

PRINCIPLE 4:

Members shall not engage in conduct that could be construed as a conflict of interest or that reflects negatively on the profession.
4.1 Members should conduct themselves personally and professionally in a manner that does not compromise their professional responsibilities or the practice of athletic training.
4.2 National Athletic Trainers' Association current or past volunteer leaders shall not use the NATA logo in the endorsement of products or services or exploit their affiliation with NATA in a manner that reflects badly upon the profession.
4.3 Members shall not place financial gain above the patient's welfare and shall not participate in any arrangement that exploits the patient.
4.4 Members shall not, through direct or indirect means, use information obtained in the course of the practice of athletic training to try to influence the score or outcome of an athletic event, or attempt to induce financial gain through gambling.

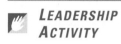

LEADERSHIP ACTIVITY

If your state regulates athletic training, use an Internet browser to find your state's athletic training regulations, or rules and laws (if your state does not regulate athletic training choose a neighboring state that does to complete the project). Once you find your state's athletic training rules, laws, and regulations read them. In your reading be sure to find any specific references to:

1. Ethics or ethical behavior
2. Offenses that require disciplinary actions
3. Procedures for administering any discipline
4. Expected professional behaviors

Be prepared to discuss those items and questions that inspire with ACI's, peers, or faculty members.

ensure the "spirit" of the principles is being honored at all times. To do this requires intentional evaluation and reflection on the NATA Code of Ethics before too many ethical situations are introduced.

CAATE Code of Ethics

The CAATE has also delineated certain principles that should guide the behavior of CAATE members (i.e., those acting on behalf of CAATE) and those institutions accredited by CAATE. Like the NATA Code, CAATE's does not have purview over all athletic trainers. These are important ethical principles and values on which athletic trainers should reflect. Hopefully, these principles will serve as a framework for athletic trainer's actions whether CAATE members or not. The CAATE ethics principles are: 1) honesty; 2) respect; 3) accountability and responsibility; 4) integrity; and 5) fairness.[2] These ethical values and emerging principles serve to guide the conduct and decision making of the Commission's practice and its members (Box 14-2). Each principle then has specific actions, steps, or behaviors that are expected in order to demonstrate that principle.

Violating a Code of Ethics

Violating a code of ethics is a serious offense that requires a thorough investigation. Because so many variables can be introduced into an alleged ethical violation, a careful review of the behaviors, intents, and reactions of several parties is necessary. However, before any ethics violation can be considered by NATA's Ethics Investigation Board, an ethics complaint form must be filled out and submitted. An ethics complaint form can be accessed by members from the NATA website (http://www.nata.org) (Fig. 14-1). All allegations must be made in writing and can be done anonymously. However, if information provided is too vague or cannot be substantiated, the investigation cannot move forward. Therefore, individuals making allegations may need to provide their names, but can ask that their name be kept confidential when possible. Once submitted, a formal process of investigation begins. Once an investigation is underway, it might become necessary for NATA to disclose confidential information supplied by the person making the allegation. If the reporting individual insists that the necessary information remain confidential, the investigation will likely be closed. Therefore, reporting an alleged ethical violation requires careful consideration and willingness to be branded a "whistleblower." A **whistleblower** is a person who reports inappropriate behavior of members to an entity or organization that presumably has the power and authority to take corrective action. However, one must also consider if the failure to report a known ethical violation is itself a violation of professional ethics.

BOC Standards of Professional Practice

The BOC Standards of Professional Practice is similar to a code of ethics. However, it is slightly more detailed and compliance is mandatory, therefore, there are no "guiding principles," but standards that must be followed. The BOC's Standards of Professional Practice consists of two sections:

1. Practice Standards
2. Code of Professional Responsibility

The practice standards delineate essential practice expectations for all athletic trainers. These standards are intended to help the public and the athletic trainer. They help the public by delineating the kinds of services they can expect from an athletic

BOX 14-2 CAATE Code of Ethics[5]

PRINCIPLE I – HONESTY

The CAATE Commissioners and its members shall be truthful and transparent in a relationship with institutions.

1. CAATE commissioners and its members shall honor explicit commitments.

2. CAATE commissioners and its members shall provide accurate and truthful information.

3. CAATE commissioners and its members shall admit and rectify errors in an expeditious manner.

4. CAATE commissioners and its members shall focus on its mission, goals, and objectives, and conduct its operations in a trustworthy manner.

PRINCIPLE II – RESPECT

The CAATE Commissioners and its members shall convey a courteous and professional regard toward institutions.

1. CAATE commissioners and its members shall acknowledge and honor the institution's autonomy, multifaceted relationships, and culture and processes.

2. CAATE commissioners and its members shall work with issues of institutional autonomy in light of the commitment to mutual accountability implied by participation in accreditation.

3. CAATE commissioners and its members shall honor ATEP diversity and its interdisciplinary nature.

4. CAATE commissioners and its members shall not discriminate against any individual based on race, religion, gender, national origin, sexual orientation, disability, age, veteran status, and will honor the institution's culture and processes.

PRINCIPLE III – ACCOUNTABILITY AND RESPONSIBILITY

The CAATE Commissioners and its members are trustworthy and shall carry out their duties within the Commission's legal and ethical limits.

1. CAATE commissioners and its members shall focus on the educational qualities of the institution, and in doing so:

    a. Recognizes that teaching and learning, not accredited status, are the primary purposes of institutions and programs.

    b. Respects the expertise and aspirations for high achievement already present and functioning in institutions and programs.

    c. Keeps the accreditation process as efficient and cost-effective as possible by minimizing the use of visits and reports, and by eliminating, whenever possible, duplication of effort between accreditation and other review processes.

    d. Works cooperatively with other accrediting bodies to avoid conflicting standards, and to minimize duplication of effort in the preparation of accreditation materials and the conduct of on-site visits.

    e. Provides the institution or programs with a thoughtful diagnostic analysis that assists the institution or program in finding its own approaches and solutions, and that makes a clear distinction between what is required for accreditation and what is recommended for improvement of the institution or program.

2. CAATE commissioners and its members shall participate in regular open communication with certified athletic trainers, athletic training students, faculty, and host institutions regarding pertinent accreditation information.

3. CAATE commissioners and its members shall focus accreditation reviews on the development of knowledge and competence, and in doing so:

    a. Concentrates on results in light of specific institutional and programmatic missions, goals, objectives, and contexts.

    b. Deals comprehensively with relationships and interdependence among purposes, aspirations, curricula, operations, resources, and results.

    c. Considers techniques, methods, and resources primarily in light of results achieved and functions fulfilled rather than the reverse.

    d. Has standards and review procedures that provide room for experimentation, encourage responsible innovation, and promote thoughtful evolution.

4. CAATE commissioners and its members shall maintain functional and operational autonomy.

5. CAATE commissioners and its members shall be current, efficient, effective, thorough with the review and accrediting process through orientations, training, and professional development.

6. CAATE commissioners and its members shall seriously take into consideration all feedback relative to standards, policies, decision making, and action

7. CAATE commissioners and its members shall make appropriate changes to standards, policies, decision making, and action when warranted.

8. CAATE commissioners and its members shall act or represent themselves as agents of the CAATE only when so charged or appointed by the CAATE.

PRINCIPLE IV – INTEGRITY

CAATE Commissioners and its members shall convey steadfast and genuine interest in upholding their duties in all places and at all times.

1. CAATE commissioners and its members shall be expected to maintain moral standards and character, and doing so: presents its materials and conducts its business with accuracy, skill, and sophistication sufficient to produce credibility for its role as an evaluator of educational quality.

2. CAATE commissioners and its members shall review the institution from the perspective of function and results, and in doing so:

    a. Maintains sufficient financial, personnel, and other resources to carry out its operations effectively.

    b. Provides accurate, clear, and timely information to the higher education community, to the professions, and to the public concerning standards and procedures for accreditation, and the status of accredited institutions and programs.

3. CAATE commissioners and its members shall base reviews and recommendations to ATEPs on existing evidence and best-practice

4. CAATE commissioners and its members shall make judgments within their assigned scope of published procedures and standards, and in doing so:

    a. Creates and documents its scope of authority, policies, and procedures to ensure governance and decision making under a framework of "laws not persons."

    b. Exercises professional judgment in the context of its published standards and procedures.

    c. Demonstrates continuing care with policies, procedures, and operations regarding due process, conflict of interest, confidentiality, and consistent application of standards.

    d. Presents its materials and conducts its business with accuracy, skill, and sophistication sufficient to produce credibility for its role as an evaluator of educational quality.

5. CAATE commissioners and its members shall avoid situations that incite questions about one's objectivity.

6. CAATE commissioners and its members shall be quick to admit errors in any part of the evaluation process, and equally quick to rectify such errors.

PRINCIPLE V – FAIRNESS

CAATE Commissioners and its members shall recognize the complexity of the accrediting process and shall be considerate and impartial in its process.

1. CAATE commissioners and its members shall avoid conflicts of interest.

2. CAATE commissioners and its members shall not receive personal gain from any affiliations that are assigned by CAATE.

3. CAATE commissioners and its members shall make decisions free of personal biases and non-sanctioned interpretations.

4. CAATE commissioners and its members shall maintain a broad perspective as the basis for wise decision making, and in doing so:
    a. Gathers and analyzes information and ideas from multiple stakeholders.
    b. Uses the results of these analyses in formulating policies and procedures that promote substantive, effective teaching and learning, that protect the autonomy of institutions and programs, and that encourage trust and cooperation within and among various components of the larger higher education community.

5. CAATE commissioners and its members shall have mechanisms to ensure that expertise and experience in the application of its standards, procedures, and values are present in members of its visiting teams, commissions, and staff, and in doing so:
    a. Works with institutions and programs to ensure that site teams represent a collection of expertise and experience appropriate for each specific review.
    b. Conducts evaluations of personnel that involve responses from institutions and programs that have experienced the accreditation process.
    c. Conducts evaluations of criteria and procedures that include responses from reviewers and those reviewed.

trainer. They help the athletic trainer evaluate quality of care and understand the ramifications of what it means to hold the ATC® credential.

The Codes of Professional Responsibility ensure that athletic trainers act responsibly in all athletic training services and activities. Failure to act responsibly, according to the code, may result is having the ATC credential revoked. There are six specific codes of professional responsibility listed by the BOC, they include:[1]

1. Patient Responsibility
2. Competency
3. Professional Responsibility
4. Research
5. Social Responsibility
6. Business Practices

Each of the codes for professional responsibility have specific behaviors associated with the code (Box 14-3).

Foundational Behaviors for Professional Practice

In addition to the Codes of Ethics of these athletic training agencies and associations, every athletic trainer is expected to abide by certain foundational behaviors for professional practice. These foundational behaviors are an explicit aspect of professional responsibility and implicit aspect of ethical behavior. These foundational behaviors are delineated in NATA's Athletic Training Educational Competencies manual.[5] Similar to the Codes of Ethics, these Foundational Behaviors are overarching and should be practiced in every area of an athletic trainer's job-specific tasks

NATA Code of Ethics Complaint Form

Please complete the following questionnaire to the best of your ability. Answers may be provided on the form or on a separate page.

A complaint is filed against:

Name of Athletic Trainer_____Title_____

Employer _____Phone No._____

Address _____

City _____ State_____

1. Please identify the section of the NATA Code of Ethics that you feel has been violated.

2. Please provide a detailed factual scenario setting forth all relevant facts in support of your assertion of a violation or violations.

3. Please provide the name(s) and contact information (phone # preferred) of any and all witnesses to the alleged violation or violations.

4. Please provide a list of all documentation (and all copies of those documents) supporting your assertion of said violation or violations.

_____ _____

COMPLAINING INDIVIDUAL   Date

Please mail to:
Ethics Investigation
National Athletic Trainers' Association
2952 Stemmons Freeway #200
Dallas, TX 75247

FIGURE 14-1 NATA Code of Ethics Complaint Form

BOX 14-3   BOC Codes of Professional Responsibility

CODE 1: PATIENT RESPONSIBILITY

The Athletic Trainer or applicant:

1.1 Renders quality patient care regardless of the patient's race, religion, age, sex, nationality, disability, social/economic status or any other characteristic protected by law

1.2 Protects the patient from harm, acts always in the patient's best interests and is an advocate for the patient's welfare

1.3 Takes appropriate action to protect patients from Athletic Trainers, other healthcare providers or athletic training students who are incompetent, impaired or engaged in illegal or unethical practice

1.4 Maintains the confidentiality of patient information in accordance with applicable law

1.5 Communicates clearly and truthfully with patients and other persons involved in the patient's program, including, but not limited to, appropriate discussion of assessment results, program plans and progress

1.6 Respects and safeguards his or her relationship of trust and confidence with the patient and does not exploit his or her relationship with the patient for personal or financial gain

1.7 Exercises reasonable care, skill and judgment in all professional work

CODE 2: COMPETENCY

The Athletic Trainer or applicant:

2.1 Engages in lifelong, professional and continuing educational activities

2.2 Participates in continuous quality improvement activities

2.3 Complies with the most current BOC recertification policies and requirements

CODE 3: PROFESSIONAL RESPONSIBILITY

The Athletic Trainer or applicant:

3.1 Practices in accordance with the most current BOC Practice Standards

3.2 Knows and complies with applicable local, state and/or federal rules, requirements, regulations and/or laws related to the practice of athletic training

3.3 Collaborates and cooperates with other healthcare providers involved in a patient's care

3.4 Respects the expertise and responsibility of all healthcare providers involved in a patient's care

3.5 Reports any suspected or known violation of a rule, requirement, regulation or law by him/herself and/or by another Athletic Trainer that is related to the practice of athletic training, public health, patient care or education

3.6 Reports any criminal convictions (with the exception of misdemeanor traffic offenses or traffic ordinance violations that do not involve the use of alcohol or drugs) and/or professional suspension, discipline or sanction received by him/herself or by another Athletic Trainer that is related to athletic training, public health, patient care or education

3.7 Complies with all BOC exam eligibility requirements and ensures that any information provided to the BOC in connection with any certification application is accurate and truthful

3.8 Does not, without proper authority, possess, use, copy, access, distribute or discuss certification exams, score reports, answer sheets, certificates, certificant or applicant files, documents or other materials

3.9 Is candid, responsible and truthful in making any statement to the BOC, and in making any statement in connection with athletic training to the public

3.10 Complies with all confidentiality and disclosure requirements of the BOC

3.11 Does not take any action that leads, or may lead, to the conviction, plea of guilty or plea of *nolo contendere* (no contest) to any felony or to a misdemeanor related to public health, patient care, athletics or education;, this includes, but is not limited to: rape; sexual abuse of a child or patient; actual or threatened use of a weapon of violence; the prohibited sale or distribution of controlled substance, or its possession with the intent to distribute; or the use of the position of an Athletic Trainer to improperly influence the outcome or score of an athletic contest or event or in connection with any gambling activity

3.12 Cooperates with BOC investigations into alleged illegal or unethical activities; this includes but is not limited to, providing factual and non-misleading information and responding to requests for information in a timely fashion

3.13 Does not endorse or advertise products or services with the use of, or by reference to, the BOC name without proper authorization

CODE 4: RESEARCH

The Athletic Trainer or applicant who engages in research:

4.1 Conducts research according to accepted ethical research and reporting standards established by public law, institutional procedures and/or the health professions

4.2 Protects the rights and well being of research subjects

4.3 Conducts research activities with the goal of improving practice, education and public policy relative to the health needs of diverse populations, the health workforce, the organization and administration of health systems and healthcare delivery

CODE 5: SOCIAL RESPONSIBILITY

The Athletic Trainer or applicant:

5.1 Uses professional skills and knowledge to positively impact the community

CODE 6: BUSINESS PRACTICES

The Athletic Trainer or applicant:

6.1 Refrains from deceptive or fraudulent business practices

6.2 Maintains adequate and customary professional liability insurance

and roles and should overlap into his or her personal, social, and civic duties and roles. There are seven foundational behaviors for professional practice for athletic trainers regardless of role or setting, and include:[5]

1. Primacy of the patient—includes being an advocate for the needs of the patient and providing the highest quality health care available.

2. Team approach—includes willingness to work on interdisciplinary health care teams, understanding the scope of practice of other health care professionals, and collaborative decision making.

3. Legal practice—includes practicing within the confines of the laws that govern athletic training.

4. Ethical practice—includes abiding by the NATA Code of Ethics and the BOC's Standards of Practice, and practice ethical behavior at all times.

5. Advancing knowledge—includes recognizing and promoting athletic training knowledge.

6. Cultural competence—includes awareness and knowledge of cultural, social, and ethnic diversity within the health care population and amongst the diversity of patients for whom athletic trainers care.

7. Professionalism—includes being an advocate for athletic training, demonstrating honesty and integrity, communicating appropriately, and demonstrating empathy toward others.

Similar to the Codes of Ethics, these Foundational Behaviors of Professional Practice for athletic trainers are the minimal expectations. When a behavior is not specifically addressed or if a principle is vague, the athletic trainer is not released from obligation to behave professionally or act ethically.

ETHICAL DECISION MAKING

Taking the time to consider and weigh all the possible outcomes in the middle of an ethical dilemma can difficult. When evaluating the values of several stakeholders (e.g., the coach's, patient's, and athletic trainer's) coming to the right decision can be an emotional roller-coaster. Making ethically correct decisions involves awareness of ethical standards and an intentional evaluation of the possible outcomes for whichever decision might be made. The most obvious and potent tool for avoiding "accidental" unethical behavior is to delineate certain ethical situations before they occur and decide in advance how you will respond. However, no matter how many situations are rehearsed there will always be ethical dilemmas that were unforeseeable.

Consequences are often considered in the ethical decision-making equation. However, a potential trap in the ethical decision-making process is to rely too much on consequences as a criteria. All consequences can never be fully foreseen or anticipated. Therefore, making decisions based purely on the severity of any perceived consequences is poor judgment. Furthermore, the sole use of perceived consequences in an ethical dilemma can lead one toward a teleological philosophy. Unfortunately, there are some for whom the lack of severe enough consequences is all it takes to justify unethical behavior. The next section will look into how motives may play a role in ethical decision making.

Motives

Any discussion of ethics is not complete without mentioning motives. Motives are the reasons and intentions behind an action. Within ethics motives are typically referred to as egoistic or altruistic. Egoism is an outcome where the individual gains the most and others experience the most harm (or least benefit). Egoistic behaviors are those that benefit the decision maker (i.e., me) the most and others may have less or no benefit. In other words, egoism is nothing more than selfishness. The opposite of egoism is altruism. Altruism is when others benefit the most and the decision maker receives the most harm (or least benefit). Altruistic behaviors are those behaviors admired by others and often considered "selfless acts." An example of altruism in athletic training might be accommodating rehabilitation for an athlete after the athletic training room has closed for the evening. One other aspect of motive can be considered, utilitarianism. **Utilitarianism** is the idea that the good of many outweighs the good of the one, i.e., the larger group benefits more than any single person or smaller group.

Deciding who benefits and how much they benefit is difficult. When a decision about who benefits the most is not obvious remember the "Golden Rule: Do unto others as you would have done unto you"… and the right answer is not far off. However, behaving ethically is not always as easy as one might hope. Furthermore, the difference between ethical and unethical behavior is not always obvious. One of the best ways to curtail unethical behavior is to seek counsel from trustworthy sources and practice regular self-reflection. In the next section we will delineate specific questions that can be asked to help make ethical decision.

Evaluating Ethical Behaviors by Asking Questions

There are informal questions that can be asked to help guide one toward the ethical action. The first question to consider is, "Is this action legal?" Within athletic training the answer must be "yes." However, even "yes" answers can be a fully loaded ethical dilemma. Within the legal framework there are informal but practical questions to ask to help make ethical decisions more easily, such questions include:

1. Are there "shushers?" (i.e., is anyone pressuring me to keep this quiet)
2. Will I have to hide this from anyone?
3. Is this something I can tell my mother?
4. Does is violate the "Golden Rule?"
5. What if everyone did this?
6. Who might this decision impact and how?

CHAPTER SUMMARY

Athletic trainers are exposed to situations that require ethical considerations, both large and small, on a daily basis. Ethical considerations transcend merely determining if an action is legal or illegal. Most ethical situations are never seen by others or discussed in public; they are usually personal and resonate with the individual after self-reflection and an examination of motives or even past behavior. Often ethics becomes a factor if providing preferential treatment to a favorite patient; even having "favorite" patients can become ethical, if it dictates or influences in any way how you treat or care for those patients. Remaining silent when knowing a colleague has violated or is violating a code or standard can also be a serious ethical consideration.

> ### Leadership
> ### Application

Let's suppose that you are required to make four visits a month to three area high schools to briefly consult with coaches and triage any athletes for possible referral to your clinic. The mileage reimbursement policy states you can claim mileage from work to the locale and back to work for each visit. The point of origin for travel reimbursement must be from work. Fortunately, one of the high schools is directly across the street from your house and you drive by it every day to and from work, whether it is necessary to visit or not.

Critical Thinking Questions

1. What factors make this an ethical situation?
2. Is it ethical to claim mileage reimbursement for visiting the school next to your house, even if entitled to claim it?
3. Does the consequence of the decision increase or decrease based on price of gas, for example, if gas is $1.79 per gallon versus $4.15 per gallon?
4. Is it "OK" to just claim my drive to the high school after work on your way home, but not the return trip back to work the next morning?
5. If the underlying purpose of the mileage reimbursement policy is to cover depreciation of your car due to work-related travel, does this travel cause depreciation that otherwise might not occur?
6. Are there any statements or principles in the NATA Code of Ethics to help you make this decision?

Being sure to know and adhere to the NATA Code of Ethics, NATA's Foundational Behaviors of Professional Practice, and the BOC's Standards of Professional Practice can help ensure ethical standards are met. Furthermore, being aware of other Codes and standards, such as the CAATE Code of Ethics and ethics codes of other professional organizations can be valuable. Violating behavioral standards or ethical codes are serious offenses and can result in loss of credentials, licenses, or dismissal from the profession. Asking straightforward and honest questions about intended actions or past behaviors is a good way to help determine the appropriateness of an action.

References

1. Board of Certification Inc. (2006). *BOC standards of professional practice.* Available at: http://www.bocatc.org/images/stories/multiple_references/standardsprofessionalpractice.pdf. Accessed September 5, 2008.

2. Commission on Accreditation of Athletic Training Education. (2008). *CAATE code of ethics.* Available at: http://www.caate.net/dynamic/CAATECoE.pdf. Accessed September 5, 2008.

3. MacDonald C, McDonald M, Norman W. (2002). Charitable conflicts of interest. *Journal of Business Ethics 39.*1–2:67–74.

4. National Athletic Trainers' Association. (2006). *Athletic training educational competencies.* Dallas, TX: NATA.

5. National Athletic Trainers' Association. (2005). *NATA code of ethics.* Available at: http://www.nata.org/codeofethics/code_of_ethics.pdf. Accessed September 5, 2008.

6. Schlabach G, Peer K. (2008). *Professional ethics in athletic training.* St. Louis, MO: Mosby.

Chapter 15

International Implications

"We all should know that diversity makes for a rich tapestry, and we must understand that all the threads of the tapestry are equal in value no matter what their color."

MAYA ANGELOU

CHAPTER RATIONALE

Role Delineation Study Components

Domain V: Organization and Administration

- Respecting diversity of opinions and positions

Educational Competencies

- Describe the theories and techniques of... cross cultural communication

Foundational Behaviors of Professional Practice

- Cultural Competence:
  - Understand the cultural differences of patients' attitudes and behaviors toward health care.
  - Demonstrate knowledge, attitudes, behaviors, and skills necessary to achieve optimal health outcomes for diverse populations.
  - Demonstrate knowledge, attitudes, behaviors, and skills necessary to work respectfully and effectively with diverse populations and in a diverse work environment.

Key Terms

Cultural competence: The capacity of an individual to incorporate ethnic and cultural considerations of diverse co-workers into their work.

Culture: Common beliefs and practices of a group of people that lead to specific habits of thought, behavior, diet, dress, music, and art.

Diversity: A complex social issue that describes differences both within cultural groups and between cultural groups.

Ethnocentric: Believing that one's own culture is superior to all others.

Globalization: The exchange and integration of cultural ideals, social ideals, values, politics, and technologies between diverse people groups as a result of increased communication and access.

Stereotype: The belief that all people from a given group are the same.

Worldview: A set of conscious or subconscious presuppositions about the basic makeup of our world; the ideas and beliefs through which an individual interprets the world and interacts with his or her surroundings.

Ethnic diversity is on the rise in the United States. *The Pew Health Professions Commission identified 21 competencies for health care professionals in the new millennium. Competency 12 states to "provide culturally sensitive care to a diverse society."[13] Underrepresented minorities are becoming the fastest-growing segment in the United States population, and racial and ethnic minorities are expected to comprise 40% of the United States population by 2030 (Fig. 15-1).[11] The challenge to all health care and allied health care providers is to increase the number of minority health care professionals.*

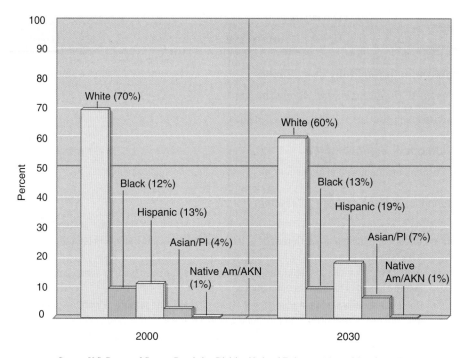

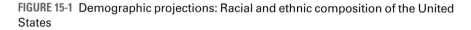

Source: U.S. Bureau of Census, Population Division National Estimates, *"Annual Population Estimates by Sex, Race, and Hispanic Origin, Selected Years from 1990 to 1998."* May 1999

FIGURE 15-1 Demographic projections: Racial and ethnic composition of the United States

Athletic training has become a profession with a global impact. In addition to the United States, athletic training is practiced in Japan, Canada, and China. Furthermore, athletic training education programs in the United States are attracting students from around the globe, who in turn are returning to their country of origin and introducing athletic training to new cultures and new populations. With such a growing profession, it is critical that athletic trainers and athletic training education promote a greater appreciation for diversity.

Diversity in athletic training is a larger issue than recognition in other countries. There are also an increasing number of differences among patient populations within the United States. **Diversity** *is a complex social issue that describes differences of individuals within cultural groups and between cultural groups. In spite of growing diversity among the patients athletic trainers serve, athletic training remains a Caucasian- dominated profession. Currently less than 8% of athletic trainers are African American, Asian American, Hispanic, or Native American.[2] As professionals, athletic trainers need to meet the challenges that accompany increasing diversity with innovation and creativity.*

We live in a global context. Access and exposure to culturally, ethnically, religiously, and politically diverse groups is at an all-time high. Never before has this level of exposure been as great as it is today. Athletic trainers are working with athletes and patients from all walks and stages of life and from a variety of different cultural and ethnic backgrounds. The advent of globalization has made cultural competence a requisite for professional behavior and advancement. It is critically important that athletic trainers understand how globalization and cultural competency influence the growth and future of athletic training. An emerging leadership competency within global health care is to embrace diversity and cultural competence.

In this chapter we will begin by addressing the concept of globalization and how it has impacted athletic training and the future challenges facing athletic training as related to globalization. After discussing globalization, we will turn our attention to international implications for athletic training as well as diversity within the profession. When discussing international implications we will cover several global athletic training organizations as well as committees dedicated to supporting and promoting international relations and diversity. Finally, we will conclude our discussion of diversity with a brief introduction to cultural competence, the importance of understanding different worldviews, and promoting cultural awareness.

GLOBALIZATION

Globalization was originally an economic phenomenon that in its simplest form meant the increased ease of movement of goods and services across international borders. Today globalization represents more than just economic fluidity; there is a "cultural globalization."[1] Globalization is not a new phenomenon; it began when Christopher Columbus discovered the new world and consequently different world-views collided. However, advances in technology and international trade have catapulted globalization to a major sociological phenomenon. With the advent of the Internet, global communications, global media, and easier international travel, the world is proverbially shrinking. This means it is easier now, more than any other time in history, to interact with people from diverse cultures. **Globalization** is then the exchange and integration of cultural ideals, social ideals, values, politics, and technologies between diverse people groups as a result of increased communication and access.

Globalization causes a fundamental shift in the concept of citizenship. It is less likely that people will hold to the notion they are only a citizen of an isolated place or to a geographic location. Everyone is now faced with the reality that values from "somewhere else" influence thoughts and decisions. It is precisely because of globalization that cultural competence is such a valuable commodity today. Leaders in a global context must strive to be culturally competent. **Cultural competence** is the capacity of an individual to incorporate ethnic and cultural considerations of diverse co-workers into their work. Therefore, globalization forces the critical examination of one's basic assumptions about themselves and about others.

For centuries, much of what validated someone's action or practice was based on local traditions.[9] The advent of globalization reduces the value of local traditions as the key measure of appropriate behavior. This fundamental change has tremendous implications for health care.

Complexities of Globalization

Globalization is not a welcome phenomenon to everyone. For example, one might argue that before "global awareness" there were adequate delivery and low cost-benefit ratios in health care. However, the context of that thinking was likely restricted to highly industrialized and generally wealthy countries. Enter globalization and suddenly one is forced to recognize health care and health care delivery on a global scale. For example, the rising awareness of health delivery and access issues in less-developed countries with poorly run infrastructures brings to light the fact that on a global level, health care may not be very advanced at all. Therefore, there are those who might argue globalization is good because it makes us aware of these issues and therefore, someone can do something about the inadequate health care in less-fortunate countries. However, this same argument may be made for globalization having a negative impact. For example, now that we are aware of global health care disparity, health care resources, delivery, and access are spread more thinly. As a result, there is an increase in the overall cost that brings down the overall health care delivery in the "developed" country.

Regardless of any one particular perspective concerning globalization, it is happening. However, leaders in the profession of athletic training are taking advantage of globalization trends by making strides to position the profession for global recognition as expert health care providers to physically active populations.

Globalization in Athletic Training

Athletic training as we know it is a relatively North American phenomenon.[5] However, athletic training has an increasing global presence; as time goes on it is likely that athletic training will have an increasing presence on the global sports scene. Only a short time ago athletic trainers could only be found in the United States, working with major sports programs, treating only athletes on those teams. Today the background and culture of the patients that athletic trainers treat are as diverse as any, and the geographic locations where athletic trainers practice extend far beyond the "sidelines" to truly span the globe. A major challenge facing athletic trainers is the necessity to become culturally competent. This challenge falls to the profession and our professional education programs to ensure a minimum level of cultural competency in practitioners at all levels.

Value of Globalization to Athletic Training

Athletic training has benefited from globalization. Because of sport's popularity, specialists in sports-based health care are highly desirable in many industrialized countries. As a relatively new profession, athletic training, with its emerging body of knowledge and professional education, is appealing to many in other countries. As a result there is a growing international population becoming athletic trainers. This has led to many international students coming to the United States for their professional education and then returning to their country of origin to practice athletic training and sports health care. Another interesting phenomenon is that some of those international students stay in the United States after they become professionals, bringing many of their values, ideas, traditions, and cultures to athletic training. For example, acupuncture, a predominately Chinese intervention, has been used in athletic training rooms to treat athletes' injuries.

Athletic training education programs have also directly benefited from globalization. This new and emerging student base has helped encourage athletic training educators and administrators to innovate new methods for delivering and facilitating athletic training education. For example, language barriers are becoming less of an issue with new technology and innovative pedagogy, such as video pod casts, downloadable mp3 lectures, and online materials available in other languages. Furthermore, challenges of international students are not only referred to the "international office" on campus; National Athletic Trainers' Association's (NATA) ethnic diversity and international committees can also serve as a resource for athletic training students.

Other changes in athletic training intended to meet the requirements of a changing student and professional makeup include the introduction of entry-level masters programs, study-abroad programs, scholarships for international students, agreements with equivalently credentialed healthcare professionals from other countries (i.e., Canadian Athletic Therapy Association); the creation of global sports health care organizations (e.g., World Federation of Athletic Training and Therapy); and the formation of professional athletic training associations in other countries. These are only a small sample of some of the initiatives undertaken to promote athletic training in our global context and make athletic training available to more students around the world. However, in spite of these and other innovations there remains much work to be done in the area of diversity and cultural competence within athletic training. There is still a small percentage of athletic trainers who come from ethnically diverse backgrounds.

Ethnic Diversity Advisory Committee

NATA has taken a proactive stance in valuing and promoting diversity within athletic training. In 1986 NATA formed the Minority Athletic Trainers' Committee (MATC). In 1991 the MATC was disbanded due to a lack of direction and was reformed later that year under a new name, the Ethnic Minority Advisory Council (EMAC); in 1999 the name was changed again to the Ethnic Diversity Advisory Council (EDAC) to reflect a broader perspective. In 2002 the EDAC began to receive funding from NATA and has since evolved into the Ethnic Diversity Advisory Committee (EDAC).

The purpose of the EDAC is to identify and address issues relevant to American Indian/Alaskan Natives, Asian/Pacific Islanders, Black, non-Hispanic and Hispanic members. Additionally, the EDAC addresses health care concerns affecting physically active individuals in these ethnic groups. It is the EDAC's goal to promote sensitivity and understanding toward ethnic and cultural diversity. To do this, EDAC offers a formal mentoring program for ethnically diverse students, the ethnic diversity enhancement grant for educational programs that promote diversity in athletic training, and the Bill Chisholm Professional Service Award. The Bill Chisholm Professional Service Award is presented to an individual who advanced athletic health care to ethnic minority individuals or the professional development and advancement of ethnic minority athletic trainers. For more information on mentoring, grants, or the Bill Chisholm Professional Service Award, visit http://www.edacweb.org.

Other efforts have been made by NATA and proactive athletic trainers that foster and create a global community of athletic trainers. Those efforts have resulted in the formation of other organizations or agencies with similar aspirations. The next few sections will detail some of these organizations.

World Federation of Athletic Training and Therapy

In 1998 the NATA Board of Directors decided it was important to begin to investigate globalization as it pertains to athletic training. As a result, in 2000, through the collaboration of several organizations, agencies, and associations, the World Federation of Athletic Training and Therapy (WFATT) was formed. The WFATT is a coalition of sports medicine-based organizations around the world. WFATT's purpose is to encourage quality health care and functional activity through the collaborative effort (Box 15-1).

WFATT has four goals within its charter:

1. Create a global forum for exchanging non-binding information about health care for active populations, including academic preparation and professional practice, through meetings and communication vehicles.

LEADERSHIP ACTIVITY

Divide the existing class into small workgroups of two to three members (i.e., team leaders). Once the class is divided, these team leaders should recruit other athletic training students from different classes or levels (i.e., observer, first-year, second-year, etc) as well as students from different majors on campus, so that each group's size ranges from five to seven members. Once a group is created, meet with the entire group and brainstorm three to five ideas that you collectively thought of on how to market and recruit minority students to the profession of athletic training. As team leaders, formally delineate these ideas on paper and present them to the class. After all the ideas have been presented in class, discuss which idea or ideas were the very best, then as an entire class develop a comprehensive strategic plan for carrying the idea out to fruition. After the plan has been evaluated by peers, ACI's/CI's, and your instructor, try to implement it.

BOX 15-1   WFATT Members

CHARTER MEMBERS

Association of Chartered Physiotherapists in Sports Medicine
Biokinetics Association of South Africa
Canadian Athletic Therapists' Association
Japan Sports Association
Japan Athletic Trainers' Organization
Taiwan (Republic of China) Athletic Trainers' Society
National Athletic Trainers' Association

MEMBERS

Board of Certification
Federazione Italiana Fisioterapisti
Japan Athletic Trainers' Association for Certification
Korean Association of Certified Exercise Professionals
Ontario Athletic Therapists' Association
Spanish Association of Sport Nurses
Society of Tennis Medicine and Science
University of Bedfordshire
Korean Athletic Trainers' Association
Japan Amateur Sports Association
The University of Texas Health Science Center at San Antonio

2. Provide opportunities for collaborative research efforts among members to improve the quality of health care to active populations.
3. Provide information on professions and organizations that deliver health care to active populations.
4. Promote the development of international and domestic relationships with sport, health care and governing bodies.

One way that WFATT is accomplishing its goals is through bi-annual world congresses. These world congresses are hosted by different nations on a revolving basis and are designed to advance a global health care agenda for the physically active. WFATT also endorses international exchange of sports medicine and sport-health-care professionals. Another aspect of WFATT's mission is to promote basic knowledge of injury prevention on a global scale. To do this WFATT has spearheaded the dissemination of athletic training information in several languages. Box 15-2 is a Chinese version of the standard R.I.C.E. (Rest, Ice, Compression, Elevation) protocol, which was developed in collaboration by NATA, WFATT, and Taiwan (Republic of China) Athletic Trainers Society. In addition to WFATT, NATA strives to promote diversity within its membership base, which led to the creation of the EDAC (mentioned earlier) and the International Committee.

NATA International Committee

The purpose of NATA's International Committee is to establish a global network of colleagues in the allied health profession to include: certified athletic trainers (ATC), certified athletic therapists (CAT(C)), physical therapists, physiotherapists,

BOX 15-2 R.I.C.E. Protocol in Chinese

运动的健康诀窍 #3：休息 - 冰敷 - 压迫 - 抬高 (R.I.C.E 米字诀)

✧ 休息(Rest)

让受伤的部位休息对使身体能有时间控制创伤与反应是必要的，以避免组织受到额外的压力或损伤。休息的时间长短会随着伤害的严重性而不同(数天到数个星期)。急性伤害(突发性或创伤性)若无适当休息，可能会因而延长发炎期与增加愈合所需的时间，进而延迟复原。

✧ 冰敷(Ice)

迅速的对伤害使用冰敷可以有效的降低与减少发炎反应。冰敷会使组织间的小动脉闭合，减少出血。局部组织的代谢也会减缓，因而降低氧气及养分的需求，以及减慢疼痛神经冲动的传导，并产生钝麻的止痛效果。 冰敷治疗的范例包括使用冰袋或是冰桶 15～20 分钟，或直接以冰块按摩 7～10 分钟。在确定出血及肿胀都已经完全停止之后才可以开始使用热敷，否则会延迟复原时间。

✧ 压迫(Compression)

压迫是利用绷带或是类似对象在受伤区域缠绕，其目的是为了帮忙控制肿胀及提供适度的支持。任何的缠绕都必须小心谨慎，过紧的绷带会限制或阻断受伤区域赖以维生的血液循环。

✧ 抬高(Elevation)

尽可能的抬高受伤区域使其高于心脏，这样可以利用重力与淋巴系统之引流来促进肿胀的减少与消除。

为了预防受伤，运动员应该：
- ✓ 维持适当的身体状况
- ✓ 参与任何运动或竞赛前都要热身与伸展
- ✓ 总是穿着合脚的鞋子，并在当鞋子的跟部或缝线出现磨损时尽快换新鞋
- ✓ 藉由均衡的饮食保养肌肉
- ✓ 使用或穿着适当的保护设备
- ✓ 维持体内水分
- ✓ 维持健康的体重
- ✓ 当疲劳或有身体疼痛时避免从事运动或比赛
- ✓ 在平坦的表面行走或运动

此运动的健康秘诀的目的在于预防伤害以及提升参予活动者的健康安全。 具认证的运动伤害防护员是一群的致力于运动者伤病之预防、评估、治疗、与复健的专业医疗人员。

and other sports medicine specialists. The international committee also has a role in evaluating and creating programs, policies, and alliances that affect international members and regular certified members living abroad. Specifically, the NATA international committee serves and promotes NATA members who live and work abroad as well as promotes the use of ATCs to international job markets. Furthermore, the NATA International Committee promotes and assists with study abroad and international internship programs for athletic training students and athletic trainers. As part of their purpose to form alliances and promote ATCs in international job markets, the international committee has helped create the mutual recognition agreement with the Canadian Athletic Therapy Association (CATA).

Canadian Athletic Therapy Association

The CATA is an association similar to NATA. In fact, the CATA was formed in 1965 by a group of Canadian Athletic Trainers who were members of NATA.[4] These vanguard leaders convened a meeting of other athletic trainers in Canada to discuss the possibility of forming a Canadian association for athletic trainers. Out of that landmark meeting, the CATA was formed. The first CATA meeting was held in Chicago in conjunction with the 1965 NATA national meeting.[4]

NATA and CATA still enjoy a great relationship. Over the years each association has promoted and supported the other. Today there is a mutual recognition agreement between CATA and BOC. BOC certified athletic trainers are eligible to sit for certification as a Canadian Certified Athletic Therapist (CAT(C)) and certified athletic therapists can sit for the BOC exam. For details on the CATA/BOC mutual recognition agreement, visit the BOC or CATA websites (http://www.bocatc.org or http://www.athletictherapy.org). In addition to CATA there are other athletic training organizations with which NATA and athletic trainers share common interests; one such organization is the Japanese Athletic Trainers Organization (JATO).

Japanese Athletic Trainers Organization

The JATO was established in June 1996 as a non-profit organization. JATO is the only organization in Japan that consists solely of NATA members. The objectives of JATO are the following.[6]

1. To educate the community [in Japan] about the value of NATA standards and to promote the athletic training profession in Japan.
2. To provide continuous education opportunities for the membership [in Japan].
3. To exchange opinions among the membership [in Japan] about the current sports medicine environment.
4. To communicate with other organizations [in Japan] to promote higher standards of care for athletes.
5. To share knowledge and experience with other health care providers in Japan.

The WFATT and NATA International committee in conjunction with JATO has developed a definition of athletic training in Japanese. To see the Japanese definition of athletic training, visit http://www.jato-trainer.org.

DIVERSITY WITHIN ATHLETIC TRAINING

As defined earlier, diversity signifies differences of individuals within a group, as well as differences between groups. These differences can range between, age, gender, politics, ability, sexual orientation, social class, ethnicity, or religion. Basically all differences in values or beliefs about any number of issues lead to diversity. Some of these differences are more overt than others. Diversity within a profession should be celebrated and not viewed as an obstacle to progress or growth.

A significant challenge for the athletic training profession is to create a workforce that is similar to the diversity of clients, families, and communities served by the profession. Practicing athletic training professionals are not as ethnically diverse as the populations they serve. Over 90% of athletic trainers are Caucasians. Contrast that to the nearly 53% of college football players in division 1A who are African American, Latino, or Asian American.[12] Clearly athletic training needs to develop and put in place systems to create interest, recruit, and educate diverse populations to be athletic trainers. Future leaders in athletic training must embrace this challenge and innovate for the future of athletic training.

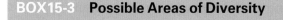

| BOX15-3 | **Possible Areas of Diversity** |

- Age
- Gender
- Geographical location
- Physical ability
- Political affiliation
- Race and ethnicity
- Religion
- Sexual orientation
- Socioeconomic status

The Essence of Diversity

The foundation of diversity is ultimately expressed in different value systems. While on the surface diversity seems to be about ethnicity, gender, or race, the deeper issue rests with different values. In other words, two people with different skin colors or backgrounds can think and behave in very similar ways. Therefore, the essence of diversity is not about different physical features per se, rather it is about how different experiences or values alter behavior. Often it is the rationale behind the behavior that constitutes the spirit of diversity.

The challenge of diversity is to avoid presuming that "different" means "competing" or "wrong" (Box 15-3). In the diversity context the temptation is to presume that other viewpoints or other values compete for preeminence with our own. When this is the mindset, there is a tendency to need to have a winner and loser. The athletic trainer must avoid this at all costs and hold to the perspective that different views or values enhance the process and enrich a situation.

People who resist diversity do so out of an irrational fear that they might lose their own identity, or they fear having to accept wholesale something they may not believe or value. Honoring diversity does not mean that every view must be accepted as correct. Honoring diversity is ultimately about two things:

1. Being willing to concede that one's own view or values are not the only views or values worthy of considering, and
2. Providing an atmosphere so that every view is able to be expressed without fear of backlash.

As diversity is given place the next step is to develop cultural competence. Religion, perhaps more than any other aspect, influences a culture's values. Religious belief is often the foundation of many people's thinking on ethics, morality, politics, relationships, global sustainability, sexual orientation, and so on. Therefore, steps toward cultural competence should include awareness of worldview issues. Another common contributor to diversity is socioeconomic class. Regardless of the reason for a difference the athletic trainer should not discount a peer's or patient's belief or make them feel irrational or silly in any way. Some general tips for increasing diversity awareness are listed in Box 15-4.

Cultural Competence

Learning specific or even isolated facts about the nuances or common beliefs of different cultures just for the sake of learning them is not the objective for developing cultural competence.[7] There is a responsibility to put that knowledge to use in the clinical context; cultural competence must inform our behavior. The basis of cultural competence can be summarized as three "essential principles:"[7]

> ### BOX 15-4 Tips for Increasing Cultural Diversity Competence
>
> - Avoid comparison of other's traditions with your own country's traditions or values.
> - Be open to new ideas and experiences.
> - Familiarize yourself with different worldviews.
> - Familiarize yourself with other customs and traditions (e.g., punctuality, greetings, meal etiquette).
> - Familiarize yourself with the customs and traditions of other religions or national holidays.
> - Foster open communication between cultural and ethnic groups.
> - Learn a foreign language.
> - Participate in study-abroad programs.
> - Subscribe to foreign media, publications, and periodicals (i.e., newspapers, journals, blogs, list-serves).

1. Acknowledging the importance of culture to individuals.
2. Respecting cultural differences
3. Minimizing any negative impact of cultural differences

The National Center for Cultural Competence[7] lists several reasons why cultural competency is important to health care. Those reasons are:

1. To respond to demographic changes in the United States
2. To eliminate long-standing disparities in the health status of diverse people groups
3. To improve quality of service and health outcomes
4. To meet legislative, regulatory, and accreditation mandates
5. To gain a competitive edge in the marketplace
6. To decrease the likelihood of liability and malpractice.

Culturally competent athletic trainers are essential to the profession's longevity and credibility. Culture is framed by what we do.[8] In other words, **culture** consists of the beliefs and practices of a group of people that lead to specific habits of thought, behavior, diet, dress, music, and art.[8] Being culturally competent requires recognizing, affirming, and valuing the worth of diverse individuals, families, tribes, and communities, so that the dignity of each is preserved and protected.[3] Becoming culturally competent is an ongoing process that does not happen simply by enacting policy or attending training sessions. Roberts[8] has outlined a three-stage model for becoming culturally competent:

- Stage 1—cultural awareness, which consists of being aware of the needs and differences among cultures.
- State 2—cultural sensitivity, which adds to cultural awareness the ability to reflect on one's practice and emotional responses to work.
- Stage 3—cultural competence, the ability to change behavior or the way we practice in order to accommodate patients from all cultural backgrounds.

Acquiring cultural competence requires the refusal to stereotype and a personal awareness of different worldviews.

Worldviews

A **worldview** is a set of conscious or subconscious presuppositions about the basic makeup of our world."[10] In other words, a worldview represents the ideas and beliefs through which an individual interprets the world and interacts with their surroundings. Knowing one's worldview is essential to successfully interacting with others and is a key component to developing cultural competence. It is in essence the belief system that informs one's values. For example, traditional Western medicine presumes that illness or injury can be traced back to some physical pathology. On the other hand, many cultures believe that physical illness or injury is a result of social or spiritual pathology. There are many medical situations where having knowledge of different patient's worldview would help inform clinical action.

Discovering one's worldview is a significant step toward awareness, understanding, and knowledge.[10] All conscientious professionals should examine their worldview in an attempt to better understand the complex world of ideas and values they live in. To do this, some philosophical and perhaps even uncomfortable questions must be asked and answered. Most people never question or think about their worldview unless it is challenged or questioned by someone from another "ideological universe."[10] To discover one's worldview, Sire[10] recommends answering seven basic questions that most people take for granted or else presume everyone else thinks the same way about. Those questions are:

1. What is real (or what is ultimate reality)?
2. What is the nature of reality?
3. What is a human being?
4. What happens to a person after death?
5. Why is it possible to know anything?
6. How do we know what is right or wrong?
7. What is the meaning of human history?

These questions are best considered and answered individually as a form of self-reflection. Ignoring these questions is something professionals in a global society cannot afford.

How can personally answering these questions enrich an athletic trainer? As athletic trainers become more prevalent within the health care industry, a larger diversity of patients is to be expected. Many of these patients may have a diverse way of thinking about injury, illness, treatment, and recovery. The more an athletic trainer or athletic training student is prepared to address his or her biases, the easier the transfer of ideas can be.

Once the process of understanding one's own worldview is undertaken, then the task of determining and defining other worldviews becomes necessary. Table 15-1 is a list of some of the dominant worldviews and a basic description of their distinctive beliefs. Knowing these worldviews may help increase the understanding of another's perspective and therefore foster greater appreciation of other's values and viewpoint. Table 15-2 is an example of how the possible answers to the worldview questions may inform health care decisions or practices.

Awareness of Cultural Differences

Being **ethnocentric** is at its worst the belief that one's own culture is superior to all others; at its best being ethnocentric is the failure to consider other culture's worldviews. Ethnocentric behavior does not happen by accident, it is often an intentional belief. Ignorance of other cultural behaviors is not in and of itself ethnocentric per se, but it is certainly irresponsible, and not fitting of an athletic trainer. Furthermore, any temptation to stereotype must be rejected. A **stereotype** is the belief that all people from a given group are the same. Athletic trainers should make an intentional effort to understand and appreciate the values and the framework behind the values from those of other cultures.

From the Field

I remember one particular post-game meal where cultural diversity became a serious issue. After a football game post-game meals were being distributed to players as they entered the bus for our return home. One of the players on the team was a devout Muslim and was accidentally handed (we had an alternative for him) a meat pizza, which included ham, sausage and other pork products. After he realized that he had nearly touched the pork, he was a little disgruntled (and this is stating it nicely; I seem to remember a pizza flying across the bus, loud yelling and profanity, and a lot of shrinking and hiding behind seats). By touching the pizza this athlete would have violated a very serious religious law, a law that had grave consequences. To make matters worse, one of the graduate assistant coaches suggested to him to stop whining and pick the toppings off. This was an obviously poor suggestion and demonstrated zero cultural competence. The issue of pork with Muslims is not convenience or preference; to eat pork is a serious transgression and abomination. The culturally correct response would have been to sincerely apologize and offer to take the pizza back. As a result of that single experience, I now understand the sincerity and conviction that religious law can play in an athletic training setting.

TABLE 15-1 A Sample of Different Worldviews†

Worldview*	Brief Description
1. Theistic	The idea there is one personal God (several religions are theistic, e.g., Judaism, Christianity, and Muslim).
2. Deism	Acknowledges the presence of a divine being, but one that does not interact with creation.
3. Naturalism	Believes that observation and reason is the sole criteria for truth.
4. Nihilism	Promotes the denial of even the possibility of knowledge or anything valuable.
5. Existentialism	Expresses how only humanity is significant in an otherwise insignificant world.
6. Eastern Pantheistic Monoism	Belief that everything is connected and that the divine can be seen anywhere in anything.
7. New Age	An eclectic hodge-podge of several different worldviews.
8. Postmodernism	Not a "true" worldview, but a framework based on the value and legitimacy of all knowledge.

*There are additional worldviews; some of these have subcategories with additional nuances.
† Adapted from Sire, 1997.

The first step in this process is to realize that there are in fact cultural differences. Followed by the step of exploring what those differences might be. Exacerbating the problem is that many people place the onus of becoming "culturally aware" on the other party. In other words, they presume it is someone else's duty to learn about "how we do it here," versus being proactive and accommodating for someone else. Athletic trainers should take on that responsibility themselves and learn about the other's culture, which can be viewed as a way to welcome diversity into the athletic training room.

A great resource for health care professionals to use to explore diversity issues within health care is Ethnomed. Ethnomed (http://www.ethnomed.org) is a joint project of University of Washington Health Sciences Library and the Harborview Medical Center's Community House Calls Program. Its primary purpose is to link patient education materials in both English and a community's native language. Ethnomed also provides a detailed "Cultural Profile" of a number of ethnic groups that

TABLE 15-2 Examples of how Worldviews may Impact Health Care

Worldview Question	Medical/Health Implication or Relevance
1. What is real (or ultimate reality)?	Determines primary source sought for help or reassurance when ill or injured
2. What is the nature of reality?	Helps to explain the existence or reason of sickness or disease
3. What is a human being?	Helps determine the amount of value and worth one may place on human life
4. What happens to a person after death?	Determines level of hope or peace one may have when injured or ill
5. Why is it possible to know anything?	Determines value of evidence and research as it pertains to epidemiology and clinical outcomes
6. How do we know what is right or wrong?	Medical and bioethics – behavior of clinicians toward patients
7. What is the meaning of human history?	Purpose and destiny of an individual – help to rationalize injury or illness

includes information on beliefs, customs, and traditional medical practices that may assist health care professionals with culturally sensitive care.

CHAPTER SUMMARY

Athletic training is quickly becoming a globally recognized profession. With the advent of advanced communication technology, the word about athletic training and value of athletic trainers is spreading quickly. As a result, athletic trainers must become much more culturally competent and aware of diversity. This includes awareness, promotion, and engagement in NATA committee activities that foster diversity and cultural awareness. Furthermore, we must be vigilant in making our athletic training programs and associated athletic departments in which individuals from diverse backgrounds feel supported, encouraged, and valued for the richness they bring to the academic environment.

Leadership Application

During the summer after your third year as an athletic training student you have an opportunity to gain a much desired clinical education experience covering an international sports competition in Japan. You have been selected for a two-week internship. You arrive in Japan and are escorted to the sports facility and begin helping immediately. In addition to a language barrier you quickly realize that the clinical supervisors allow you much more autonomy than you are used to in the United States; in fact, they expect you to perform at a level higher than you believe you are able. With the conviction that you should not go beyond your boundaries and stay within what you believe are the appropriate boundaries for your level and experience, you decide it is necessary to tell the main supervisor that you are not comfortable doing all that is being expected. You compose the dialogue and rehearse it over and over in your mind. The next morning you approach the supervisor and as succinctly and humbly as you can state your case. After you state your case, he bows and nods as if he agrees with you. You leave feeling satisfied that you did the right thing and remained humble. Later that week you find out that you received a very negative and even harsh evaluation from that supervisor. After a little investigation you find out your athletic training skills are perceived to be excellent, however the evaluation was not based on your clinical skills, it was based on some other standard, which no one can satisfactorily articulate to you. Talking with some of the other native students you realize it was a major mistake to approach a supervisor without being summoned, address him directly, and look him in the eye while doing so. In Japan, these traits, which are respected in the United States (i.e., showing assertiveness and initiative), are frowned upon if done by subordinates.

Critical Thinking Questions

1. Why is looking a superior in the eye considered disrespectful?
2. How should you have handled the situation?
3. What information would have been useful to know in advance?
4. Where could such information have been found and how would you even know to look for it?
5. Investigate and describe the Asian concept of "saving face," how might that have been an issue?

References

1. Berger P. (1997). Four faces of global culture. *National Interest 49*(fall):23–29.
2. Board of Certification. (2004). *Role delineation study.* Omaha, NE: BOC, Inc.
3. Child Welfare League of America. Retrieved September 19, 2008 from http://www.cwla.org/newsevents/terms.htm.

4. DeConde C. (1990). The C.A.T.A. – Historical perspective 1965 – 1990. *The Journal of the Canadian Athletic Therapy Association* 6–10.

5. Ferrara M. Globalization of the Athletic Training Profession. (2006). *JAT 41*(2):135–136.

6. Japanese Athletic Trainers' Organization. Retrieved November 20, 2007 from http://jato-trainer.org/english/index.html.

7. Paasche-Orlow M. (2004). The ethics of cultural competence. *Academic Medicine* *79*(4):347–350.

8. Roberts JH. (2006). Cultural competence in the clinical setting. *The Clinical Teacher 3*:97–102.

9. Shenk WR. (2006). Foreword. In: Ott C, Netland H, eds. *Globalizing theology.* Grand Rapids, MI: Baker Academics; 9–11.

10. Sire J. (1997). *The universe next door: A basic worldview catalog.* Downers Grove, IL: Intervarsity Press.

11. Sofia-Lopes A. Student *National Medical Association: Cultural competency position statement.* Retrieved September 26, 2008 from http://www.snma.org/downloads/snma_cultural_competency.pdf.

12. The Institute for Diversity and Ethics in Sport. (2007). *Decisions from the top: Diversity among campus, conference leaders at Division IA institutions: All-time high for diversity among athletics directors.* Retrieved September 19, 2008 from http://www.bus.ucf.edu/sport/public/downloads/2007_Division_IA_Demographics_Study.pdf

13. The Pew Health Professions Commission. *Recreating health professional practice for a new century.* Retrieved January 5, 2008, from http://www.futurehealth.ucsf.edu/pdf_files/recreate.pdf

Student-Athlete Health History Questionnaire Form

ATHLETIC TRAINING UNIVERSITY
Student-Athlete Health History Questionnaire Form

The information contained in this medical history form will only be used by the Sports Medicine Department at XYZ University for purposes of determining if you pose a health threat / risk to yourself on the athletic field. This information will be discussed with you in detail later in your physical examination by an Athletic Trainer and/or Team Physician. This information will remain **CONFIDENTIAL** at all times.

(please print clearly)

Name _____ Date _____

Social Security # _____ Gender: ☐ Male ☐ Female Date of Birth _____

Race: ☐ Caucasion ☐ Afro-American ☐ Hispanic ☐ Asian/Pacific ☐ Alaskan/Indian ☐ Other _____

Sport(s) _____ Position(s) _____

Height _____ Weight _____ ☐ Right Handed ☐ Left Handed

PERMANENT ADDRESS:

_____
STREET

_____
CITY   STATE   ZIP CODE

_____
PHONE 1   PHONE 2 (CELLULAR)   E-Mail

LOCAL ADDRESS:

_____
STREET

_____
CITY   STATE   ZIP CODE

_____
PHONE 1   PHONE 2 (CELLULAR)   E-Mail

Father's Name _____ Age ____ If Deceased, Cause of Death _____

Age @ Death _____ Father's Occupation _____

Address (if different from permanent address):

_____
STREET   CITY/STATE   ZIP CODE

_____
HOME PHONE   WORK PHONE

Mother's Name _____ Age _____ If Deceased, Cause of Death _____

Age @ Death _____ Mother's Occupation _____

Address (if different from permanent address):

_____
STREET   CITY/STATE   ZIP CODE

_____
HOME PHONE   WORK PHONE

ORTHOPEDIC HISTORY:

I. Head Injuries / Concussion:

History of Head Injury / Concussion Injury?   ☐ YES   ☐ NO

◆   List Dates/Time Missed _____

◆   Please Describe _____

Were Any Diagnostic Tests Performed?   ☐ YES   ☐ NO   (check all that apply)

☐ MRI   ☐ CT-Scan   ☐ Neuropsychological Testing   ☐ Other _____

Have You Ever Been Hospitalized, Knocked Out, Become Unconscious, and/or Lost Your Memory Due To A Head Injury / Concussion?   ☐ YES ☐ NO

◆   Please Describe _____

Do You Suffer From Headaches?   ☐ YES   ☐ NO

◆   When?   ☐ Every Day   ☐ 1-2 Times/Week   ☐ 1-2 Times/Month

◆   Where Are Your Headaches Located?   ☐ Left Side of Head   ☐ Right Side of Head

☐ Front of Head   ☐ Back of Head   ☐ All Over Your Head

Do You Have A History of Migraine Headaches?   ☐ YES   ☐ NO

◆   How Often _____   Please Describe _____

◆   Medications Taken for Migraines? _____

Have You Had Headaches For More Than Three (3) Months?   ☐ YES   ☐ NO

◆   If yes, please explain _____

II. Cervical Spine / Neck:

History of Cervical Spine / Neck Injury?   ☐ YES ☐ NO

◆   List Dates/Time Missed _____

◆   Please Describe _____

Were Any Diagnostic Tests Performed? (check all that apply)   ☐ X-Rays   ☐ Bone Scan

☐ MRI   ☐ CT-Scan   ☐ Other _____

Have You Ever Been Hospitalized For A Cervical Spine / Neck Injury?   ☐ YES ☐ NO

◆   When? _____   Where? _____

◆   Please Describe _____

Have You Ever Had "Burners", "Stingers", or Any Bracial Plexus Injury?   ☐ YES   ☐ NO

◆   How Many? _____   Date(s)/Time Missed? _____

Have You Ever Had Surgery of Any Kind on Your Cervical Spine / Neck?   ☐ YES   ☐ NO

◆   When? _____   Surgeon? _____

◆   Please Describe _____

Do You Presently Wear A Neck Roll or Neck Collar?   ☐ YES   ☐ NO

Do You Presently Wear A "Cowboy Collar" or Helmet Restrictor Plate?   ☐ YES   ☐ NO

Have You Ever Worn or Been Advised To Wear a Neck Roll, Neck Collar, "Cowboy Collar", and/or Helmet Restrictor Plate?

☐ YES   ☐ NO   If yes, please explain _____

III. Shoulder / Upper Arm:

History of Shoulder / Upper Arm Injury? ☐ YES ☐ NO

  ◆ List Dates/Time Missed _____

  ◆ Please Describe _____

Were Any Diagnostic Tests Performed? (check all that apply) ☐ X-Rays ☐ Bone Scan

  ☐ MRI ☐ CT-Scan ☐ Other _____

Have You Ever Been Hospitalized For A Shoulder / Upper Arm Injury? ☐ YES ☐ NO

  ◆ When? _____ Where? _____

  ◆ Please Describe _____

Have You Ever Had Surgery of Any Kind on Your Shoulder / Upper Arm? ☐ YES ☐ NO

  ◆ When? _____ Surgeon? _____

  ◆ Please Describe _____

Have You Ever Experienced Numbness and/or Tingling in Your Arms/Fingers? ☐ YES ☐ NO

  ◆ Date(s)? _____

  ◆ Please Describe? _____

IV. Elbow / Forearm:

History of Elbow / Forearm Injury? ☐ YES ☐ NO

  ◆ List Dates/Time Missed _____

  ◆ Please Describe _____

Were Any Diagnostic Tests Performed? (check all that apply) ☐ X-Rays ☐ Bone Scan

  ☐ MRI ☐ CT-Scan ☐ Other _____

Have You Ever Been Hospitalized For An Elbow / Forearm Injury? ☐ YES ☐ NO

  ◆ When? _____ Where? _____

  ◆ Please Describe _____

Have You Ever Had Surgery of Any Kind on Your Elbow / Forearm? ☐ YES ☐ NO

  ◆ When? _____ Surgeon? _____

  ◆ Please Describe _____

V. Wrist, Hand, & Fingers:

History of Wrist, Hand, and/or Finger Injury? ☐ YES ☐ NO

  ◆ List Dates/Time Missed _____

  ◆ Please Describe _____

Were Any Diagnostic Tests Performed? (check all that apply) ☐ X-Rays ☐ Bone Scan

  ☐ MRI ☐ CT-Scan ☐ Other _____

Have You Ever Been Hospitalized For A Wrist, Hand, and/or Finger Injury? ☐ YES ☐ NO

  ◆ When? _____ Where? _____

  ◆ Please Describe _____

Have You Ever Had Surgery of Any Kind on Your Wrist, Hand, and/or Finger(s)? ☐ YES ☐ NO

  ◆ When? _____ Surgeon? _____

  ◆ Please Describe _____

III. Shoulder / Upper Arm:

History of Shoulder / Upper Arm Injury?   ☐ YES   ☐ NO

  ◆ List Dates/Time Missed _____

  ◆ Please Describe _____

Were Any Diagnostic Tests Performed? (check all that apply)   ☐ X-Rays   ☐ Bone Scan

     ☐ MRI   ☐ CT-Scan   ☐ Other _____

Have You Ever Been Hospitalized For A Shoulder / Upper Arm Injury?   ☐ YES   ☐ NO

  ◆ When? _____   Where? _____

  ◆ Please Describe _____

Have You Ever Had Surgery of Any Kind on Your Shoulder / Upper Arm?   ☐ YES   ☐ NO

  ◆ When? _____   Surgeon? _____

  ◆ Please Describe _____

Have You Ever Experienced Numbness and/or Tingling in Your Arms/Fingers?   ☐ YES   ☐ NO

  ◆ Date(s)? _____

  ◆ Please Describe? _____

IV. Elbow / Forearm:

History of Elbow / Forearm Injury?   ☐ YES   ☐ NO

  ◆ List Dates/Time Missed _____

  ◆ Please Describe _____

Were Any Diagnostic Tests Performed? (check all that apply)   ☐ X-Rays   ☐ Bone Scan

     ☐ MRI   ☐ CT-Scan   ☐ Other _____

Have You Ever Been Hospitalized For An Elbow / Forearm Injury?   ☐ YES   ☐ NO

  ◆ When? _____   Where? _____

  ◆ Please Describe _____

Have You Ever Had Surgery of Any Kind on Your Elbow / Forearm?   ☐ YES   ☐ NO

  ◆ When? _____   Surgeon? _____

  ◆ Please Describe _____

V. Wrist, Hand, & Fingers:

History of Wrist, Hand, and/or Finger Injury?   ☐ YES   ☐ NO

  ◆ List Dates/Time Missed _____

  ◆ Please Describe _____

Were Any Diagnostic Tests Performed? (check all that apply)   ☐ X-Rays   ☐ Bone Scan

     ☐ MRI   ☐ CT-Scan   ☐ Other _____

Have You Ever Been Hospitalized For A Wrist, Hand, and/or Finger Injury?   ☐ YES   ☐ NO

  ◆ When? _____   Where? _____

  ◆ Please Describe _____

Have You Ever Had Surgery of Any Kind on Your Wrist, Hand, and/or Finger(s)?   ☐ YES   ☐ NO

  ◆ When? _____   Surgeon? _____

  ◆ Please Describe _____

☐ MRI ☐ CT-Scan ☐ Other _____

Have You Ever Been Hospitalized For A Thigh Injury? ☐ YES ☐ NO

♦ When? _____ Where? _____

♦ Please Describe _____

Have You Ever Had Surgery For A Thigh Injury? ☐ YES ☐ NO

♦ When? _____ Surgeon? _____

♦ Please Describe _____

XII. Knee:

History of Injury? ☐ YES ☐ NO

♦ List Dates/Time Missed _____

♦ Please Describe _____

Were Any Diagnostic Tests Performed? (check all that apply) ☐ X-Rays ☐ Bone Scan

☐ MRI ☐ CT-Scan ☐ Other _____

Have You Ever Been Hospitalized For A Knee Injury? ☐ YES ☐ NO

♦ When? _____ Where? _____

♦ Please Describe _____

Have You Ever Had Surgery For A Knee Injury? ☐ YES ☐ NO

♦ When? _____ Surgeon? _____

♦ Please Describe _____

Have You Ever/Do You Presently Wear A Knee Brace? ☐ YES ☐ NO

♦ Which Knee? _____ Brand / Model of Brace? _____

♦ Reason for Wearing ? _____

XIII. Ankle / Lower Leg:

History of Ankle / Lower Leg Injury? ☐ YES ☐ NO

♦ List Dates/Time Missed _____

♦ Please Describe _____

Were Any Diagnostic Tests Performed? (check all that apply) ☐ X-Rays ☐ Bone Scan

☐ MRI ☐ CT-Scan ☐ Other _____

Have You Ever Been Hospitalized For An Ankle / Lower Leg Injury? ☐ YES ☐ NO

♦ When? _____ Where? _____

♦ Please Describe _____

Have You Ever Had Surgery For An Ankle / Lower Leg Injury? ☐ YES ☐ NO

♦ When? _____ Surgeon? _____

♦ Please Describe _____

Do You Presently ☐ Tape Your Ankle(s) ☐ Use Ankle Brace(s) ☐ Other

♦ Please Describe _____

XIV. Foot / Toes:

History of Foot / Toe Injury? ☐ YES ☐ NO

♦ List Dates/Time Missed _____

◆ Please Describe _____

Were Any Diagnostic Tests Performed? (check all that apply) ☐ X-Rays ☐ Bone Scan

☐ MRI ☐ CT-Scan ☐ Other _____

Have You Ever Had Surgery For A Foot / Toe Injury? ☐ YES ☐ NO

◆ When? _____ Surgeon? _____

◆ Please Describe _____

XV. Prescription Medications:

Please List **ALL** Prescription & Over-the-Counter Medications That You Are **CURRENTLY** Taking or **Have Taken** In The PAST, & For What Purpose:

MEDICATION	PURPOSE	DOSAGE	DATE(S)

XVI. Medical Testing:

Have you ever been tested for HIV/AIDS, that you are aware of? ☐ YES ☐ NO

◆ Date(s) of Test(s)? _____ Location(s) of Test(s) _____

Have you ever contracted any type of Hepatitis? ☐ YES ☐ NO

◆ Date(s)? _____ Treatment? _____

Have you ever been tested for Sickle Cell Anemia, that you are aware of? ☐ YES ☐ NO

◆ Date? _____ Result? _____

XVII. Heat Related Problems:

Have You Ever Experienced (check all that apply):

◆ ☐ Heat Cramps- Date(s)? _____

◆ ☐ Heat Exhaustion- Date(s)? _____

◆ ☐ Heat Stroke- Date(s)? _____

Have You Ever Received Intravenous Fluids (IV) For A Heat Related Problem? ☐ YES ☐ NO

◆ Date(s)? _____

Have You Ever Been Hospitalized For a Heat-Related Problem? ☐ YES ☐ NO

◆ Date(s)? _____ Where? _____

XVIII. Allergies:

Have You Ever Been Diagnosed With Any Allergies? ☐ YES ☐ NO

♦ Please Describe _____

Are You Presently Taking/Have You Previously Taken Any Allergy Medications? ☐ YES ☐ NO

♦ Please Describe _____

Are you allergic to and/or ever had an unfavorable / allergic reaction to any medications? ☐ YES ☐ NO

♦ Please Describe _____

Are you allergic to and/or ever had an unfavorable / allergic reaction to any food items? ☐ YES ☐ NO

♦ Please Describe _____

Are you allergic to and/or ever had an unfavorable / allergic reaction to bee stings, insect bites, etc.? ☐ YES ☐ NO

♦ Please Describe _____

XIX. Asthma:

Have You Ever Been Diagnosed With Asthma and/or Exercised Induced Asthma? ☐ YES ☐ NO

♦ Date(s)? _____

♦ Please Describe _____

Are You Presently Taking / Have You Previously Taken Any Allergy Medications / Use an Inhaler? ☐ YES ☐ NO

♦ Date(s)? _____

♦ Please Describe _____

How Many Acute Asthma Attacks Have You Had In The Past 24 Months? _____

♦ Date(s)? _____

♦ Please Describe _____

XX. Diabetic History:

Have You Ever Been Diagnosed With Diabetes? ☐ YES ☐ NO

♦ Date? _____

Are You Presently Taking or Have You Taken Any Diabetic Medications? ☐ YES ☐ NO

Medication	**Form**	**Dosage**	**Frequency**

Do You Daily Monitor Your Blood Sugar Level? ☐ YES ☐ NO

♦ Please Describe _____

Please List Any Precautions That You Take and/or Additional Information Not Mentioned Above:

_____

_____

XXI. Eyes:

Do you routinely wear glasses? ☐ YES ☐ NO

Do you routinely wear contact lenses? ☐ YES ☐ NO

♦ What Type? _____

Do you require any special devices / equipment? ☐ YES ☐ NO

♦ Please Describe _____

XXII. Cardiovascular Risk Factors:

Have you ever had chest pain and/or shortness of breath during or after exercise / practice? ☐ YES ☐ NO

♦ Please Describe _____

Have you ever felt dizzy, lightheaded, and/or passed out during or after exercise / practice? ☐ YES ☐ NO

♦ Please Describe _____

Have you ever had the feeling of your heart racing or skipping beats during or after exercise / practice? ☐ YES ☐ NO

♦ Please Describe _____

Do you get tired more quickly than your teammates / friends do during exercise / practice? ☐ YES ☐ NO

♦ Please Describe _____

Have you ever been told that you have a heart murmur? ☐ YES ☐ NO

♦ Please Describe _____

Has any family member or relative died or heart problems and/or of sudden death before age 35? ☐ YES ☐ NO

♦ Please Describe _____

Has a physician ever denied or restricted your participation in sports due to any heart problems? ☐ YES ☐ NO

♦ Please Describe _____

Have you ever had an electrocardiogram (EKG) of your heart? ☐ YES ☐ NO

♦ Dates / Please Describe _____

Have you ever been told that you have / had high blood pressure? ☐ YES ☐ NO

♦ Please Describe _____

Have you even been told that you have / had high blood cholesterol? ☐ YES ☐ NO

♦ Please Describe _____

XXIII. Please Answer: *{All questions are strictly **CONFIDENTIAL** & will not be shared with parents or coaches!}*

☐ YES ☐ NO   Have you ever had any injury or illness other than those already noted?
☐ YES ☐ NO   Do you have any ongoing or chronic illnesses?
☐ YES ☐ NO   Have you ever been hospitalized overnight?
☐ YES ☐ NO   Have you ever been told by a physician to restrict your sports activity or not to participate in a sport?
☐ YES ☐ NO   Are you currently under a physician's care for any medical conditions?
☐ YES ☐ NO   Have you ever been under the care of a psychiatrist and/or psychologist?
☐ YES ☐ NO   Have you consulted and/or been under the care of a chiropractor, hypnotist, acupuncturist, massage therapist, spiritual healer, and/or other such practitioner in the past five (5) years?

☐ YES ☐ NO   Do you take any vitamins or supplements?
☐ YES ☐ NO   Have you ever had a rash or hives develop during and/or after exercise?
☐ YES ☐ NO   Do you have any skin problems? (itching, rashes, acne, herpes, eczema, warts, fungus, or blisters)
☐ YES ☐ NO   Do you cough, wheeze, or have trouble breathing during or after exercise / practice?
☐ YES ☐ NO   Do you have only one of two paired, functioning organs (eyes, kidney, ovary, etc.)?
☐ YES ☐ NO   Have you ever been told that you have kidney disease?
☐ YES ☐ NO   Have you had a viral infection (i.e. mononucleosis, myocarditis, etc.) within the past six (6) months?
☐ YES ☐ NO   Have you ever had seizures or convulsions?
☐ YES ☐ NO   Do you have recurrent or frequent headaches?
☐ YES ☐ NO   Do you have ringing in your ears or trouble hearing?
☐ YES ☐ NO   Do you have frequent ear infections or nosebleeds?
☐ YES ☐ NO   Do you require any special equipment (braces, neck rolls, dental, orthotics, hearing aids, etc.)?
☐ YES ☐ NO   Have you ever had the chickenpox? If yes, when? _____
☐ YES ☐ NO   Do you or anyone in your family have sickle cell trait or disease?

☐ YES ☐ NO   Do you have any body piercing or tattoos?
☐ YES ☐ NO   Are you aware of any reasons why you should not participate in intercollegiate athletics at ATU at this time?
☐ YES ☐ NO   Have you had a tetanus booster within the past five (5) years? If yes, when? _____
☐ YES ☐ NO   Have you ever received the Hepatitis B (HBV) Vaccination series (all 3 shots)? If yes, when? _____

☐ YES ☐ NO   Do you smoke cigarettes, use smokeless tobacco, or use tobacco in any form?
☐ YES ☐ NO   Do you use alcohol? If yes, how often? _____
☐ YES ☐ NO   Have you ever used / tried marijuana, cocaine, or any other illicit "street" drugs?
☐ YES ☐ NO   Do you have any questions regarding drugs, tobacco, or alcohol?
☐ YES ☐ NO   Do you feel stressed out? If yes, do you feel as though you get the necessary support to deal with your stress?
☐ YES ☐ NO   Have you had a weight change (loss or gain) of greater than 10 pounds in the past year?
☐ YES ☐ NO   Are you a vegetarian? If yes, what type? _____
☐ YES ☐ NO   Do you regularly lose weight to participate in your sport?
☐ YES ☐ NO   Do you want to weigh more or less than you presently do?
☐ YES ☐ NO   Have you ever felt forced to limit your food intake due to concerns about your weight and/or body size?
☐ YES ☐ NO   Have you had a history of anorexia, bulimia (forced vomiting), and/or any other eating disorders?
☐ YES ☐ NO   Would you like to meet with a dietitian to discuss your nutritional needs or eating habits?

For Females Only-

When was your first menstrual period? _____
☐ YES ☐ NO   Have you had menstrual periods within the past 12 months?
   ◆ If yes, how many? _____   When was your most recent menstrual period? _____
   ◆ How much time do you usually have from the start of one period to the start of another? _____
   ◆ What was the longest time between menstrual periods within the past year? _____
☐ YES ☐ NO   Do you have painful or heavy menstrual periods?
☐ YES ☐ NO   Do you take any medications during your menstrual periods? If yes, what? _____
☐ YES ☐ NO   Do you take birth control pills? If yes, what brand? _____
☐ YES ☐ NO   Have you ever had any problems with your breasts?
☐ YES ☐ NO   Have you had a pelvic examination within the last year?

If you have answered **YES** to any of the above, please explain: _____

_____

_____

_____

_____

_____

_____

_____

_____

_____

_____

I, the undersigned, hereby acknowledge, affirm, and represent that all statements on pages one (1) through ten (10) are true and accurate to the best of my knowledge; and that no answers or information have been withheld. If any information and/or statements are false and/or have been omitted in reference to my past and/or present medical history, I fully understand that the **ATU**, its agents, servants, trustees, and employees disclaim liability, and will not be held liable for any injuries and/or illnesses not noted.

_____   _____
Student-Athlete Signature   Date

_____
Student-Athlete Print Name

_____   _____
Parent/Guardian Signature _(if under 18 years of age)_   Date

_____
Parent/Guardian Print Name

_____   _____
Witness   Date

Please describe below any further injury information, which is knowledgeable to you and not required on this form.

Reviewed By:

_____   _____
Reviewer's Signature   Date

_____
Reviewer Print Name

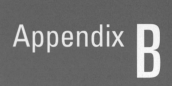
Athlete Information Form

ATHLETE INFORMATION FORM
(All information contained within is confidential)

Last Name: _____ First Name: _____ M.I. _____

Gender: _____ Age: _____ Birth date: _____ Social Security Number: _____-_____-___

Campus Address: _____ Phone/Ext.: _____

Class: _____ Participated in sport at C.L.U. last year: (Circle) <u>Yes / No</u>

Home Address: _____

City: _____ State: _____ Zip: _____ Phone: (_____) _____-_____

<u>Known</u> allergies: _____

Personal Physician: _____ Address: _____

_____ Physician Telephone: (_____) _____-_____

In case of emergency contact:

Name: _____ Relationship: _____

Address: _____

City: _____ State/Country: _____ Zip: _____

Work Phone: (_____) _____ Home Phone: (_____) _____

I, _____, do certify that all information contained on this form is accurate to the best of my knowledge and agree to update information, as needed based on current circumstances.

Signed: _____ Date: _____

Student Signature

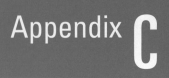

Daily Treatments Log

DAILY TREATMENTS
ATHLETIC TRAINING UNIVERSITY

No. _____

Date: _____

NAME	SPORT	Ice Pack	Whirlpool	Ice Bath	Ultra Sound	Elec. Stim.	Contrast	Hydrocollator	A.I. Compression	Cryo Cuff	Massage	Bike	Exercise	Orthotron	Leg Massage	Bapes Board	Other	ANATOMICAL SITE	INJURY	TIME

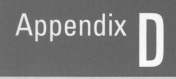
NATA Organization Chart

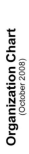
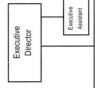
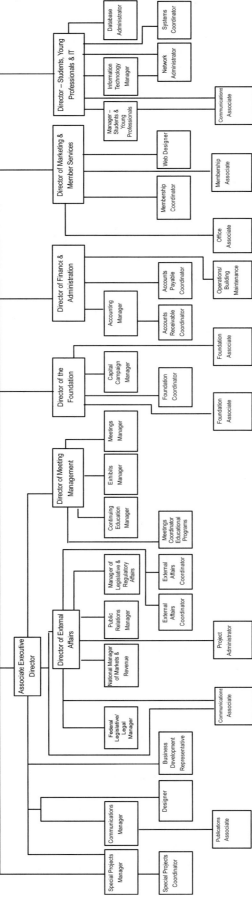

Allied Health, Medical, and Professional Organizations

- International Federation of Sports Medicine (FIMS): http://www.fims.org
- American Academy of Family Physicians (AAFP): http://www.aafp.org
- American College of Sports Medicine (ACSM): http://www.acsm.org
- American Orthopaedic Society for Sports Medicine (AOSSM): http://www.sportsmed.org
- American Academy of Pediatrics, Sports Committee (AAP): http://www.aap.org/sections/sportsmedicine/
- American Physical Therapy Association (APTA): http://www.apta.org
- American Medical Association (AMA): http://www.ama-assn.org/
- National Strength & Conditioning (NSCA): http://www.nsca-lift.org
- American Massage Therapy Association (AMTA): http://www.amtamassage.org/
- American Nurses Association (ANA): http://www.nursingworld.org/
- American Chiropractic Association (ACA): http://www.amerchiro.org/
- World Federation of Athletic Trainers and Therapists (WFATT): http://www.wfatt.org
- American Kinesiotherapy Association (AKTA): http://www.akta.org/
- American Dental Association (ADA): http://www.ada.org/
- American Dietetic Association (ADA): http://www.eatright.org
- American Occupational Therapy Association (AOTA): http://www.aota.org/
- American Speech-Language-Hearing Association (ASHA): http://www.asha.org

List of NATA Position Statements

Note: Position statements can be accessed at http://www.nata.org.

NATA POSITION STATEMENT DISCLAIMER

The NATA publishes its position statements as a service to promote the awareness of certain issues to its members. The information contained in the position statement is neither exhaustive nor exclusive to all circumstances or individuals. Variables such as institutional human resource guidelines, state or federal statutes, rules, or regulations, as well as regional environmental conditions, may impact the relevance and implementation of these recommendations. The NATA advises its members and others to carefully and independently consider each of the recommendations (including the applicability of same to any particular circumstance or individual). The position statement should not be relied upon as an independent basis for care, but rather as a resource available to NATA members or others. Moreover, no opinion is expressed herein regarding the quality of care that adheres to or differs from NATA's position statements. The NATA reserves the right to rescind or modify its position statements at any time.

POSITION, OFFICIAL, CONSENSUS, AND SUPPORT STATEMENTS

1. Emergency planning in athletics
2. Exertional heat illnesses
3. Fluid replacement for athletes
4. Head down contact and spearing in tackle football
5. Lightning safety for athletics and recreation
6. Management of asthma in athletes
7. Management of sport-related concussion
8. Management of the athlete with Type 1 diabetes mellitus
9. Preventing, detecting, and managing disordered eating in athletes
10. Automated external defibrillators
11. Commotio cordis
12. Communicable and infectious diseases in secondary school sports
13. Community-acquired MRSA infections
14. Full-time, on-site athletic trainer coverage for secondary school athletic programs
15. Steroids and performance enhancing substances
16. Use of qualified athletic trainers in secondary schools
17. Youth football and heat related illness
18. Appropriate medical care for secondary school-age athletes
19. Recommendations on emergency preparedness and management of sudden cardiac arrest in high school and college athletic programs
20. Inter-association task force on exertional heat illnesses
21. Prehospital care of the spine-injured athlete
22. Spine care supplement
23. Sickle cell trait and the athlete
24. The Coalition to Preserve Patient Access to Physical Medicine and Rehabilitation Services
25. American Academy of Family Physicians' support of athletic trainers for high school athletes
26. American Medical Association's support of athletic trainers in secondary schools
27. Appropriate medical care for secondary school-age athletes
28. Endorsement of NATA Lightning Position Statement by the American Academy of Pediatrics
29. Recommendations and guidelines for appropriate medical coverage of intercollegiate athletics
30. NCAA support of recommendations and guidelines for appropriate medical coverage of intercollegiate athletics

Glossary

Accident: The direct result of a documented trauma that has an identifiable time and place.

Accreditation: The process of assessing the rigor of the training and education for an institution or program of study in accordance with pre-established criteria.

Actual cause: Explicit proof that a breach of duty was the actual cause of damage to an individual.

Actual harm: Literal and real damage or loss (as opposed to potential damage or loss).

Ad hoc: Latin, meaning "for this purpose;" typically refers to a committee that is assembled for a specific purpose and that is disbanded once that committee's purpose is completed.

Adjudication: The decision of the court regarding a specific case or defendant.

Administering: Giving medications in a dose that is to be consumed within 24 hours.

Agreement: The ancient belief that dialogue, and not sharing a common opinion, was the most important aspect of working together.

Altruism: An approach in which an individual is more concerned with benefiting others than himself or herself.

Ambition: The use of available resources (intrinsic and extrinsic) and other effective strategies to promote professional and personal development.

Analytic jurisprudence: The philosophy of law that asks specific questions such as, "what is law?" or "what is the relationship between law and ethics or morality?" It seeks to analyze any differences between legal behaviors and other behaviors, such as ethical or moral behaviors.

Applied ethics: The study of the use of ethical values and actual behaviors.

Assertiveness: The quality of being proactive about new ideas, innovations, and change initiatives while maintaining respect for personal boundaries and rights of others.

Asynchronous: Not occurring at the same time; in this case, in reference to electronic communications.

Authority: The degree to which power is accepted or acknowledged by a subordinate.

Bandwidth: The rate or speed of data transfer; often used synonymously with data transfer rate.

Battery: A tort that involves deliberately bringing about a harmful or offensive contact without consent that is likely to cause an injury or bodily harm.

Benchmarking: Determining best practices by measuring one's performance against the best organizations in one's industry.

Bid sheet: A list of needed supplies and equipment for the upcoming year that is sent to multiple vendors. Each vendor then estimates the cost of all or some of the supplies and returns a proposal for the total cost of the supplies to the athletic trainer for consideration.

Board of Certification (BOC): The professional body that sets the standards for the practice of athletic training.

Brainstorming: A technique used to generate new ideas, in which the context is such that there are no "right" or "wrong" ideas.

Breach of duty: A finding that any duty or obligation owed to a harmed individual was in fact violated.

Budget freeze: Suspension or stoppage of spending.

Business plan: A document that spells out the expected course of action of an existing or new enterprise for a certain period of time.

Capital budget: Money that is set aside and disbursed for expensive equipment that is intended to last for more than one budget cycle.

Capitation: A reimbursement system in which the providers are paid a set amount for a certain number of patients in a given time frame regardless of number of visits or services to those patients.

Case law: The decisions made by judges in previous cases that are recorded and used as precedent for other cases.

Causation: A finding that a breach of duty was the actual or proximate cause of any alleged harm, damage, or loss.

Central processing unit (CPU): The part of a computer that includes the circuits controlling the processing and execution of instructions.

Certification: A form of credential that is awarded by a national association or organization.

Chronological resume: A resume that lists all education and work experience in chronological order (present to past) and is the "traditional" resume format preferred by many employers.

Civil law: The most common form of law in the world, based on abstract rules or notions, which require a judge to interpret and apply to each case individually.

Clinical proficiencies: A common set of skills that entry-level athletic trainers should possess.

Co-acting teams: Teams with members who function with a high degree of autonomy.

Code of ethics: The rules, standards, or principles that dictate proper behavior among members of a profession.

Cognitive competencies: The knowledge and intellectual skills necessary for an athletic trainer to possess.

Collaborating: Effectively participating with other professionals within the local or global community in achieving similar goals.

Collaborative teams: Teams that share common values and goals but have diverse experiences and backgrounds.

Commission on Accreditation of Athletic Training Education (CAATE): The agency responsible for accrediting entry-level (undergraduate and graduate) athletic training educational programs.

Commission: Performing an act that one is not legally permitted to perform.

Common law: Deals with the rights and responsibilities of individuals toward each other.

Communication: The use of a variety of different means to convey information.

Comparative negligence: Assignment of negligence among multiple parties by considering all parties whose negligence contributed to a tort. The negligence is then allocated among the parties at fault and damages are assigned to the level each contributed toward the negligent action(s).

Competency: A demonstrated behavior or skill an athletic trainer is required to possess.

Computer network: Two or more computers connected together using a telecommunication or wireless system for communicating and sharing resources.

Computer technology: The application of computers for manipulation and management of information or data.

Computer virus: A program introduced from an external source that replicates within a computer's system and can render it useless and can destroy data files.

Conflict of interest: A situation in which a person has a private or personal interest that appears to influence or does influence the objective exercise of his or her official duties as an allied health care professional.

Conflict: A state of disagreement or incompatibility between two or more people or groups of people.

Construction management: An approach in which a general contractor is involved early on in the design process.

Context: The background information to an event; the integration of any number of external and internal variables, such as attitudes, belief systems, values, cultural bias, and symbols that make up a circumstance.

Contextual intelligence: The ability to recognize, assess, and assimilate multiple external and internal variables that constitute any context.

Continuing education: Education and or training activities earned by a certified or licensed professional that are acquired post-credential in order to maintain that credential.

Contrast: The degree of difference between the lightest and darkest elements in a room; poor contrast makes it difficult to distinguish details of an object or room as a result of paint colors that are too similar in the background or foreground or poor lighting.

Co-payment: The amount of money paid by the insured at the time any service is rendered; typically, a nominal fee for a doctor visit, emergency room visit, or prescription.

Core competency of an organization: The collective talent, experience, and creativity of the people within that organization that differentiates them from others.

Counterpower: Influence that a subordinate has over a supervisor.

Cover letter: A tool used to introduce oneself to potential employers and highlights important aspects of one's resume.

Creativity: The willingness and ability to produce plausible ideas when asked or needed.

Credentials: Official statement or recognition of a governing body that an individual has demonstrated pre-established competency in an area.

Critical thinking: The cognitive ability to make connections, integrate, and make practical application of different actions, opinions, and information.

Cultural competence: The capacity of an individual to incorporate ethnic and cultural considerations of diverse co-workers into their work.

Cultural sensitivity: The quality of promoting diversity by aligning diverse individuals and creating opportunities for diverse members to interact in non-discriminatory manner.

Culture: Common beliefs and practices of a group of people that lead to specific habits of thought, behavior, diet, dress, music, and art.

Cyberspace: The virtual world accessible via the Internet.

Data mining: The process of examining a large pool of information and summarizing it into more useful information.

Deductible: The amount of money the insured (first-party) is responsible to pay for any covered health-related expenses.

Deontology: A branch of moral philosophy that underscores the duty or obligations of an individual to act; it is what a person ought to do regardless of outcome.

Design-bid-build: A construction process in which the design and building of a project is completed by several different groups (or sub-contractors).

Design-build: A construction process in which a single entity is used for all of the construction processes.

Discipline: The quality of demonstrating consistent and steady behavior.

Dispensing: Giving medications in a dose that is to be consumed in a period of time greater than 24 hours.

Diversity: A complex social issue that describes differences both within cultural groups and between cultural groups.

Domains: One of six general practice areas in which an athletic trainer needs to have competency and proficiency.

Download: The transfer of data from an external source unit (i.e., server, network, internet, or software program) to a personal unit (i.e., personal computer).

Duty of care: Proving that there is a responsibility to provide care based on the relationship between parties.

Education: The process of equipping an individual to perform undefined functions in unpredictable situations.

Egoism: Behaviors based solely on self-interest and personal gain.

Empathy: Awareness of another's feelings from remembering or imagining being in similar circumstances.

Ergonomics: The science of increasing work productivity by designing work stations that are comfortable for any person.

Ethical behavior: Behavior characterized by reporting incompetent, unethical, and illegal practice objectively, factually, and according to current standards/procedures. Treating people equitably and fairly.

Ethics: A systematic inquiry and judgment about the moral dimensions of human conduct.

Ethnocentric: Believing that one's own culture is superior to all others.

Evidence-based practice: The integration of individual clinical expertise with the best available external clinical evidence from systematic research.

Exclusions: Health-related conditions that are not covered under the insurance policy.

Exemption: A type of state regulation that allows a professional to practice without having to comply with the standards of practice of other professionals.

Explicit knowledge: Knowledge that has been or can be articulated, codified, and stored in media and that is easily transmitted to others.

Family Educational Rights and Privacy Act (FERPA): A federal statute that delineates how to disseminate educational data.

Fee-for-service: The traditional reimbursement model in which the health care provider is paid by the patient when service is performed.

Firewall: A software program that inspects and regulates the traffic into a network and either allows files to pass through or restricts access based on predefined rules.

First party: The insured individual (or patient).

Foot-candle: The amount of light that a candle generates one foot away.

Formula budget: A budget model that uses a ratio of full-time employees to students as a means to determine total disbursement of funds.

For-profit organization: A legal corporate entity that distributes any profit to shareholders and investors.

Functional resume: A resume designed around skills and experiences and that is used when there have been frequent job changes or long lay-offs between jobs.

Glare: Inability to distinguish details or focus eyes on an object as a result of too much light or too many reflective surfaces.

Globalization: The exchange and integration of cultural ideals, social ideals, values, politics, and technologies between diverse people groups as a result of increased communication and access.

Groupthink: A social phenomenon in which members of a team remain silent when a point is open for discussion and debate out of an assumption that everyone either already knows or shares a similar opinion.

Health insurance: A policy held that will pay specified sums of money for medical expenses or treatments incurred as a result of covered injuries or illnesses.

Health maintenance organization (HMO): A group of health care providers intentionally organized to offer predefined services to members.

Health savings accounts: A form of self-coverage in which money can be saved for medical expenses in a tax-deferred status.

Health care common procedure coding system (HCPCS): Codes for items not covered in the CPT codes, such as, ambulance service, orthotics, and supplies.

Heroes or heroines: The people (alive or dead, real or imagined) who represent the ideals of the organization.

Homogeneous teams: Teams that are composed of individuals who share common experiences and backgrounds.

Hoshin Kanri (or planning): A Japanese phrase that is translated "direction setting" and is the systemic process by which an organization sets and achieves specific long-term goals with respect to quality.

Human capital: The experience, education, and background that people bring to a job or role that contribute toward organizational success.

Hygiene factors: Variables that when absent contribute toward job dissatisfaction, such as status, job security, salary, and fringe benefits.

Incident to billing: Billing under a licensed physician (or other health care provider).

Influence: The ability to affect the behavior of others in a particular direction.

Information: Data that has been sorted, analyzed, and displayed and typically has been communicated through text, figures, or tables.

Informed consent: The process of ensuring a patient is aware of all risks of having or not having a procedure or treatment, benefits, and any other possible outcomes associated with a given procedure.

In-group: A supervisor-subordinate relationship based on trust, respect, close interaction, and mutually developed objectives.

Initiative: Willingness to embark on a new venture.

Innovation: Implementation of a brand new idea or a different application of an existing product or idea.

Input: The information or data received from an external source.

Insurance: A system created to minimize financial losses to an individual or organization by transferring risk of loss from the insured to the insurer.

Interdependent teams: Teams whose members rely heavily on other members of the team for accomplishing goals and objectives.

Intranet: A private computer network used to foster communication and data sharing within an organization.

Intuition: A compressed expertise; instinctive knowledge that comes from instantly accessing and assimilating years of experience or a lot of experiences in a moment.

Inventory: All of the goods and materials available for use by an athletic training program.

Jurisprudence: The theory and philosophy of law.

Knowledge management: Practices that identify, create, represent, and distribute knowledge for reuse, awareness, and learning.

Knowledge workers: Specialized professionals who have a unique skill set.

Leadership: The ability to facilitate and influence superiors, peers, and subordinates to make recognizable strides toward shared or unshared objectives.

Licensure: A form of credential that is awarded by a state or federal agency. Licensure is often more restrictive than certification.

Line-item budget: A budget model that distributes a fixed amount of funds for each function within a program.

Litigation: A dispute between parties that is argued in a court of law under the purview of a judge.

Lump sum budget: A budget model that distributes funds in a single amount for the entire budget cycle without delineating specific expenditures.

Management: The ability to use organizational resources to accomplish predetermined objectives.

Material safety data sheet (MSDS): A form from manufacturers that contains all the necessary data (including handling and storage, hazards, chemical ingredients, and exposure care) regarding the properties of a particular substance.

Medical insurance: Insurance that covers only medical expenses related to a diagnosed illness.

Meta-ethics: The study of the philosophy or concept of ethics, dealing with relativism and the meaning of "good," "bad," "right," and "wrong."

Minutes: Notes or the records from the proceedings of a meeting.

Mission statement: The athletic training program's statement of its reason for existence in respect to present-day clientele, distinct services offered, philosophy, and geography.

Moral agent: An individual who takes personal responsibility for actions and is genuinely committed to other's wants, needs, aspirations, and values.

Morals: The values or principles rooted in an individual's philosophy, culture, or religion used to determine right or wrong conduct.

Motivator factors: Variables that when present increase job satisfaction, such as challenging work, recognition, and responsibility.

National Athletic Trainers' Association (NATA): The membership-based professional association that represents the needs of athletic trainers and profession of athletic training.

Natural law: The philosophy that there are unchangeable laws of nature that govern human behavior.

Negligence: The failure to act prudently or in a way that a reasonable person would act under the same or similar circumstances.

Netiquette: Network etiquette; acceptable behaviors for electronic communications.

Normative ethics: The study of how to determine ethical values and concerned with what "ought to be."

Normative jurisprudence: The field of law that considers obedience to the law and how law-breakers might be suitably punished within the proper uses and limits of regulations.

Not-for-profit organizations: A legal corporate entity that reinvests any profits back into the organization.

Omission: The failure to perform a duty.

Out-group: A supervisor-subordinate relationship based on predefined roles, job descriptions, and formal contracts.

Output: Data or information that has been converted into a usable form.

Performance budget: A budget model similar to program based, but money is allocated based on athletic training functions (i.e., record keeping, inventory, etc).

Physician extender: Any allied or health care professional who acts on the behalf of or in conjunction with a licensed physician by providing time with patients that the physician is unable to spend.

Planning: The act of delineating behaviors intended to bring about a predetermined or expected course of actions.

Policy: A written statement intended to encourage a specific behavior.

Pooled bidding: Bidding in which several organizations join their resources so that a larger order can be placed, in an attempt of receiving a reduced price on certain items.

Power: The degree to which influence is exercised by an individual.

Precedent: The prior decision of a judge that is used if another case has identical or similar legal questions.

Preferred provider organization (PPO): A group of medical providers (similar to an HMO) who have contracted to provide care to a specific population.

Premium: A fee (usually monthly) paid by the first party to the insurance company for health care coverage.

Privacy: The right to protection against unreasonable and unwarranted interference with the patient's solitude.

Procedure: A written course of action, usually in sequential steps, intended to accomplish a certain outcome.

Profession: An organized body of educated people who have specialized knowledge.

Professional: An individual who has acquired a highly specialized education within a defined body of knowledge.

Program budget: A budget model in which funds are distributed based on services provided to patients; i.e., based on organizational goals and objectives.

Proximate cause: An action that leads to or ultimately ends in harm.

Psychological barriers: Barriers in communication that result from skepticism or cynicism.

Psychomotor competencies: The manipulative and motor skills necessary for an athletic trainer to possess.

Purchase order (PO): The securing of permission (or pre-approval) for a payment to a vendor.

Random access memory (RAM): The physical memory used to store data while a computer is operating. More RAM will normally contribute to a faster PC.

Rapport: A relationship of mutual understanding and trust.

Referral: A written recommendation from one health care provider for a patient to receive medical care from another health care provider.

Regional investigations: Evaluations that include data about the surrounding environment and local community and that outline possible interactions.

Registration: A form of state credential that protects the public by requiring professionals to notify the state of their intent to practice.

Regulatory law: The federal authorization necessary to establish rules and regulations to make a law effective.

Reimbursement: The amount of money a third-party payer is willing to pay for services rendered.

Resilience: The ability to recover from and adjust to misfortune or change.

Return on investment (ROI): A measure of the total benefit or outcome of an expenditure.

Revenue: The total amount of money generated by a business before any deductions are taken out.

Rider: An addendum to an insurance policy that expands coverage to include certain exclusions.

Risk: The probability or potential for harm as a result of some action.

Rituals: Those actions that fill social needs within an organization.

Role Delineation Study (RDS): The athletic training job analysis authorized by the Board of Certification that identifies essential knowledge and skills for the athletic training profession and is used for exam development.

Scope of practice: Established practice boundaries of a profession that delineate to whom can a service be provided and where those services are rendered.

Second party: The health care provider.

Semantic barriers: Barriers in communication as a result of industry-specific jargon and personal or cultural meanings.

Site investigations: Evaluations of different geographical sites or locations for the facility.

Social loafing: When members of a team significantly decrease their effort, forcing other members to "pick up the slack."

Spam: unsolicited junk e-mail or other electronically transmitted propaganda.

Specifications: Facility drawings with all of the details included, such as outlet locations, drainage, plumbing, ventilation, etc.; everything that is supposed to be in the final product should be included in the specifications.

Stakeholders: Any person or party that has a vested interest in what is being done.

Standard of care: The level at which a reasonable and prudent health care provider in a given community or context would practice.

Standards of professional practice: A document published by the Board of Certification that outlines behaviors expectations of athletic trainers.

Standing committees: Committees organized by NATA that have perpetual existence.

Standing orders: A physician's (or other qualified, licensed health provider's) orders pre-established and approved for use by an athletic trainer under specific conditions in the absence of their physician.

Statutory law: Rules and regulations imposed by regulatory bodies such as Congress, legislatures, or local governments.

Stereotype: The belief that all people from a given group are the same.

Strategic planning: The process of diagnosing the organization's external and internal environments, articulating values, vision, and mission, developing overall goals, implementing action steps, and allocating resources to achieve goals and promote values.

Submission: The voluntary yielding to the authority of another person.

Supply chain management: An approach that involves organizing details of all activities involved in forming supply and service agreements, obtaining supplies and services, and paying for supplies and services.

SWOT analysis: The thorough assessment of a program's specific strengths, weaknesses, opportunities, and threats.

Symbols: The words or objects used to communicate ideas within an organization.

Synergy: The compounding impact of group effort, which results in more being accomplished than what individual efforts might have produced.

Tacit knowledge: The knowledge, typically based on personal experiences, that individuals may or may not be aware of and that, therefore, is difficult to disseminate and share.

Team: An interdependent group formed for an express purpose that must rely on mutual collaboration and insist on accountability.

Teamwork: An action of a group who have agreed to work together for the sake of a common goal.

Technological barriers: Barriers in communication as a result of a lack of face-to-face interaction.

Technology: The beneficial application of scientific advances or discoveries.

Teleology: A branch of moral philosophy that underscores the importance of the outcome. Appropriate actions are based on the outcome; i.e., the end justifies the means.

The Health Insurance Portability and Accountability Act (HIPAA): A law enacted by the U.S. Congress in 1996 that ensures health care coverage for employees who change or lose their jobs and ensures confidentiality and that minimum technical standards of those records are met as they are transferred.

Third party: The person who is contracted to pay.

Tolerance: Acknowledging others' differences of opinion, values, and beliefs without allowing those differences to affect team dynamics or productivity.

Tort: A private wrong or injury suffered by an individual because of another individual's conduct.

Traffic flow: The relationship between the different services or designated spaces within the facility.

Training: The process of preparing individuals to perform a specific task within a defined or predictable situation.

Universal serial bus (USB): A computer port that is compatible with many devices.

Upload: The transfer of data from a smaller unit (i.e., PC) to a larger unit (i.e., server or network).

Usual, customary, and reasonable (UCR): Signifies the reimbursement rate a third-party payer pays to a health care provider.

Utilitarianism: An approach in which the good of the many outweighs the good of the one; i.e., the larger group benefits more than any single person or smaller group.

Values: Priorities held by the organization.

Vendor: A seller or distributor of athletic training supplies and equipment.

Vision statement: An ideal image of the future one seeks to create.

Whistleblower: A person who reports inappropriate behavior of members to an entity or organization who presumably have the power and authority to take corrective action.

Worldview: A set of conscious or subconscious presuppositions about the basic makeup of our world; the ideas and beliefs through which an individual interprets the world and interacts with his or her surroundings.

Zero-based budget: A budget model that does not take into consideration previous spending patterns. Therefore, each expense must be justified annually.

Zone of indifference: The tolerance of or adherence to commands or requests because they fall beneath an individual's threshold of what is consequential.

Index

Page numbers followed by "f" denote figures; those followed by "t" denote tables

360° Feedback, 93–94